KETO for Foodies

NICOLE DOWNS

VICTORY BELT PUBLISHING

Las Vegas

First published in 2019 by Victory Belt Publishing Inc.
Copyright © 2019 Nicole Downs
All rights reserved

ISBN-13: 978-1-628603-65-1

The author is not a licensed practitioner, physician, or medical professional
and offers no medical diagnoses, treatments, suggestions, or counseling. The
information presented herein has not been evaluated by the U.S. Food and Drug
Administration, and it is not intended to diagnose, treat, cure, or prevent any
disease. Full medical clearance from a licensed physician should be obtained
before beginning or modifying any diet, exercise, or lifestyle program, and
physicians should be informed of all nutritional changes.
The author claims no responsibility to any person or entity for any liability, loss,
or damage caused or alleged to be caused directly or indirectly as a result of the
use, application, or interpretation of the information presented herein.

Cover photography by Tatiana Briceag
Back cover photography by Hayley Mason and Bill Staley
Cover design by Justin-Aaron Velasco
Interior design by Yordan Terziev and Boryana Yordanova

Printed in Canada
TC 0119

To the absolute loves of my life,

Makenzie Leigh
&
Cameron Alexander

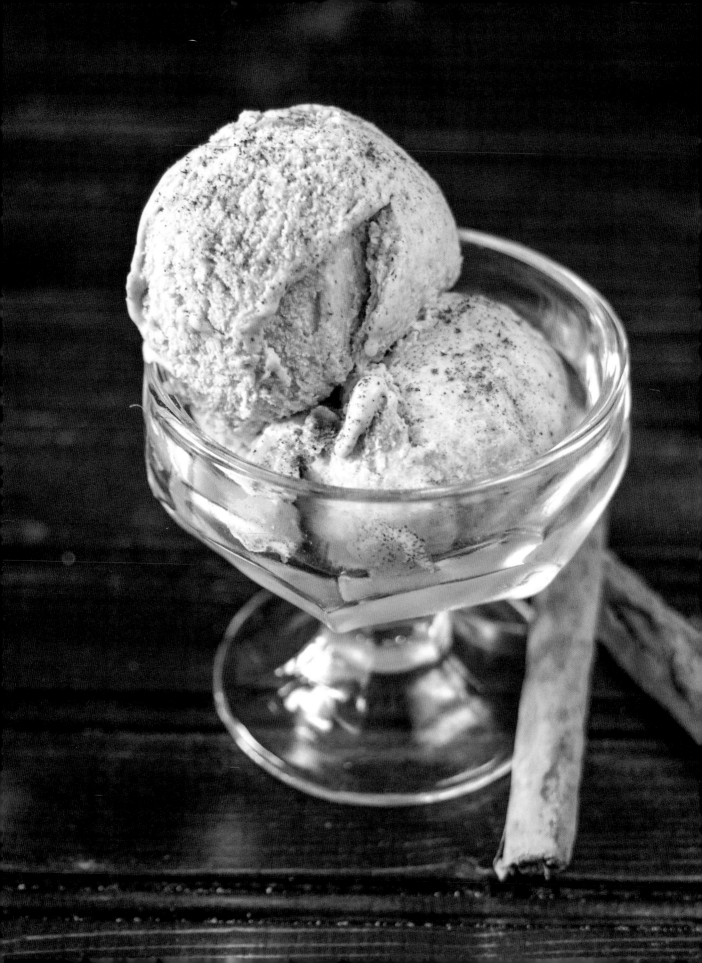

Contents

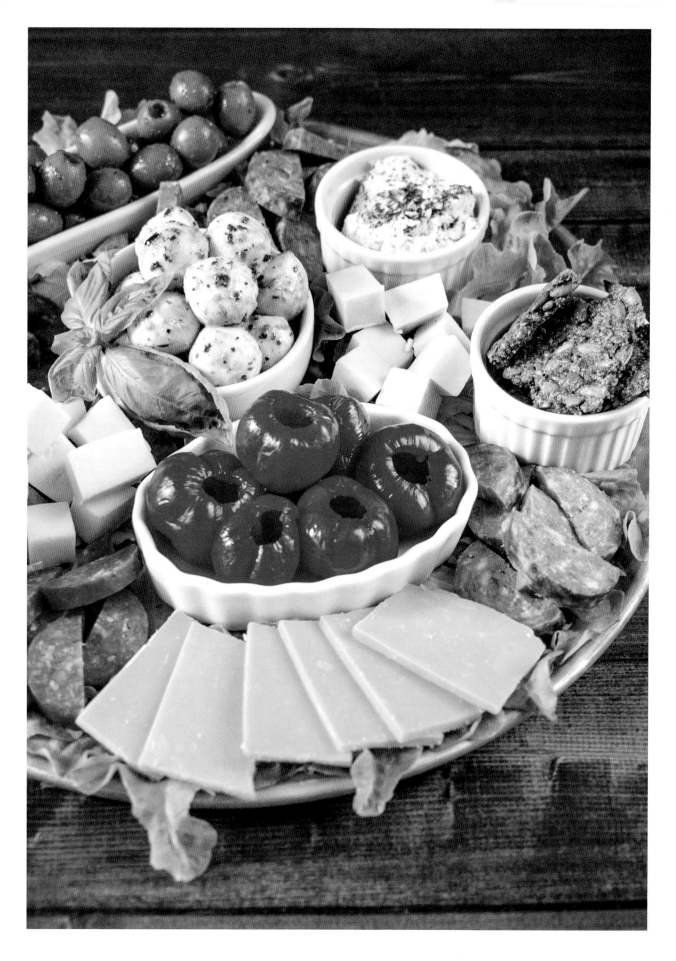

PREFACE

Ever since I was a little girl, I've been obsessed with food. I love eating it, watching it being made, eating it, watching others enjoy it, and did I mention eating it?

Once I was old enough to make my own meals, I was always putting different flavor combinations together, and I remember being so proud when people would taste my dish and their faces would light up. There is nothing that makes me happier than someone gushing over how wonderful a meal I made was and how much they enjoyed it.

Cooking for a low-carb, high-fat keto diet requires a little bit more creativity in the kitchen, and it's really allowed my cooking and innovation skills to flourish. My kids like to suggest different foods for me to make keto-friendly, and so far, they've all been winners! And that's why I wrote this book: to show that low-carb meals don't have to be boring or tasteless. One of the main reasons I have been able to stick with keto and enjoy its amazing benefits is that I never feel like I'm missing out. I truly enjoy everything that I eat!

I'm very excited to share so many of my favorite recipes with all of you. Whether you're just starting to adapt to a low-carb, high-fat diet or you're a seasoned pro, this book is full of mouthwatering recipes that will make you love eating keto. All my dishes are toddler-, teenager- and even carb eater–approved. I've taken the time to test each and every one to make sure they are perfectly seasoned and absolutely delicious—you won't need to make any guesses about how much salt or other seasonings to add. Most of the recipes in this book can be made within 30 to 45 minutes, but if a recipe has a longer cook time, don't let that scare you off—it's just as easy to make! And it will be worth the extra time, I promise.

Thank you for being a part of my journey and for allowing me to be a part of yours.

Nicole

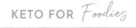

MY STORY

I started eating keto in May 2016 as a last-ditch effort to lose the excess weight I had been carrying around for three decades. Yes, three decades! I started gaining weight around the age of seven, even though I wasn't allowed to have sugary drinks or cereal and all our meals were home-cooked and "healthy." Of course, now we know that mashed potatoes and corn aren't really part of a healthy meal, but back then no one knew that.

I never really knew that I was overweight, or at least I didn't acknowledge it. The first time I ever realized I was overweight was when I was twelve years old and my mom took me shopping for my uncle's rehearsal dinner. Nothing I tried on was really working, so she took me to the *maternity section*. As I reluctantly tried on clothes meant for pregnant women, I vowed that I was going to lose weight so I would never have to feel so ashamed and embarrassed again.

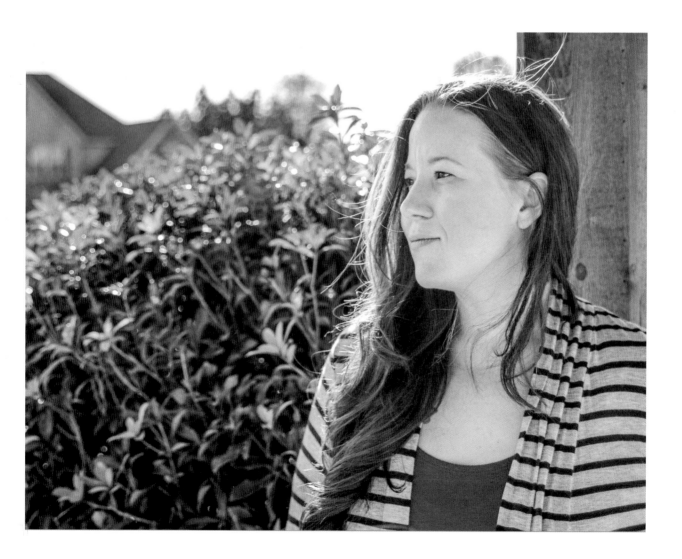

That vow lasted until my parents said that I was not allowed to diet because I had already been measured for my bridesmaid's dress and it couldn't be altered. For some reason, in my mind, that gave me a free pass for the rest of my childhood, which was spent eating carb-filled school lunches followed by carb-filled dinners. To me, unhealthy food was fast food, which I ate very rarely—until I started working at Burger King and Baskin-Robbins at the same time! We were allowed free meals and free ice cream, and boy, did I take them up on that. I must have put on thirty pounds within two months. After I graduated high school and moved out on my own, it didn't get any better; with two jobs, I didn't have any extra minutes in my day to cook, so I was eating two meals of fast food every day. The only thing that kept me from becoming obese then was the high-activity job I had at FedEx. I actually started to lose weight and look pretty good after a few months of working there.

Then I got pregnant with my daughter. I was no longer able to work in the same department at FedEx while pregnant, so while my eating stayed pretty much the same, my activity level plummeted. I gained close to eighty pounds with that pregnancy, and I never got much of it off. Once my daughter was eating solid food, I was making home-cooked meals every day that included mashed potatoes and corn several times a week. I would always eat two very full plates of food along with two large glasses of milk (close to 50 grams of carbs on their own!), and yet I thought I was doing the right thing.

Once my daughter was a toddler, I dabbled in different weight-loss programs like Weight Watchers, but I never saw any results and I was always hungry. I tried killing myself at the gym, but again, no results. I then started to do more drastic things to lose weight, like the lemonade diet, which was just plain silly. No matter what I tried, I always felt hungry, lethargic, and completely let down.

Then, in 2006, I found out about Atkins and cut my carbs way down. That was great for a few months—I lost around twenty-five pounds. I celebrated with a few cheat meals, which turned into cheat days and then cheat weeks and sometimes even months. This continued for several years—I just ate whatever I wanted, gained weight, went back to Atkins and lost weight, cheated again, and repeat.

I tried raw vegan and vegan diets for two years. That was a miserable existence. I lost almost a hundred pounds, but it was mostly due to starvation. I love salad, but only when it's covered in blue cheese or ranch dressing, and ranch made from cashews isn't gonna cut it! In my vegan years, I basically just consumed fruit, fruit juice, and spinach smoothies with hemp protein.

In 2013, I needed emergency neck and spinal cord surgery, and in my research on quick healing, I found that eating additional protein was important. At that time, I was getting very low amounts of protein, and there was no way I could handle more plant protein. Then I discovered Paleo. That was just fantastic. I was eating whole fresh foods and meat! I was thrilled; life was good. Then I started making Paleo breads and using plentiful amounts of maple syrup and honey. Then white potatoes found themselves on the Paleo accepted-foods list, and my brain said, *Mmm, fried potatoes*. It was all downhill from there.

All the carbs I was consuming were quickly adding up, and before I knew it, I had gained sixty-five pounds! And, as I found out later, I'd developed insulin resistance. I started working out twice a day for two months straight, and guess what, no results (aside from aching feet)! I was ready to give up. I had been fighting to lose weight for over a decade at this point, and nothing was working.

Then I heard about keto. It reminded me of Atkins, which had worked for me in the past for a little while, though I'd had trouble sticking with it—but the hope that this time would be different was enough to get me to try keto. I found that with keto, I ate more fat—Atkins put more emphasis on protein—and that difference was enough that I had no problem sticking to keto. I was happy with what I was eating, always satiated, and I was finally losing weight! I truly believe it is the extra fat intake that makes this way of eating so amazing. Fat is delicious and satiating, so you never feel deprived, and that makes it easy to stick with keto.

Within a year of eating keto, and with the addition of intermittent fasting, which keto makes so easy, I lost ninety-two pounds and a total of forty inches from my body. I've never felt this amazing in my life. I'm constantly bursting with energy (without the use of any caffeine), my sleep is perfect, and I started kickboxing this year, which is my absolute new love! It amazes me every day that keto completely gave me my life back. I went from breathlessly struggling to tie my shoes to kickboxing five days a week! I'm so thankful to keto for making my life and my family's lives 100 percent better.

I also love that keto lets me be creative in the kitchen again. I just love to cook, so dieting was always a struggle for me—I hated losing that creative outlet. With keto, I've been able to turn all the favorites I enjoyed before into keto-friendly dishes without compromising any flavor! Both my eighteen-year-old daughter and seven-year-old son eat keto as well, and they love everything I put in front of them. I have had countless non-keto people try my recipes, and they all say they'd never have known the dishes were keto, which fills my heart with joy!

The friendships I have formed within our loving and supportive keto community are absolutely priceless, and I'm so thankful for each and every one of them. It was the overwhelming support and encouragement of this community that led me to create Keto Transformations, an Instagram account that celebrates all of the hard work we all put in and the amazing results it leads to. I admire all of you, and your successes motivate me every single day.

Now, let's eat!

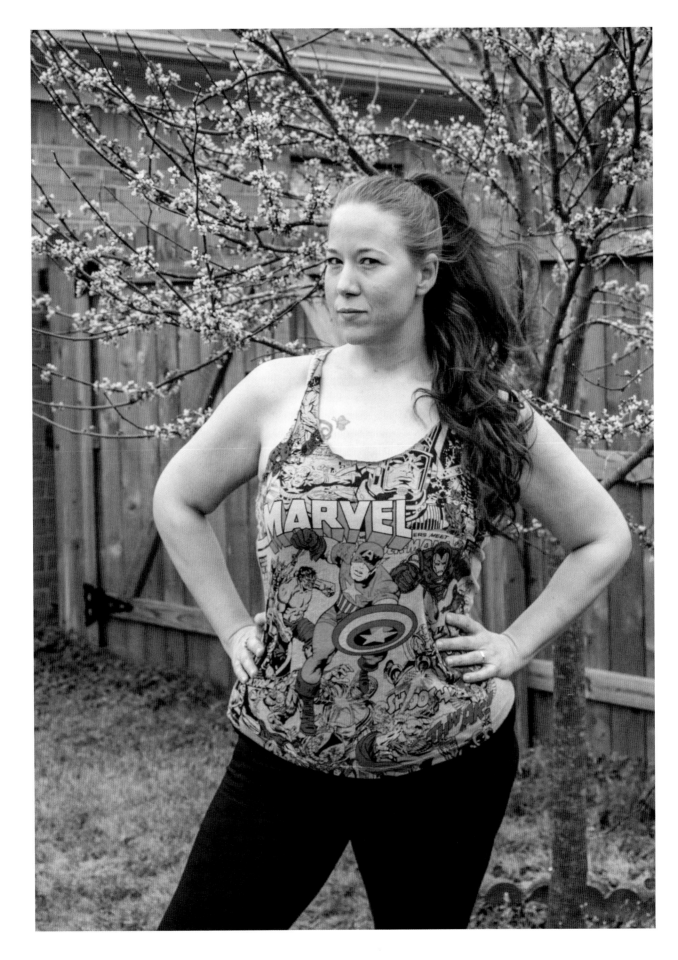

THE NUTS and BOLTS of KETO

If you are reading this, you probably have some idea what the keto diet is all about. My purpose in writing this book is not to give you a comprehensive education in keto; it's about delicious keto recipes! There are countless books, websites, blogs, and videos that explain in very technical terms what ketosis is and how it works, so I won't do that here. What I would like to do is give you a brief understanding (or reminder) of what keto is and how it works, without getting into any of the technical jargon.

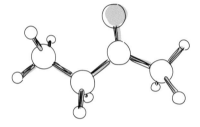

WHAT'S A KETONE?

If you've ever attempted to research what a ketone is, you've probably noticed two things: there is a lot of information about the subject, and you may need a degree in organic chemistry to understand it all.

So let's break it down to the basics. When people refer to "ketones," they're talking about a group of three molecules called "ketone bodies" that are produced by your liver. For our purposes, there are three important things to know about ketones:

1. They are by-products of fat-burning.
2. They are an alternative fuel source to glucose.
3. Their production is triggered by the absence of glucose.

That absence of glucose is a key part of the ketogenic diet. The ketogenic diet itself is designed to increase the production of ketones (the name literally means "ketone-generating"). Since carbs break down into glucose and the absence of glucose is what allows ketones to be produced, the ketogenic diet is low in carbs. And because ketones are produced when fat is burned, keto is also high in fat.

Ketones are not only an alternative fuel source to glucose; they are the preferred fuel source of your body and a much more efficient fuel for your brain and heart as well. They're even better for your metabolism.

Ketones are usually associated with a very-low-carb diet, but they also are produced during pregnancy, infancy, fasting, and exercise.

KETOSIS VS. SUGAR-BURNING

Ketosis is simply the state of having a certain amount of ketones in your blood. To understand why that's desirable, first we need to look at the typical American diet and how it affects the body.

Most Americans today consume a highly processed, high-sugar diet. Even when we try to eat healthy, we typically fuel our bodies with foods that quickly convert to glucose—sugar. For example, on the glycemic index, which measures how foods affect blood sugar levels, wheat bread is nearly equal to a can of sugary soda.

To process all that glucose, the body produces an abundance of insulin, which moves glucose from the bloodstream into cells. Insulin also causes the body to store excess glucose that you're not using as body fat, so that you can use that fat for energy later.

But as long as you're eating a high-glucose diet, this fat is never utilized. Although it's not the best or most efficient fuel source for your body, glucose is the easiest molecule for the body to convert to energy. Because of this, when glucose is present, your body chooses glucose first as its fuel. So when your body is constantly stocked with glucose, it becomes accustomed to using it and never uses that stored body fat. After a while, eating a glucose-heavy diet (which means a carb-heavy diet) can lead to excess body weight, insulin resistance (the forerunner to type 2 diabetes, in which your body no longer responds to insulin's signals), type 2 diabetes, and many other health problems.

So that's what's going on for most of us. When you're on a low-carb, high-fat ketogenic diet, though, you can use fat as fuel instead of sugar and shift into ketosis, which is actually your natural metabolic state. Newborns produce a massive number of ketones, even when they're primarily fed breast milk, which has a fair amount of carbs in it.

To generate more ketones and get into ketosis, the general idea is to eat a low-carb, moderate-protein, high-fat diet. On this diet, your liver uses fat to produce ketones, which are used for energy. You are essentially using fat rather than glucose for fuel—quite the opposite of the typical high-glucose diet. Over time, your body adapts to using fat as its primary fuel and becomes more efficient at it. When your body is completely used to fat and no longer craves glucose, you're "fat-adapted."

Getting into ketosis generally takes anywhere from a few days to a few weeks (depending on what your previous diet was) and typically requires eating 30 grams of net carbs or less per day. Some people may find that they need to eat as few as 20 grams of net carbs per day to achieve ketosis. This usually means eliminating or greatly reducing sugary foods like candy, soda, many fruits, grains (bread, cereal, pasta, and the like), and starchy vegetables, like potatoes.

While it may take you up to six weeks to achieve true ketosis, that does not mean you will not see benefits much sooner. In fact, it is not uncommon to see a significant weight loss in the first few weeks. While some of this is attributed to shedding excess water weight (a high-carb diet is known to cause water retention), it's still very nice to see the scale move in the right direction!

BENEFITS OF THE KETOGENIC DIET

On a low-carb diet, you won't have such a high demand for insulin, giving your pancreas a much-needed rest and allowing your body to become more sensitive to insulin, especially if you were insulin resistant. You also won't experience the well-known energy crash about an hour or so after eating—since your body is accustomed to burning fat, not carbs, it can use body fat as a steady supply of fuel that's always available.

Since keto means consuming less glucose (so there's less to be turned into body fat) and actually burning stored body fat (since your body is used to relying on fat for fuel), many people find they lose a significant amount of weight on keto. A recent study found a keto diet to be 2.2 times more effective for weight loss than a low-fat or low-calorie diet.*

You may also notice that you feel less hungry and more satisfied on keto, and because a healthy high-fat diet is very satiating, you may need smaller portions than you did before—which is also great for weight loss.

Many people on the keto diet also report improved energy, improved physical performance, better cognitive function, improved digestion, much less heartburn, clearer skin, and an increase in muscle density.

Other conditions that a keto lifestyle have been reported to improve include the following:

- Acne
- Alzheimer's disease
- Cancer
- Heart disease
- Metabolic syndrome
- Parkinson's disease
- Polycystic ovary syndrome
- Type 2 diabetes

TOTAL CARBS OR NET CARBS?

Fiber is a carbohydrate, but it's not digestible, so it doesn't contribute to blood sugar levels and doesn't provide fuel for the body. With that in mind, you can subtract the amount of fiber from the total amount of carbohydrate in a food. The result is the food's net carbs.

Whether you count your total carb intake or net carb intake is up to you. I prefer counting net carbs—I find that it's easier to stay on keto when you give yourself an allowance for those carbs you're not getting fuel from. But each recipe in this book tells you the amount of total carbs, net carbs, and fiber, so you can choose whatever works best for you!

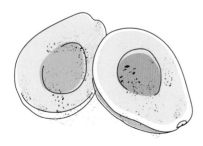

---

* *Bonnie J. Brehm, Randy J. Seely, Stephen R. Daniels, and David D'Alessio, "A Randomized Trial Comparing a Very Low Carbohydrate Diet and a Calorie-Restricted Low Fat Diet on Body Weight and Cardiovascular Risk Factors in Healthy Women,"* Journal of Clinical Endocrinology and Metabolism *88, no. 4 (April 2003): 1617–1623.*

BALANCING YOUR KETO DIET

The keto diet is high in fat, moderate in protein, and low in carbs. That balance is an important part of getting your body to consistently burn fat as its main fuel. It's not just about eating low-carb, as important as that is—you need to eat high-fat, too!

The usual rule of thumb for keto is 75 percent fat, 20 percent protein, and 5 percent carbs. But that's just a ballpark guideline. You may find that you feel better and stay in ketosis when you eat more carbs and less fat. Test your ketone level with a blood ketone meter (the most accurate method) and see how different foods affect your levels. You may find that you do great on 65 percent fat, 20 percent protein, and 15 percent carbs. Just keep in mind the figure I mentioned earlier: to get into ketosis, it's best to stay under 30 grams of net carbs per day, although some may find that staying under 20 grams of net carbs is best.

To calculate your intake of fat, protein, and carbs, there's a bit of math involved. Every gram of protein contains 4 calories, as does every gram of carb. Every gram of fat contains 9 calories. With those figures in mind, you can add up your total calories for the day and figure out the percentage of fat, protein, and carb.

For example, let's say that your goal is to consume 2,000 calories per day, with 120 of those calories coming from carb (30 grams of carb). To get 75 percent of those calories from fat, you'd need to eat 167 grams of fat (167 grams x 9 calories per gram = 1503 calories). To get 20 percent of those calories from protein, you'd need to eat 100 grams of protein (100 grams x 4 calories per gram = 400 calories).

But again, you might find that a different balance works better for you. Try different percentages and see how you feel—always keeping your carb intake very low.

Personally, I've found that tracking macros is difficult to sustain over the long term, but you may find it helpful, especially as you're transitioning to keto and getting into ketosis. Eventually you'll get a feel for the kinds and amounts of foods that work best for you, and you may find that you don't need to track your intake as closely. The most important thing is to stay under 30 grams of net carbs each day.

KETO FLU

While many people can transition to keto with no ill effects, it is also not uncommon to have some minor symptoms as your body adapts to relying on fat instead of carbs for fuel. These symptoms have become widely known as the "keto flu."

Keto flu has many of the same symptoms as the regular flu, including low energy, headache, and stomach discomfort. These symptoms usually last only a few days.

If you experience the keto flu, first, replenish your electrolytes! With the drop in insulin as you transition from a high-carb to a low-carb diet, your body releases more water, and with it go electrolytes. Sodium, magnesium, and potassium are particularly important, so consider supplementing these or eating whole foods that contain more of these electrolytes, like spinach and avocados—and don't forget to drink plenty of water! I've found success in adding electrolytes with sole solution (see page 16 for instructions).

Another option for handling keto flu is to eat a normal low-carb diet (under 50 grams of net carbs daily) for a week or so and then decrease your carbs to ketogenic levels (under 30 grams of net carbs daily).

TIPS FOR KETO SUCCESS

I've found through trial and error that there are things you can do to improve your success on keto. These are my top tips.

1. Add sole to your daily routine.

Keto is a diuretic, especially in the early days—it causes your body to stop retaining water, and when that water goes, so do important electrolytes. So it's of the utmost importance to replenish your electrolytes on keto, especially when you are first transitioning to a keto diet and may be experiencing keto flu. While you can always eat foods that contain more sodium, potassium, and magnesium, or take supplements, I've found the most success with sole (pronounced "so-lay").

Sole is a solution in which the water is fully saturated with natural salt such as pink Himalayan, which contains all eighty-four essential trace elements your body needs. It's made at home, and simply adding a bit of this solution to a glass of fresh water each morning provides your body with much-needed electrolytes. I personally have found that drinking sole each morning has helped heal several problems:

- **Leg cramps:** I used to have horrendous leg cramps every single night for years. Once I added sole to my daily routine, they went away completely!
- **Dry skin:** My skin used to be so dry that it flaked and peeled, but since I started taking sole, my skin has been bright, clear, and hydrated.
- **Insomnia:** I would sometimes lay in bed for hours trying to fall asleep, but sole has fixed that as well. I'm sound asleep as soon as my head hits the pillow every night.

Here's how to make sole:

1. Fill a 16-ounce mason jar a quarter of the way full with pink Himalayan salt (either coarse or fine will work).
2. Fill the jar with *filtered* water, leaving a bit of space at the top.
3. Cover tightly with a plastic lid. Metal will deionize the solution, so look for plastic mason jar tops in stores—they can be found right next to the mason jars.
4. Shake the mixture, then let it sit on the counter for twenty-four hours.
5. When the solution is clear and has a layer of undissolved salt at the bottom, it's ready! If there is no salt on the bottom, just add a little more salt, shake, and leave it for another twenty-four hours to be sure the solution is fully saturated with salt.

Each morning, pour 8 ounces of fresh water into a glass and add a small amount of sole solution. The amount of solution you add will depend on your body's needs, and your tongue will tell you what's right. Start with ¼ teaspoon, stir, and taste.

Keep adding sole in small increments until it tastes just like salt water. Most people find that about 1 teaspoon works for them, but it's best to start small and add more if needed. Personally, I needed a full tablespoon when I started out; now, two years later, I'm down to 2 teaspoons each morning.

Be sure to only use plastic measuring spoons for the solution so that no deionizing takes place. If you use fine-grind pink salt, try not to slosh the solution, so the salt at the bottom remains undisturbed. (You don't want to drink grains of salt in addition to what's dissolved in the solution!) Don't put sole into a bottle in order to pour the solution out; this will disturb the salt at the bottom and make the solution overly salty.

And here's one more tip: I add 1 teaspoon of apple cider vinegar to my morning cup of sole. I can't say I've noticed any benefits from the vinegar itself, but I love the sour-and-salty flavor!

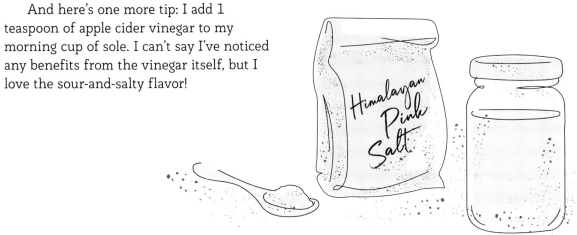

2. Embrace intermittent fasting.

Fasting has truly been one of the biggest factors in my weight-loss success, and I encourage everyone to at least give it a try. Intermittent fasting is basically an eating pattern where you cycle between eating and fasting. Often there's an "eating window" each day—for instance, you could eat in an eight-hour window, between, say, 11 a.m. and 7 p.m., and fast for the sixteen hours from 7 p.m. to 11 a.m. This is often called a 16/8 fast. You could also fast for eighteen or twenty hours—18/6 or 20/4 fasts. Another popular pattern is to eat normally five days a week and then limit yourself to 500 to 600 calories for two consecutive days.

If you've never considered fasting, I'm sure it sounds crazy! *Going without eating— won't I be starving?*

Not if you do it correctly! That's the great thing about keto. Once your body is accustomed to using fat as its primary fuel instead of glucose, fasting allows it to easily burn stored body fat for energy! And because you have a ready supply of body fat, hunger pangs are milder and don't last as long—your body doesn't need to urge you to eat in order to get fuel. Fasting also dramatically increases human growth hormone, which assists in healthy cell renewal, speeds up healing after an injury, boosts metabolism, and even slows down the aging process.

I didn't start intermittent fasting until I was six weeks into keto and fully fat-adapted, and I recommend that you do the same. Being completely fat-adapted before trying any type of fasting will reduce stress on your body and allow you to get the maximum benefits of fasting.

Easing into a new way of eating is always your best bet, so I recommend starting fasting by simply having your first meal of the day an hour later each day, until your first meal is at the beginning of your planned eating window. Then eat as you normally would (no bingeing!) until the end of your eating window. For example, if you're following a 16/8 fast and you want your eating window to be from 11 a.m. to 7 p.m., start by pushing your normal 7 a.m. breakfast back to 8 a.m. and stop eating at 7 p.m. The next day, have your first meal at 9 a.m. and, again, stop eating at 7 p.m. Continue this pattern until your first meal is at 11 a.m. (If you're going for a six-hour or four-hour eating window, you'll want to push back lunch as well as breakfast.) That's it!

When you're first starting out with fasting, drinking carbonated water helps a ton! The bubbles fill your tummy and make it easier to push yourself a little further each day. You can also have black coffee, tea, and water during your fasting window. However, I recommend consuming zero calories while on your fast. There are multiple schools of thought on this—some say you can have up to 100 calories and still not break your fast. That doesn't work for me, though. As soon as my body gets one calorie, it's ravenous for more, which makes it very difficult for me to continue my fast.

I did a twenty-hour fast with a four-hour eating window (during which I had two meals) for about six months. Then I took the plunge into a one-hour eating window, which is also known as OMAD ("one meal a day"). It turned out to be one of the best decisions I ever made! Before, I was always obsessing about food, always thinking about my next meal, even when I was eating. Taking food out of the equation for the entire day completely eliminated the constant thoughts about food. It also gave me a huge increase in energy because I wasn't spending calories just to digest food.

I have been eating OMAD for about a year now, and I'll never go back. I eat around 7 or 8 p.m. each night, which completely knocks out the need for late-night snacking, something that had been a problem my entire life. I *always* listen to my body, though, and if I feel like I need to eat earlier in the day, then I eat. Sometimes I have a small snack and then my main meal later if I had an extra-hard workout that day. The only times I eat multiple meals in a day are holidays. I still always keep it keto, but I do eat a little extra!

Don't try to prove to yourself that you're a superhero—if you feel like you need to eat, then eat! Listen to your body and make sure you're getting what you need. But once you're fat-adapted, you'll be amazed at how long you can go without food and how good you'll feel when fasting.

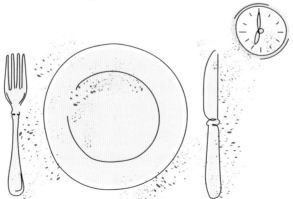

3. Take pictures and measurements before you start.

The scale will not always reflect the progress you are making, and the last thing you want is to be discouraged. So I recommend taking "before" and "after" pictures of every angle, so you can see just how far you've come. Photos in too-tight clothing are fantastic because they'll really show the change when you start losing inches all over. Take "after" photos once a month or so—when you're looking in the mirror every day, it's easy to miss small changes that add up over time, but if you take pictures once a month, you'll easily be able to see your progress.

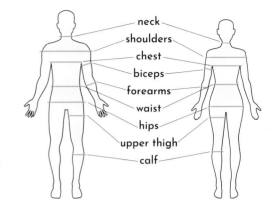

    In addition to photos, take measurements from head to toe. That will give you concrete numerical evidence of how your body is changing over time.

4. Research more about the keto diet.

There is so much information about keto all over the internet and in so many wonderful books. Go the extra mile to do the research and learn how to be successful with this way of eating. Google can be your best friend, and I found all the keto information I needed on the site Ruled.me. This amazing keto website has been the starting point for countless people who've been successful on the keto diet. Social media is also a great place to find other keto lovers and get inspired. You can find all the motivation that you need on my Keto Transformations page on Instagram. Thousands of people from all walks of life who are finding success with keto are sharing their stories and tips there.

5. Celebrate your victories!

You can't see every achievement on the scale or even in "after" photos. Sometimes you'll find that you're suddenly able to do or wear something you never have before—celebrate that!

    My own early victories were being able to tie my shoes without becoming out of breath, not obsessing over food, and noticing that my anxiety was getting better. My biggest non-scale victory was having the courage to join a kickboxing gym and pushing myself harder and harder with each class. Seeing all the improvements I made, the ease with which I could do exercises that had once seemed impossible, gave me the most incredible feeling of accomplishment.

    Celebrate yourself and the hard work you're putting in as often as possible. You deserve it!

KETO FOODS

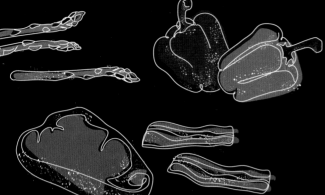

MEAT

MEAT	SERVING SIZE	NET CARBS (g)
Bacon	4 oz (113g)	0
Beef (ground, steaks, roasts)	4 oz (113g)	0
Deli meat (no sugar added)	4 oz (113g)	1
Fish (cod, flounder, halibut, salmon, sea bass, tilapia, tuna, etc.)	4 oz (113g)	0
Lamb (ground, chops)	4 oz (113g)	0
Organ meat (heart, liver, etc.)	4 oz (113g)	<1
Pork (ground, chops, loin, no-sugar-added ham, sausage)	4 oz (113g)	0
Poultry (chicken, turkey, duck)	4 oz (113g)	0
Shellfish (clams, crab, lobster, scallops, shrimp, etc.)	4 oz (113g)	0-3 *

VEGGIES

VEGGIES	SERVING SIZE	NET CARBS (g)
Artichokes	½ cup (84g)	5.2
Asparagus	1 cup (134g)	2.4
Bell peppers	1 cup (92g)	3.6
Broccoli	1 cup (91g)	3.6
Brussels sprouts	1 cup (88g)	4.6
Carrots	1 medium (78g)	5.0
Cauliflower	1 cup (107g)	3.2
Celery	1 cup (101g)	1.4
Cucumbers	½ cup (52g)	1.6
Eggplant	1 cup (82g)	2.3
Garlic	1 clove (3g)	0.9
Green beans	1 cup (100g)	4.3
Jalapeño peppers	1 pepper (14g)	0.5
Jicama	1 cup (130g)	5.1
Leeks	½ cup (45g)	5.5
Mushrooms	1 cup (86g)	2.2
Onions	½ cup (58g)	4.3
Poblano peppers	1 pepper (17g)	1.9
Radishes	1 cup (116g)	2
Scallions	1 cup (100g)	4.7
Shallots	1 cup (10g)	1.4
Spaghetti squash	1 cup (101g)	5.5
Yellow squash	1 cup (113g)	2.6
Zucchini	1 cup (113g)	2.4

Most shellfish are at the low end of this range. The ones that are higher in carbs are clams, scallops, mussels, and oysters.

FRUIT

FRUIT	SERVING SIZE	NET CARBS (g)
Avocados	½ fruit (100g)	1.8
Blackberries	½ cup (72g)	3.1
Blueberries	½ cup (74g)	8.9
Coconut meat	½ cup (40g)	2.5
Lemons	1 medium (58g)	5.4
Limes	1 medium (67g)	5.2
Olives	½ cup (67g)	2.2
Raspberries	½ cup (61.5g)	3.3
Strawberries	½ cup (76g)	4.3
Tomatoes	1 cup (180g)	4.8

DAIRY

DAIRY	SERVING SIZE	NET CARBS (g)
Cheese (all kinds)	1 oz (28g)	<1
Cottage cheese (full-fat)	½ cup (112g)	4.0
Cream cheese (full-fat)	1 Tbsp (14.5g)	0.8
Eggs	1 large (56g)	0
Greek yogurt (full-fat, plain)	1 cup (112g)	4.5
Half & half	1 Tbsp (15g)	0.7
Heavy cream	1 Tbsp(15g)	0.4
Ricotta cheese	½ cup (124g)	3.8
Sour cream	1 Tbsp (12g)	0.6

NUTS & SEEDS

	SERVING SIZE	NET CARBS (g)
Almonds	¼ cup (28g)	3
Brazil nuts	¼ cup (33g)	1.4
Chia seeds	1 oz (28g)	2.1
Flax seeds	2 Tbsp (20.5g)	0.4
Hazelnuts	¼ cup (34g)	2.3
Hemp seeds	3 Tbsp (30g)	1.4
Macadamia nuts	¼ cup (33g)	1.7
Peanuts	¼ cup (36g)	2.8
Pecans	¼ cup (36g)	1
Pine nuts	¼ cup (36g)	3.2
Pistachios	¼ cup (31g)	5
Pumpkin seeds	¼ cup (32g)	1.6
Sunflower seeds	¼ cup (11.5g)	1.3
Walnuts	¼ cup (30g)	2

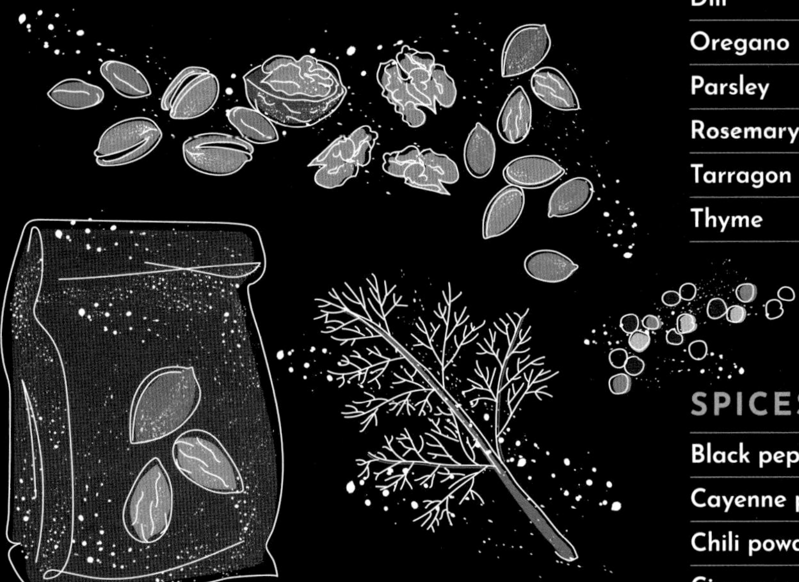

CONDIMENTS

	SERVING SIZE	NET CARBS (g)
Coconut aminos	1 Tbsp (15ml)	6
Horseradish	1 tsp (5g)	0.5
Mayonnaise	1 Tbsp (13g)	0.1
Mustard	1 tsp (5g)	0.1
Vinegar (balsamic)	1 Tbsp (15ml)	2.7
Vinegar (white, apple cider)	1 Tbsp (15ml)	0

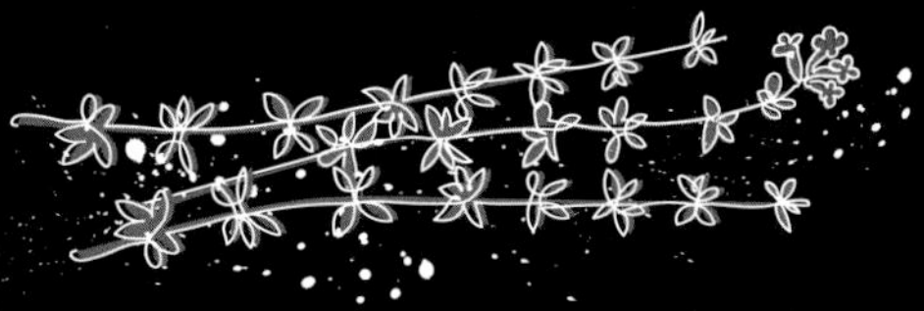

FRESH HERBS

	SERVING SIZE	NET CARBS (g)
Basil	2 Tbsp (5g)	0
Chives	1 Tbsp (3g)	0.1
Cilantro	1 Tbsp (1g)	0.1
Dill	1 Tbsp (0.5g)	0.1
Oregano	1 Tbsp (3g)	0.3
Parsley	1 Tbsp (4g)	0.1
Rosemary	1 Tbsp (2g)	0.2
Tarragon	1 Tbsp (0.5g)	0.3
Thyme	1 Tbsp (2.5g)	0.3

BAKING INGREDIENTS

	SERVING SIZE	NET CARBS (g)
Almond flour	¼ cup (28g)	3
Cocoa powder	1 Tbsp (5.5g)	1.1
Coconut flour	2 Tbsp (14g)	4
Flaxseed meal	2 Tbsp (11g)	1
Psyllium husk powder	1 tsp (4g)	0
Pure flavor extracts	1 tsp (4g)	0.1
Xanthan gum	½ tsp (0.5g)	0

SPICES

	SERVING SIZE	NET CARBS (g)
Black pepper, ground	1 tsp (2g)	0.9
Cayenne pepper	¼ tsp (0.5g)	0.2
Chili powder	1 Tbsp (8g)	1.2
Cinnamon, ground	1 tsp (2.5g)	0.7
Crushed red pepper	1 tsp (2g)	0
Cumin, ground	1 tsp (3g)	0
Dry mustard	1 tsp (2g)	0.4
Fennel seed	1 Tbsp (6g)	0.7
Garlic powder	1 tsp (3g)	2
Onion powder	1 tsp (2g)	1.5
Paprika (regular or smoked)	1 tsp (2g)	0.4
Salt	1 tsp (6g)	0
Turmeric	1 tsp (3g)	1.3

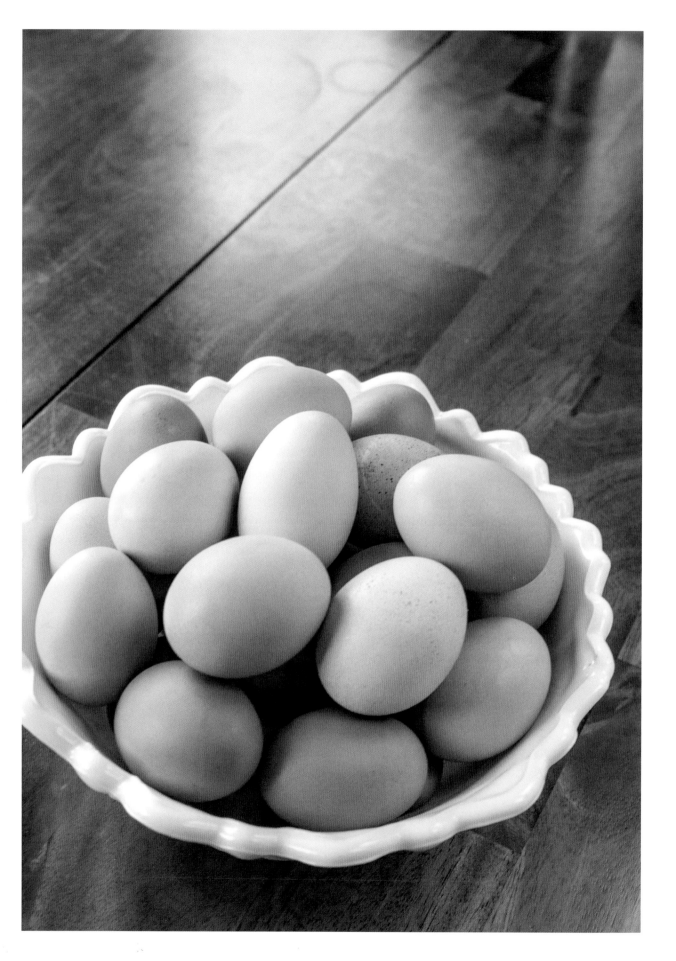

KETO COOKING TIPS & TRICKS

When you're eating keto, you'll probably find that you're spending more time in the kitchen. Not to worry, I'm here with my best tips and tricks for excellent keto meals!

Save on marked-down meat

Check your local grocery store for a clearance meat area. If it doesn't have one or you can't find it, ask the meat department when they mark down their meat selection. I check my store almost daily, and I find the most amazing steals—even upward of 75 percent off! Just use this meat within a day or freeze it immediately for later use. I love my vacuum sealer for this reason; it saves me a ton of money! The vacuum seal prevents ice crystals from forming, so I can store meat for longer periods of time without the risk of freezer burn.

Pick the best heads of lettuce

I love lettuce wraps, and I've found that there are heads of iceberg lettuce that work great and some that don't. Look for a large head that feels light for its size and seems loose—it'll be much easier to remove the leaves in one piece.

And one more tip for iceberg lettuce: whenever you're using a fresh head for lettuce wraps, hold it in your hands and hit the core of the lettuce down on the counter once or twice, then remove the core (it should release easily). It makes separating the lettuce leaves even easier!

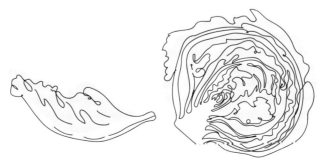

Use pork rinds generously!

OK, I get it! You either love pork rinds or hate them. But if you think you hate them, I'm here to change your mind!

I rarely eat pork rinds on their own (with the exception of pork rind nachos—see the box below), but I use them *all the time* in my cooking. Crushed pork rinds make the best keto breading, hands down! Not only are they zero-carb and high in fat, but nothing compares to the crispiness that a crust of pork rind crumbs imparts. And when toasted, they work perfectly as a binder to make the most tender and delicious meatloaf and meatballs.

Having crushed pork rinds on hand makes cooking with them super easy. Just put half of a 5-ounce bag of plain pork rinds in a food processor and pulse into fine crumbs. I crush two bags at a time; they'll keep in an airtight container in the fridge for several months. It takes 5 minutes, and you're set for a while!

If you find that the smell of bagged pork rinds bothers you, just open the bag and let it sit for a bit; the smell will be virtually gone.

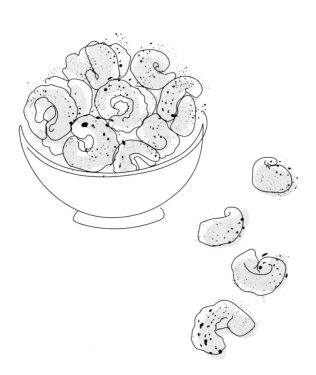

PORK RIND NACHOS

Making these nachos is so easy you don't really need a recipe!

1. Place pork rinds on a plate in a single layer and top with shredded cheese (cheddar, mozzarella, Monterey Jack, Colby Jack, pepper Jack—any kind works great).

2. Microwave on high just until the cheese melts, about 30 to 45 seconds.

3. Top with cooked meat—shredded chicken, ground beef, grilled steak, pulled pork, etc.

4. Drizzle with any sauce—Buffalo sauce, taco sauce, chipotle mayo, spicy mayo, etc.

5. If you like, add veggies, such as sautéed peppers and onions, chopped raw onions, even salsa or pico de gallo.

6. Add a dollop of goodness, like sour cream, blue cheese dressing, ranch dressing, or horseradish, and serve!

Make perfect hard-boiled eggs

To make hard-boiled eggs, I used to just let them boil for I don't even know how long! I thought it was a guessing game, and I didn't want them to not be fully cooked. Let's just say I suffered through green-ringed, rubbery, overcooked hard-boiled eggs for a good long time.

I know better now! This method for making hard-boiled eggs really couldn't be easier, and you will have perfect eggs every single time!

1. Place the eggs in a single layer at the bottom of a large pot. Fill the pot with enough cool water to cover the eggs by 1 inch.

2. Bring to a boil. Cover, remove from the heat, and set a timer for 12 minutes.

3. While the eggs cook, fill a large bowl with ice water.

4. After the time is up, transfer the eggs to the ice water and let cool for about 5 minutes. Ta-da! Perfect hard-boiled eggs.

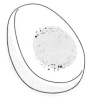

Make lardons in advance

Lardons should be called bacon crumbles 2.0—they're small pieces of fatty bacon, and they are delicious and so easy to make!

Making lardons is great for meal prep so you have crumbled bacon for the week. You can also use the bacon grease for cooking other dishes—just store it in a mason jar in the fridge. And making lardons couldn't be easier:

1. Heat a skillet over medium-high heat.

2. Slice 1 pound of thick-cut bacon in half lengthwise, then cut the strips crosswise into 1-inch pieces.

3. Sauté the bacon pieces, stirring occasionally, until browned and crispy, about 15 minutes.

4. Use a slotted spoon to transfer the crispy bacon to a paper towel–lined plate and let cool.

Serve lardons on top of everything you can think of, or store them in an airtight container in the fridge for up to a week. You can also use this method to cook salt pork or pork belly instead of bacon.

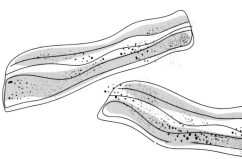

Save your meat trimmings for homemade stock

WHAT TO SAVE

- Seafood shells (lobster, shrimp, crawfish)
- Steak bones and any gristle (I always pick up a pack or two of marrow bones to add to the trimmings for beef stock—you can find these just about anywhere these days, but your local butcher will probably give you the best deal)
- Trimmings from boneless, skinless chicken breasts
- Bones and gristle from bone-in chicken thighs
- Wing tips, removed from chicken wings
- Carcass of a whole cooked chicken

This is my best tip of all!

We all know how wonderful and therapeutic stock is. It's fatty and delicious, and filled with vitamins and minerals. I'm not talking about boxed stock here, although that works in a pinch to make your favorite soup—homemade stock is on an entirely different level in both flavor and nutrition.

Making your own stock may sound daunting, but I assure you, it really couldn't be simpler. You can even make it in your slow cooker overnight!

Here's the key: Every time you're prepping meat—cutting off the fat, removing the bones, shelling seafood—save the trimmings, bones, and shells in gallon-size freezer bags. Just make sure you keep different meats separate from each other—poultry in one bag, beef in another, seafood in a third. Once a gallon bag is nearly full of bones and trimmings, you're ready to make stock!

CHICKEN STOCK

Here's my favorite recipe for homemade chicken stock.

4 pounds chicken bones and trimmings

12 cups water

1 tablespoon black peppercorns, or ½ tablespoon black peppercorns and ½ tablespoon white peppercorns

1 tablespoon dried minced onion (see Note)

1 tablespoon celery flakes (see Note)

1 tablespoon dried parsley

2½ teaspoons fine sea salt

Note : Feel free to use fresh chopped onion instead of dried minced onion and fresh chopped celery instead of celery flakes.

- Put the chicken bones and trimmings in a large stockpot and pour in the water. Bring to a boil, then turn the heat down to medium-low. Add the spices and stir well. Simmer for 4 to 5 hours.

- Strain the stock through a fine-mesh sieve into a large pot; discard the solids. Stir in the salt until it's completely dissolved.

- Let the stock cool, then store it in an airtight container in the fridge for 1 week or in the freezer for 2 months.

SLOW COOKER INSTRUCTIONS

- Place all the ingredients except the salt in a slow cooker and cook on low for at least 8 hours or up to 24 hours. Strain the stock through a fine-mesh sieve into a large pot; discard the solids. Stir in the salt until it's completely dissolved.

- Let the stock cool, then store it in an airtight container in the fridge for 1 week or in the freezer for 2 months.

Roast spaghetti squash for perfect low-carb noodles

I've been eating spaghetti squash since I was a kid, and I've always loved the lightly sweet flavor and the noodle-like texture. It's such a wonderful replacement for pasta, and it's excellent with just about any sauce you can imagine.

I have cooked spaghetti squash just about every way possible, and I've found that the very best results come from roasting your squash whole. Here's how:

1. Preheat the oven to 350°F. Prick the spaghetti squash all over with a small sharp knife. (These are vents for the steam, so the squash won't explode in the oven.)

2. Place the squash on a sheet pan and roast it in the oven until it's tender to the touch when you press on it, 1 to 1½ hours. Remove from the oven and let cool.

3. Once the squash is cool enough to handle, slice it in half crosswise (this gives you the longest strands) and remove the seeds with a spoon. Gently pull the strands of squash from the rind with a fork.

4. Alternatively, you can serve the squash in the rind: slice it lengthwise, remove the seeds, use a fork to pull apart the strands of squash, and top it with your favorite sauce.

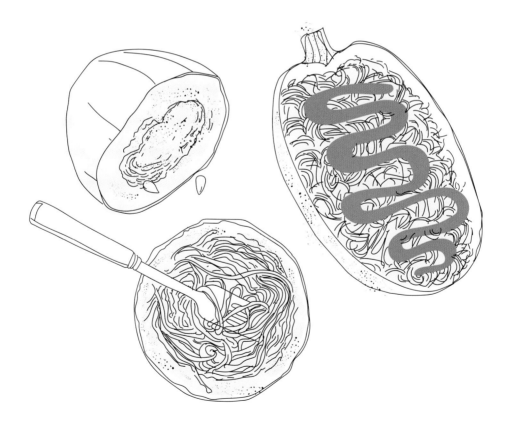

Poach chicken for the week in advance

Poaching several chicken breasts at once is a wonderful time-saver—in 15 minutes, you can have perfectly cooked chicken to use in recipes throughout the week! Truth be told, though, I poach chicken because I'm super weird about food textures, and I have found that poached chicken always has a great texture, no matter what.

Here's how to do it:

1. Place as many chicken breasts as possible in a single layer at the bottom of a large pot. Add enough water to cover the chicken by about an inch.

2. Add any seasonings you like, such as peppercorns, bay leaves, whole peeled garlic cloves, celery flakes, or dried minced onion.

3. Bring to a boil over medium-high heat, then turn the heat down to low. Cover and simmer for 10 minutes, or until the chicken's internal temperature reaches 165°F and it's no longer pink in the middle.

4. Transfer the chicken to a plate to cool and either use immediately or tightly wrap in plastic wrap and store in the fridge for up to a week.

With poached chicken made in advance, the following recipes will come together quickly:

170	238	166	236	128	244	172	144
Avgolemono	Chicken Bacon Swiss Lasagna	Chicken Bacon Poblano Soup	Chicken Pot Pie	Crispy Personal Pizzas	Green Chile Chicken Casserole	Gumbo	Lemon Tarragon Chicken Salad

You can also add poached chicken to the following dishes to make quick and easy meals:

      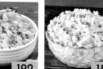

102	162	182	190	202	192	184
Queso Fundido	Golden Mushroom Soup	Gruyère Spinach Gratin	Spaghetti Squash Alfredo	Cilantro Lime Cauli Rice	Cashew Fried Cauli Rice	Cauli Risotto

And here are two of my favorite tricks for making quick no-recipe meals with poached chicken:

- *Simmer poached chicken with equal parts chicken stock (see page 26) and heavy cream until thickened, about 15 minutes, and serve over Best-Ever Cauli Mash (page 188).*

- *Sprinkle poached chicken with salt and pepper, add a little mayonnaise, and wrap it in a large lettuce leaf. Always reminds me of after-Thanksgiving turkey sandwiches!*

MEAL PREP *for* AN EASY WEEK

Meal prepping is a great tool for saving time and money. Simply set aside one afternoon or evening at the beginning of your week to cook a few entrées and sides, and all your meals are ready for you to grab and go for the rest of the week. It's a must for anyone with a jam-packed schedule, and it's also great for those who don't like to spend much time in the kitchen. Plus, when you're eating keto, it allows you to put together meals that have the right balance of fat, carbs, and protein for you, so you don't need to count and track your macros every single time you eat.

There are different ways of meal prepping, but here's what I've found to be the easiest method.

First, pick your entrées, keeping in mind the number of servings each recipe makes. If you're feeding two people for four meals, you'll want to select enough entrées that you have eight servings—probably two entrées that each make four servings.

Next, pick side dishes to go with each entrée. Look at both the number of servings the recipe makes and the amount of carbs in the dish—you'll want to add it to the amount of carbs in the entrée you're pairing it with and make sure you're staying at your goal. (Remember, on a keto diet, you want to stay under 30 grams of net carbs each day.)

On the following pages are a few of my favorite make-ahead dishes for meal prep. They can all be mixed and matched, so you have lots of options for the week!

BENEFITS OF MEAL PREPPING

- **Save time:** No more chopping and cooking every meal, every day.

- **Save money:** Less last-minute eating out, and you can shop sales when planning menus.

- **Get the perfect macros:** All components are balanced for your needs.

- **Stop overeating:** Food is ready when you are, so you don't get hungrier as you wait to eat.

- **End temptation:** You have healthy options on hand so you don't turn to junk food.

- **Reduce stress:** By cooking several meals in advance, you'll have less stress during the week—all you have to do is heat and eat.

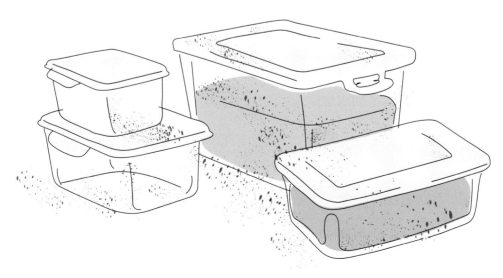

Pick Your Entrée(s)

CHICKEN

30 MINUTES or LESS

Pecan Chicken
SERVINGS 4
CALORIES 655
NET CARBS 2g

Chicken Pot Pie
SERVINGS 4
CALORIES 554
NET CARBS 9g

1 HOUR or LESS

French Country Stew
SERVINGS 4
CALORIES 687
NET CARBS 4g

Chicken Bacon Swiss Lasagna
SERVINGS 4
CALORIES 840
NET CARBS 9g

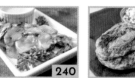

Fully Loaded Chicken
SERVINGS 4
CALORIES 430
NET CARBS 6g

Chipotle Lime Chicken
SERVINGS 4
CALORIES 473
NET CARBS 1g

Lemon Tarragon Chicken Salad
SERVINGS 4
CALORIES 354
NET CARBS 1g

Kung Pao Chicken
SERVINGS 4
CALORIES 384
NET CARBS 2g

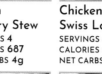

Chicken Bacon Poblano Soup
SERVINGS 4
CALORIES 441
NET CARBS 6g

Green Chile Chicken Casserole
SERVINGS 4
CALORIES 714
NET CARBS 11g

BEEF

30 MINUTES or LESS

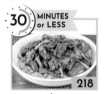

Mongolian Beef
SERVINGS 4
CALORIES 463
NET CARBS 3g

Beef Stroganoff
SERVINGS 4
CALORIES 409
NET CARBS 10g

1 HOUR or LESS

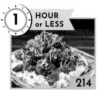

Cheesy Meatball Marinara
SERVINGS 4
CALORIES 552
NET CARBS 8g

Salisbury Steak
SERVINGS 4
CALORIES 466
NET CARBS 4g

BBQ Bacon Mini Meatloaves
SERVINGS 4
CALORIES 421
NET CARBS 4g

Bolognese Zucchini Lasagna
SERVINGS 4
CALORIES 620
NET CARBS 11g

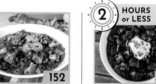

Albondigas Soup
SERVINGS 6
CALORIES 313
NET CARBS 6g

2 HOURS or LESS

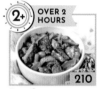

Chili con Carne
SERVINGS 4
CALORIES 514
NET CARBS 9g

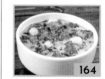

Creamy Steak Soup
SERVINGS 4
CALORIES 342
NET CARBS 5g

2+ OVER 2 HOURS

Beef Bourguignon
SERVINGS 4
CALORIES 833
NET CARBS 5g

Barbacoa
SERVINGS 6
CALORIES 635
NET CARBS 4g

PORK

30 MINUTES or LESS

Gumbo
SERVINGS 4
CALORIES 611
NET CARBS 9g

Szechuan Meatballs
SERVINGS 4
CALORIES 454
NET CARBS 1g

Spicy Garlic Pork with Stir-Fried Broccoli
SERVINGS 4
CALORIES 361
NET CARBS 3g

1 HOUR or LESS

Quiche Lorraine
SERVINGS 4
CALORIES 687
NET CARBS 5g

Loaded Cauli Leek Soup
SERVINGS 6
CALORIES 387
NET CARBS 7g

2+ OVER 2 HOURS

Carnitas
SERVINGS 6
CALORIES 537
NET CARBS 2g

Pick Your Side(s)

30 MINUTES or LESS

202

Cilantro Lime Cauli Rice
SERVINGS 6
CALORIES 69
NET CARBS 4g

182

Gruyère Spinach Gratin
SERVINGS 4
CALORIES 173
NET CARBS 1g

184

Cauli Risotto
SERVINGS 6
CALORIES 202
NET CARBS 5g

188

Best-Ever Cauli Mash
SERVINGS 6
CALORIES 146
NET CARBS 4g

1 HOUR or LESS

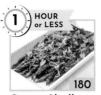

180

Crispy Shallot & Bacon Asparagus
SERVINGS 4
CALORIES 72
NET CARBS 4g

2 HOURS or LESS

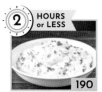

190

Spaghetti Squash Alfredo
SERVINGS 6
CALORIES 199
NET CARBS 7g

194

Lemon Garlic Baby Bok Choy
SERVINGS 4
CALORIES 122
NET CARBS 2g

192

Cashew Fried Cauli Rice
SERVINGS 6
CALORIES 162
NET CARBS 7g

138

Bacon Broc-Cauli Salad
SERVINGS 6
CALORIES 259
NET CARBS 4g

146

Sweet Dijon Coleslaw
SERVINGS 4
CALORIES 259
NET CARBS 3g

SUGGESTED PAIRINGS

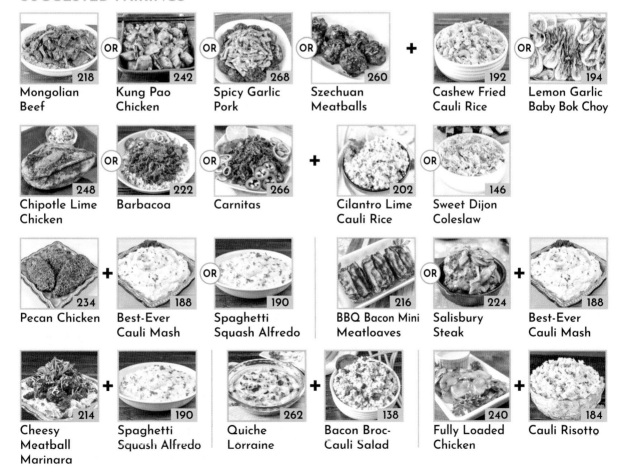

Mongolian Beef — **218**
OR Kung Pao Chicken — **242**
OR Spicy Garlic Pork — **268**
OR Szechuan Meatballs — **260**
+ Cashew Fried Cauli Rice — **192**
OR Lemon Garlic Baby Bok Choy — **194**

Chipotle Lime Chicken — **248**
OR Barbacoa — **222**
OR Carnitas — **266**
+ Cilantro Lime Cauli Rice — **202**
OR Sweet Dijon Coleslaw — **146**

Pecan Chicken — **234**
+ Best-Ever Cauli Mash — **188**
OR Spaghetti Squash Alfredo — **190**

BBQ Bacon Mini Meatloaves — **216**
OR Salisbury Steak — **224**
+ Best-Ever Cauli Mash — **188**

Cheesy Meatball Marinara — **214**
+ Spaghetti Squash Alfredo — **190**

Quiche Lorraine — **262**
+ Bacon Broc-Cauli Salad — **138**

Fully Loaded Chicken — **240**
+ Cauli Risotto — **184**

KETO SWAPS

Missing your old carby go-tos? These keto-friendly swaps are just what you're looking for!

Bread

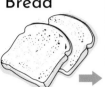

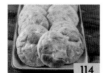 **112** Best-Ever Flax Buns

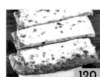 **114** Buttery Slider Buns

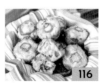 **120** Cheesy Garlic Butter Breadsticks

 116 Three-Cheese Jalapeño Muffins

118 White Cheddar Chive Biscuits

Crackers

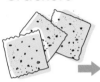 **122** Bacon Seed Crackers

124 Chewy Cheese Bites

Chocolate

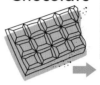 **302** Chocolate Chips

312 Dark Chocolate Pots de Crème

Potatoes

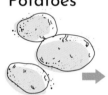 **188** Best-Ever Cauli Mash

198 Cauli Puree with Crispy Shiitake Mushrooms

204 Garlic Roasted Radishes

ADDITIONAL SWAPS

Tortillas and taco shells → Crispy cheese shells (see page 222)

Bread-crumbs → Crushed pork rinds (see page 42)

Milk → Heavy cream, unsweetened nut milk

Flour → Blanched almond flour, coconut flour, pecan flour

Sugar → Blended erythritol-stevia sweetener (see page 46)

Rice

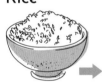 **184** Cauli Risotto

 192 Cashew Fried Cauli Rice

 202 Cilantro Lime Cauli Rice

Pasta

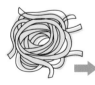 **226** Bolognese Zucchini Lasagna

 190 Spaghetti Squash Alfredo

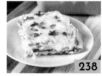 **238** Chicken Bacon Swiss Lasagna

Cake

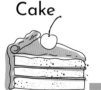 **322** Lemon Cake

 324 German Chocolate Cake

 320 Banana Cupcakes with Sweet Brown Butter Frosting

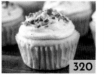 **318** Coconut Cupcakes

SPECIAL OCCASION MENUS

Celebration / Holiday

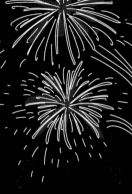

Menu #1

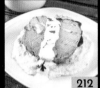 212

 188

 200

 312

Garlic Roast Beef with Horseradish Cream

Best-Ever Cauli Mash

Garlic Butter Roasted Mushrooms

Dark Chocolate Pots de Crème

Menu #2

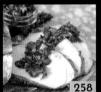 258

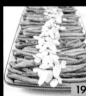 196

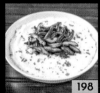 198

 324

Roast Pork Loin with Bacon Onion Jam

Toasted Almond Haricots Verts

Cauli Puree with Crispy Shiitake Mushrooms

German Chocolate Cake

Menu #3

 232

 184

 162

 310

French Country Stew

Cauli Risotto

Golden Mushroom Soup

Lemon-Lime Posset

Menu #4

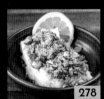 278

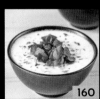 160

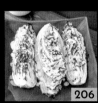 206

 322   298

Crispy Pistachio-Crusted Cod

Bacon Clam Chowder

Grilled Napa Cabbage with Creamy Dressing

Lemon Cake with Blueberry Compote

Date Night

Menu #1

 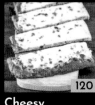 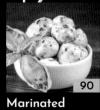

226 — Bolognese Zucchini Lasagna

120 — Cheesy Garlic Butter Breadsticks

90 — Marinated Mozzarella

316 — Snickerdoodle Frozen Custard

Menu #2

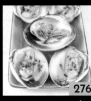 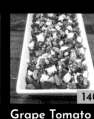 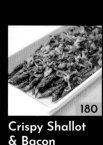 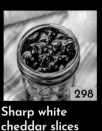

276 — Oven-Roasted Clams with Garlic Butter Sauce

286 — Brown Butter Scallops

140 — Grape Tomato Salad with Feta & Pistachios

180 — Crispy Shallot & Bacon Asparagus

298 — Sharp white cheddar slices topped with Blueberry Compote

Menu #3

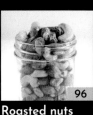 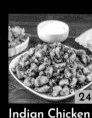 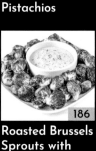 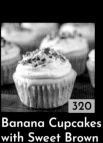

96 — Roasted nuts

246 — Indian Chicken

186 — Roasted Brussels Sprouts with Balsamic Mayo

320 — Banana Cupcakes with Sweet Brown Butter Frosting

Menu #4

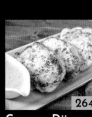 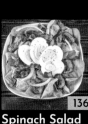 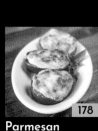 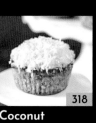
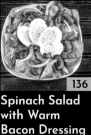

264 — Creamy Dijon Pork Chops

136 — Spinach Salad with Warm Bacon Dressing

178 — Parmesan Broiled Tomatoes

318 — Coconut Cupcakes

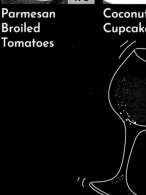

Party Time

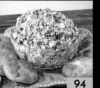
Spinach Dip — 94

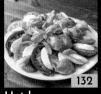
Heirloom Caprese Salad — 132

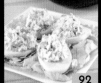
Ham & Chive Stuffed Eggs — 92

Classic Shrimp Salad — 142

Bacon Seed Crackers — 122

Garlic Chive Cheese Spread — 106

Szechuan Meatballs — 260

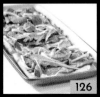
Steak Pizza with Zesty Aioli — 126

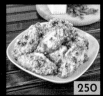
Parmesan Garlic Wings — 250

Thumbprint Cookies — 314

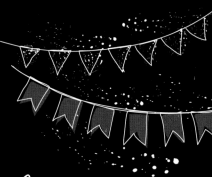

Family Game Night

Queso Fundido — 102

Crispy Personal Pizzas — 128

BBQ Bacon Mini Meatloaves — 216

Cookies & Cream Parfait — 308

Patio Dining

Menu #1

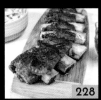
Oven-Roasted Beef Ribs — 228

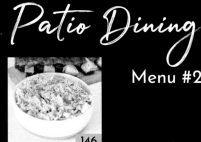
Sweet Dijon Coleslaw — 146

Menu #2

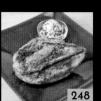
Chipotle Lime Chicken with Charred Scallion Butter — 248

Bacon Broc-Cauli Salad — 138

Casual Get-Together

Menu #1

166 270

Chicken Bacon Poblano Soup | **Cuban Sandwiches**

Menu #2

 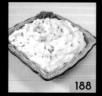

224 188

Salisbury Steak | **Best-Ever Cauli Mash**

Menu #3

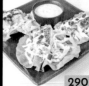

290 202

Baja Fish Tacos | **Cilantro Lime Cauli Rice**

Sunday Dinner

Menu #1

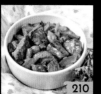 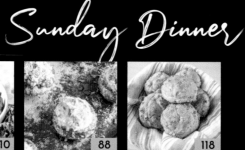

210 88 118

Beef Bourguignon | **Stuffed Mushrooms** | **White Cheddar Chive Biscuits**

Menu #2

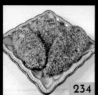 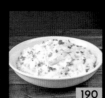

234 158 190

Pecan Chicken | **French Onion Soup** | **Spaghetti Squash Alfredo**

Menu #3

 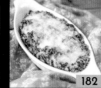 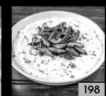

272 182 198

Bacon-Wrapped Pork Medallions with Maple Chipotle Cream | **Gruyère Spinach Gratin** | **Cauli Puree with Crispy Shiitake Mushrooms**

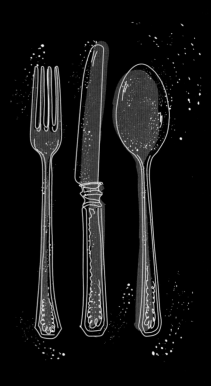

Theme Night

Asian Food

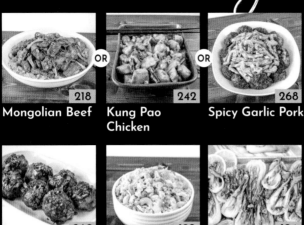

218 OR	242 OR	268
Mongolian Beef	Kung Pao Chicken	Spicy Garlic Pork

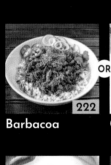

260	192	194
Szechuan Meatballs	Cashew Fried Cauli Rice	Lemon Garlic Baby Bok Choy

Mexican Food

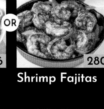

222 OR	266 OR	280
Barbacoa	Carnitas	Shrimp Fajitas

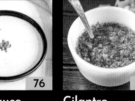 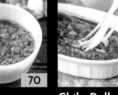 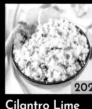 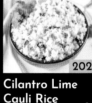

76	70	176	202
Baja Sauce	Cilantro Chimichurri	Chile Rellenos	Cilantro Lime Cauli Rice

Italian Food

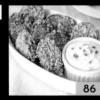 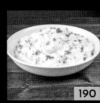 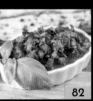

86	214	190	120	82
Zucchini Fritte	Cheesy Meatball Marinara	Spaghetti Squash Alfredo	Cheesy Garlic Butter Breadsticks	Italian Salsa

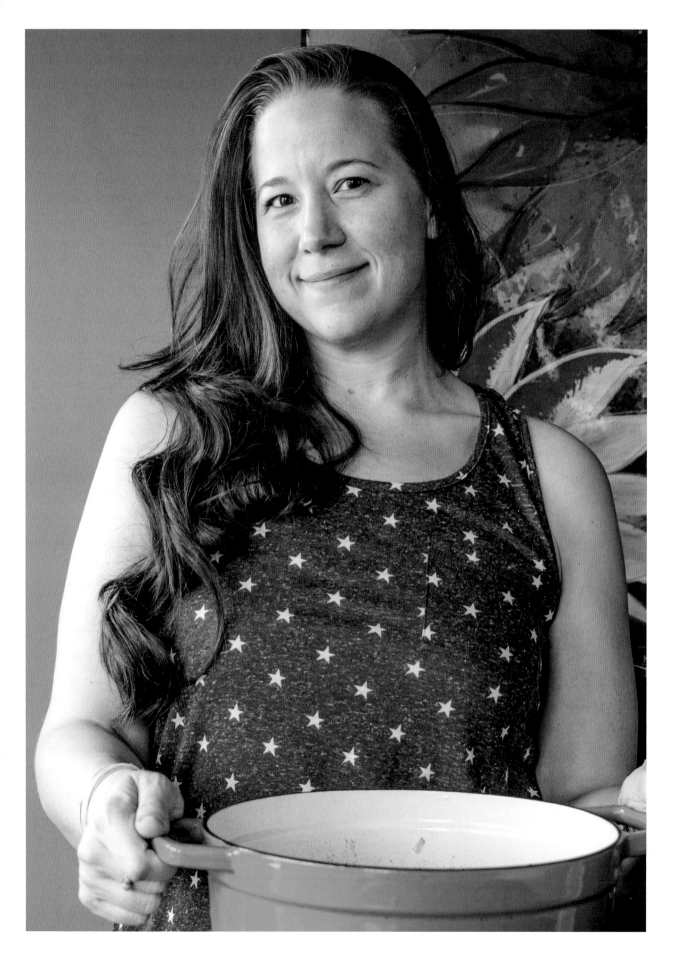

YOUR KETO KITCHEN

Although I rarely use specialty ingredients, you'll have more success with the recipes in this book if you know a little bit about the ingredients I use. This chapter will help you know what to look for at the grocery store and what common ingredients are keto-friendly. I'll also talk about my favorite kitchen tools and give a basic overview of common cooking terms.

MEAT

FISH AND SHELLFISH: I most often use cod, flounder, shrimp, clams, and scallops.

GROUND BEEF: I opt for the higher-fat packages, 85 percent lean.

CHICKEN AND TURKEY: I always have boneless breasts, thighs, and wings on hand.

LAMB: Ground lamb is great to have on hand for an exotic burger option.

PORK: I opt for loin roasts, shoulders, tenderloin, St. Louis ribs, and thick boneless chops.

PROCESSED MEATS: When you buy bacon, ham, deli meats, hot dogs, and sausages, make sure they have no added sugar. For brands, I like Wellshire Farms, Applegate, and Pederson's Natural Farms.

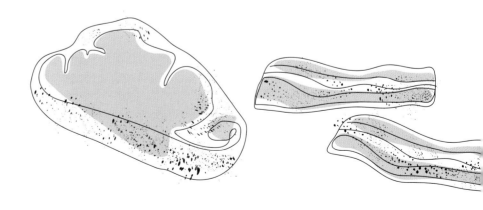

EGGS & DAIRY

Always use full-fat dairy. (The nutritional information in each recipe is calculated using full-fat dairy.)

CREAM CHEESE: Philadelphia is my go-to brand because it has the fewest ingredients.

COTTAGE CHEESE: I only buy this occasionally as a snack due to the higher carb content.

EGGS: I buy fresh eggs from local farmers when I can because I find the flavor to be much richer.

RICOTTA CHEESE: I love this stuff, especially in my Bolognese Zucchini Lasagna (page 226).

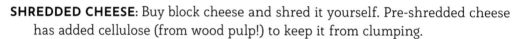

SHREDDED CHEESE: Buy block cheese and shred it yourself. Pre-shredded cheese has added cellulose (from wood pulp!) to keep it from clumping.

SOUR CREAM: Read the labels and look for brands without fillers or additives. I stick with Daisy brand for that reason.

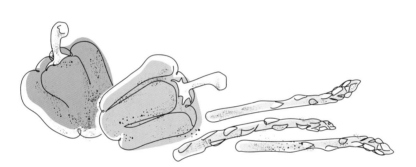

VEGGIES

I always recommend washing and drying produce before using.

ASPARAGUS: This is probably my favorite veggie. If you want to save money, as I do, look for sales, when it can go down to $1.99 per pound or less.

BELL PEPPERS: I only buy red, yellow, and orange peppers because I prefer them to green. They're great for sautéing, but I also love to make stuffed peppers. *(There's a sausage dip recipe on my website that works perfectly—www.ohmyketo.com/2017/06/18/sausage-dip).*

BROCCOLI: I generally only buy the fresh crowns.

BRUSSELS SPROUTS: I only buy these fresh so that I can roast them in the oven until crispy! (See the recipe for Roasted Brussels Sprouts with Balsamic Mayo, page 186.)

CABBAGE: I stick with shredded green cabbage for coleslaw and noodles, but I also love to pick up bok choy, baby bok choy, napa cabbage, and savoy cabbage from my local Asian market.

CARROTS: I'm not advocating eating carrot sticks for a snack—they do tend to be higher in carbs than other veggies—but I find that carrots impart a wonderful flavor in soups and stews. Since 1 medium carrot has only 5 grams of net carbs, and that will usually be split among four servings, adding a carrot is worth it in my opinion.

CAULIFLOWER: Fresh cauliflower is a must for making amazing cauli rice at home—frozen riced cauliflower will work in a pinch, but fresh is best. I also prefer fresh for cauli mash and puree, but for these, frozen cauliflower florets are a good stand-in.

CELERY: This is one veggie I always have on hand. The inside leaves are perfect for soups!

JALAPEÑO PEPPERS: I always have these on hand for making Fried Jalapeño Mozzarella Bites (page 98).

LEEKS: To clean a leek, cut off the dark green end, leaving the stem. Slice down the leek lengthwise, starting ¼ inch from the stem (so the two parts are still connected). Rinse the inside leek layers while fanning them gently under cool running water. These are a must for my Loaded Cauli Leek Soup (page 154) and French Country Stew (page 232).

LETTUCE (ALL TYPES): I always have iceberg on hand, and usually romaine as well. I'll grab a head of butter lettuce when they're on sale—perfect for wrapping my Baja Fish Tacos (page 290).

MUSHROOMS: Button, baby bellas, and shiitakes are my go-tos.

ONIONS, SHALLOTS, AND GARLIC: My kitchen is always stocked with scallions, white and yellow onions, shallots, and fresh garlic.

POBLANO PEPPERS AND GREEN CHILI PEPPERS: Roast these peppers before using for maximum flavor (be sure to remove the skin after roasting). I use these both quite often in my Queso Fundido (page 102).

RADISHES: I like to add these to salads, chop them into large chunks and eat them with a sprinkle of pink Himalayan salt, and roast them in the oven as a side dish (see my recipe for Garlic Roasted Radishes on page 204). They're also wonderful thinly sliced in an au gratin, as long as you don't mind the sauce turning pink!

SPAGHETTI SQUASH: This is a truly amazing veggie. You don't have to do anything special to turn it into perfect long strands of veggie noodles. (See page 27 for roasting instructions.)

SPINACH: I always have frozen on hand, and I grab fresh baby spinach for salads.

ZUCCHINI: I almost always have zucchini on hand, but if yellow squash looks better at the supermarket, it's a safe substitute.

FRUIT

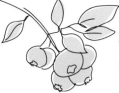

AVOCADOS: I have the best luck with large avocado varieties, like Hall or Choquette.

BERRIES: These are a great keto-friendly sweet treat, delicious on their own or added to a salad or cheese plate. My personal favorites are strawberries and blueberries.

TOMATOES: I stick with Roma tomatoes most of the time, but if you see heirloom tomatoes, grab them!

SNACKS

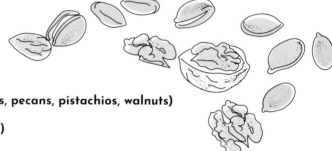

NUTS (almonds, macadamia nuts, pecans, pistachios, walnuts)

OLIVES (black, green, Kalamata)

PICKLES (dill chips, dill spears)

PORK RINDS: While I may be the self-appointed Queen of Pork Rind Breading, I'm also a pork rind snob.

Unseasoned store-brand pork rinds are the best for breading and frying. They break down into a very fine crumb and fry better than any others. I generally don't like their texture or flavor in their whole form, but that's not an issue when they're crushed for breading.

Mac's brand pork rinds (unseasoned) are great for eating whole with a dip or as nachos (see page 24), but they do not make good crumbs, for some reason—they will work in a pinch, but the results are not quite the same.

Fancy-pants brands of pork rinds—like Pork King Good, Bacon's Heir, EPIC, Southern Recipe Small Batch, and 4505—are almost always seasoned and generally have pretty clean ingredients. They're basically gourmet pork rinds. *Eat these!* These pork rinds don't need a dip or anything; they're amazing all by themselves. They are pricier than other pork rinds, but if you're looking for something to replace a crunchy high-carb snack like chips, they're well worth it.

Pork cracklings are pork rinds with fat attached, and they are crispy, fatty, and delish! Great for dips or eating alone, but don't use them for breading.

SEEDS: Pumpkin seeds, sunflower seeds, and toasted hemp seeds (in the shell) make for a quick and filling snack. I like to mix 2 tablespoons of toasted hemp seeds with 1 tablespoon of melted butter and a pinch of pink Himalayan salt. It's crunchy and fatty, and it reminds me a lot of popcorn! Hemp seeds are high in antioxidants, vitamins, minerals, and fatty acids.

CONDIMENTS

MARINARA SAUCE: Look for a jarred sauce without added sugar or sweeteners. I used to use pizza sauce for everything red sauce–related, but then I found Rao's Homemade Marinara, and it is wonderful! It doesn't have any added sugar, and the flavor is just like homemade.

MAYONNAISE: Homemade is best (see below), but if that's not an option for you, try to get your hands on Duke's brand mayo, which is sugar-free. If you're avoiding soy, your best bet is to opt for an avocado oil mayo, though be warned that they can have a strong avocado flavor.

HOMEMADE MAYONNAISE

If you have an immersion blender, making your own mayonnaise couldn't be easier. Just remember not to use extra-virgin olive oil, which will make the mayo bitter. This mayo can be flavored with anything you like: a clove of minced garlic, Sriracha, or even horseradish!

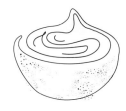

1 cup extra-light olive oil

1 large egg

1 large egg yolk

1 tablespoon fresh lemon juice or red wine vinegar

1 teaspoon Dijon mustard

⅛ teaspoon fine sea salt

Pinch of ground white pepper

- Put all the ingredients into a 16-ounce widemouthed mason jar (make sure the mouth is only slightly wider than the head of the immersion blender). Place the head of the immersion blender at the bottom of the jar and turn it on, then very slowly pull it up and watch as your mayo emulsifies!

- Cover tightly with a lid and store in the fridge for up to a week.

WINE

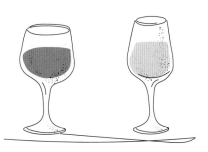

I'm not a wine drinker, but I do love the flavor it imparts in a dish. If you only need a small amount for one dish, try using a mini bottle of wine from Sutter Home, which I've found to be the most widely available. I also keep a bottle of cooking sherry on hand for a few things, like a super-quick French onion soup.

WINES LOWEST IN CARBS

Reds
Cabernet
Merlot
Pinot Noir

Whites
Chardonnay
Pinot Blanc
Pinot Grigio

PANTRY ITEMS

ALMOND FLOUR: I always use blanched almond flour, in which the skin is removed from the almonds before grinding. It's lighter and smoother than unblanched almond flour.

BAKING POWDER (aluminum-free)

BAKING SODA

COCOA POWDER: Do yourself a favor and get quality Dutch process cocoa powder. The difference in flavor and color is night and day. The only brands of cocoa powder I use in my recipes are Guittard and Droste.

COCONUT FLOUR: I've tried several brands, and they're all about the same. Be sure to sift before using.

FLAVOR EXTRACTS: I love using different flavor extracts in my baking to give a punch of flavor without any excess carbs. These can be found in the baking aisle of the grocery store next to the vanilla extract.

FLAXSEED MEAL: I like using flaxseed meal because it imparts a flavor very reminiscent of wheat bread. Be sure to get the meal or you'll have to grind the flax seeds yourself.

NATURAL NUT BUTTERS: Always be sure that any nut butter you purchase has only nuts or nuts and salt listed as the ingredients. You don't want any of the unhealthy oils or sweeteners that are commonly added. The jar will say "natural" on the front, but check the ingredients to be 100 percent sure.

PSYLLIUM HUSK POWDER: This powder makes for a great binder in baked goods. Be sure to get the powder or you'll have to grind the husks yourself.

PURE VANILLA EXTRACT: Make sure it says "pure vanilla extract" for the best flavor, but if you're avoiding alcohol, then look for imitation vanilla extract.

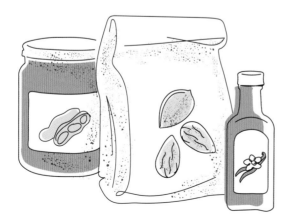

FATS

ANIMAL FAT (bacon grease, tallow, lard, schmaltz): Bacon grease and schmaltz are my two favorite animal fats, and I like to use them when I'm looking to add more flavor to my meal. I use bacon grease for the smoky flavor it gives a dish, and I reach for the schmaltz when I want a rich, roasted flavor. I use them both with meats, veggies, and eggs.

AVOCADO OIL: I personally don't care for the flavor of avocado oil, though I have used it for roasting and grilling. But if you like it, feel free to use it in most of my recipes, except when frying.

COCONUT OIL: I keep coconut oil on hand specifically for frying Coconut Shrimp (page 292). Otherwise, I rarely use it.

EXTRA-VIRGIN OLIVE OIL: I find the flavor of extra-virgin olive oil a bit strong, so the only time I use it is when I'm roasting or grilling veggies. If you're a fan of extra-virgin olive oil, it can easily be used in most of my recipes, except when frying.

GHEE: Ghee is butter with all of the milk solids removed. With ghee, you can cook at a higher temperature than you can with butter, plus it has a delicious nutty flavor, almost like brown butter! I always use Tin Star brand ghee.

GRASS-FED BUTTER: I prefer to use grass-fed butter because it has a very rich and buttery flavor, and I even think the texture is more velvety. I use unsalted for cooking and baking and salted for serving. Kerrygold is my favorite brand. For stovetop cooking, I enjoy using a combination of grass-fed butter and light olive oil. It gives you better flavor and lets you cook at a higher temperature without burning the butter.

LIGHT OLIVE OIL: This is my go-to oil. I use it for virtually everything, from making salad dressings to frying. It is basically flavorless and works great over higher heat.

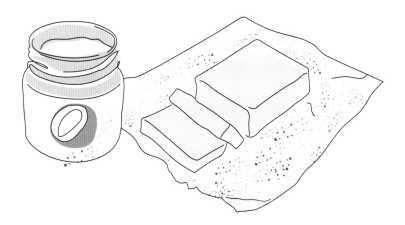

SUGAR-FREE SWEETENERS

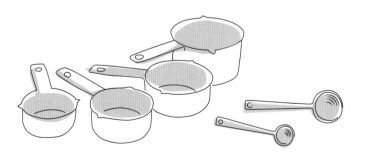

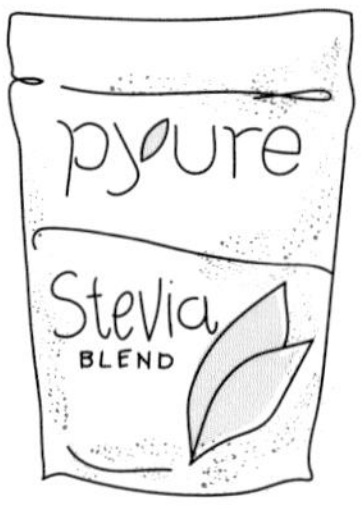

I have tried many different sugar-free sweeteners, and while xylitol is my personal favorite, I refuse to use it because it's extremely toxic for dogs. Through trial and error, I've found that I like to use a blended sweetener made of erythritol and stevia. This is available in a few different brands, but I almost always use Pyure Organic Stevia Blend. Most of my recipes have been created using this sweetener, and I've found that certain recipes, like my Sweet Chili Sauce (page 78) will only work with this sweetener. It's also one of the most cost-effective sugar-free sweeteners I've found. It's only available in granulated form right now, so if I need a powdered sweetener, I just powder it myself in a spice grinder or blender. Please note, however, a few recipes call for granulated erythritol rather than an erythritol-stevia blend.

If you decide to use a different blended sweetener, keep in mind that they don't all have the same level of sweetness. Below is a useful chart for converting sweetener amounts.

SUGAR-FREE SWEETENERS	SUGAR, GRANULATED					
	1 tsp	1 Tbsp	¼ cup	⅓ cup	½ cup	1 cup
Pyure Organic Stevia Blend, granulated	½ tsp	1½ tsp	2 Tbsp	2 Tbsp + 2 tsp	¼ cup	½ cup
Erythritol, granulated	1¼ tsp	1 Tbsp + 1 tsp	⅓ cup	⅓ cup + 2 Tbsp	⅔ cup	1⅓ cup
Xylitol, granulated	1 tsp	1 Tbsp	¼ cup	⅓ cup	½ cup	1 cup
Swerve, granulated	1 tsp	1 Tbsp	¼ cup	⅓ cup	½ cup	1 cup
SweetLeaf, Sweet Drops, Liquid Stevia	3-5 drops	⅛ tsp	½ tsp	⅔ tsp	1 tsp	2 tsp
Lakanto Monkfruit Sweetener, granulated	1 tsp	1 Tbsp	¼ cup	⅓ cup	½ cup	1 cup

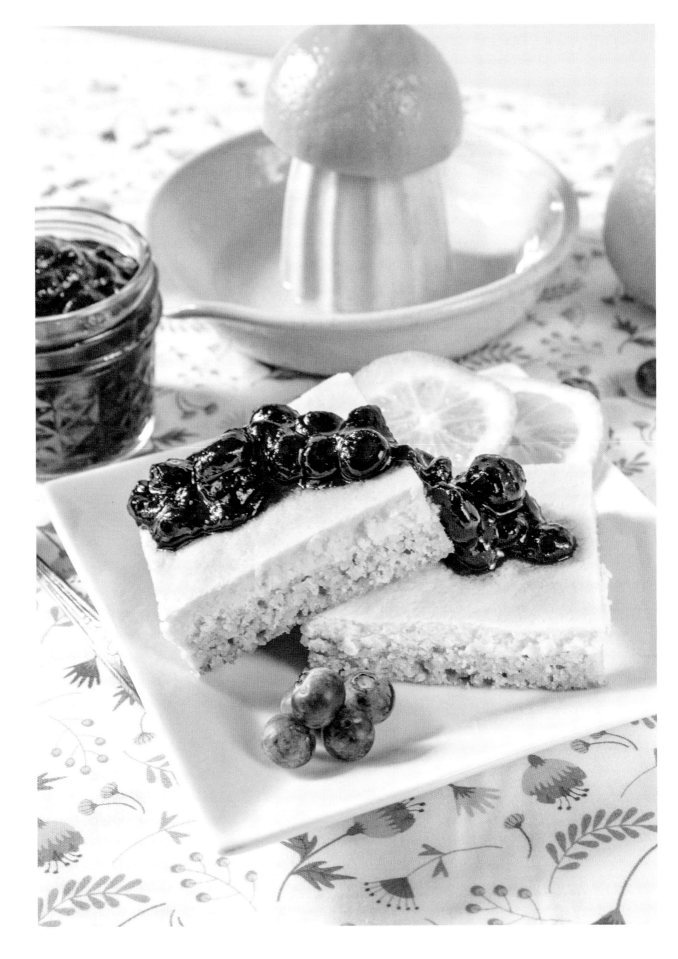

MUST-HAVE TOOLS

These kitchen tools make prep work and cooking a breeze, and I use them weekly, if not daily!

GOOD SET OF KNIVES: I've tried several different high-end knives, but my favorite knives are inexpensive and functional: the Pure Komachi 2 line. They all have a hard plastic sheath for the blade, so they can be safely stored, and they come in an array of bright colors! My favorites are the santoku (a 6½-inch all-purpose blade, similar to a chef's knife) and the nakiri (a 5½-inch blade designed for vegetables)—I use them both daily. They hold an edge longer than any knife I've used, but for best results, splurge and get yourself a great knife sharpener as well, like the Ken Onion Edition Work Sharp Knife Sharpener.

WOODEN CUTTING BOARD: Do yourself a favor and treat yourself to a nice heavy-duty wooden cutting board. It really makes a big difference when you're chopping veggies or slicing roast meat, and it won't dull your knives as quickly as a plastic cutting board. Bonus: it will double as a great charcuterie board!

CAST-IRON SKILLET: Everyone needs a cast-iron skillet! Once seasoned, cast iron is naturally nonstick, and its heat retention makes it a must for a good reverse seared steak. A cast-iron skillet will last forever, which is great news because the more you cook with it, the better it gets!

ENAMELED CAST-IRON DUTCH OVEN: I never understood the need for an enameled cast-iron pot until I used one. They heat evenly and retain the heat for a long time. I love making all of my soups and slow-roasted meats in my cast-iron pots.

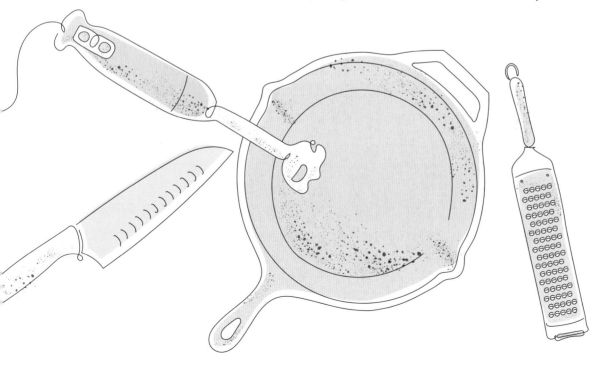

IMMERSION BLENDER: While my main reason for having an immersion blender is that they're great for making keto milkshakes, they're also wonderful for blending soups like my Loaded Cauli Leek Soup (page 154), and they're essential for making homemade mayo.

MICROPLANE GRATER: I use this all the time for zest, and it's perfect for grating everything from Parmesan cheese to sugar-free chocolate to fresh ginger. Grab one of these and never mince your garlic again—you can grate it in seconds instead.

SILICONE SPATULAS: These are so handy for so many things, and silicone is a must to avoid scratching nonstick pans. They are perfect for cooking and even better for scraping every bit of your food out of a container—no food left behind!

COOKIE SCOOPS: I cannot live without these! They are wonderful for quickly scooping up equal amounts of anything, like dough, batter, and even meatballs. I use my 2-tablespoon scoop most often, but a 4-tablespoon one is great to have as well.

SHEET PANS: Large sheet pans are the best! Their raised edges make them more versatile than flat baking sheets (though sometimes these are handy, as with my Chewy Cheese Bites on page 124)—when you're roasting veggies, the juices don't drip onto the bottom of the oven and the veggies don't roll off. They also give you ample space to bake all your cookies or rolls at once, and they make roasting veggies a dream because they all caramelize instead of steaming in the hot oven.

INSTANT-READ THERMOMETER: I really don't know what I was doing before I had one of these! Instant-read thermometers take all the guesswork out of figuring out when meats are done, so say goodbye to over- and undercooking!

FINE-MESH SIEVES, SMALL AND LARGE: Fine-mesh sieves are perfect for sifting baking flours and adding a decorative cascade of powdered sweetener to baked treats. I also use these for straining liquids to remove solids (like seeds, skins, peels, etc.).

SMALL ROASTING RACK: Just pop one into a cast iron-skillet or enameled cast-iron pot, put the seared meat on it, and you're ready for roasting.

VACUUM SEALER: I use this almost as much as my knives! I love saving money, so I'm always buying in bulk and grabbing items from clearance sales to freeze for later use. Using a vacuum sealer ensures that all your foods stay fresh and never get freezer burn.

FOOD PROCESSOR: This makes fast work of turning pork rinds into crumbs, ricing cauliflower, blending up the perfect cauli mash, and even breaking down chunks of cheese into small shred-like pieces.

GLASS MASON JARS: Not only are these a must for collecting and storing bacon grease (perfect for stovetop cooking), but they are absolutely perfect for keeping spice blends fresh.

And finally, as my cooking idol Ina Garten says,
clean hands are always your best tool!

GLOSSARY OF TECHNIQUES

I've never been to cooking school and I'm not a trained chef. Every recipe in this book is designed to be easy to follow, even for a novice. That being said, there are some techniques that may be new to you, so this glossary will make sure we're all on the same page.

Let's level up with some knife skills!

In this book, I mainly focus on chopping, dicing, and mincing, but there's a little chiffonading and bias cutting floating around.

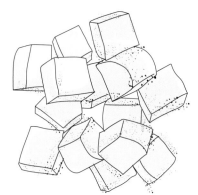

CHOP:
Cut into large ½-inch chunks

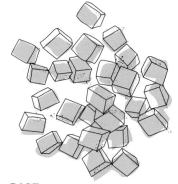

DICE:
Cut into small ¼-inch chunks

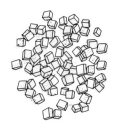

MINCE:
Cut into tiny ⅛-inch chunks

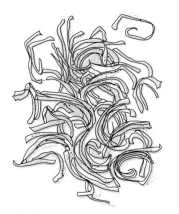

CHIFFONADE:
Roll leaves (such as basil leaves) tightly and cut crosswise to form long thin strips

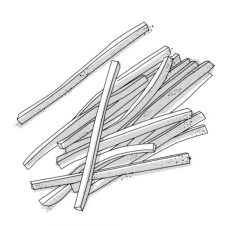

JULIENNE:
Cut into long thin strips (think matchsticks)

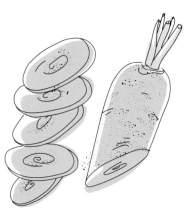

SLICE ON THE BIAS:
Cut at a 45-degree angle

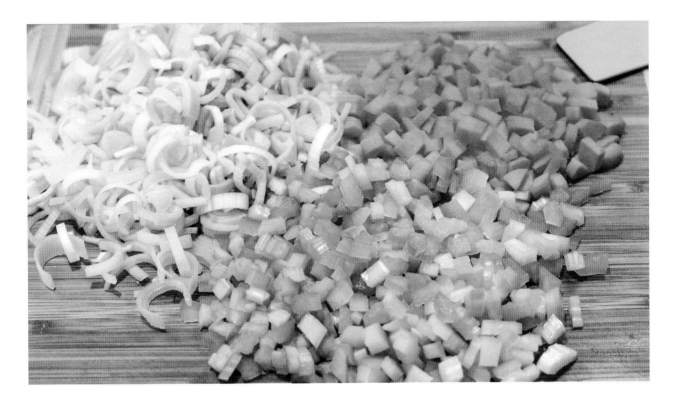

Prep work

BREADING: If you're used to using breadcrumbs for breading, you may need to adjust your technique a bit for low-carb breading, especially crushed pork rinds. You want to make sure foods are heavily coated while still knocking off the excess. After dipping the food in beaten eggs, lay it on a pile of crumbs and, using a dry hand, scoop crushed pork rinds on top of it, then press the crushed pork rinds into the food. Flip the food and repeat on the other side, then knock it gently onto the side of the plate to get rid of any excess. Always use one hand for dipping the food into the eggs and the other hand for the breading—it makes the process so much quicker and less messy!

PUREEING: The purpose of pureeing is to transform cooked foods, like a soup or sauce, into a luscious, velvety, creamy liquid. This can be done with an immersion blender, a regular jar blender, or a food processor—as a rule of thumb, use either kind of blender for liquids like smoothies and soups, and use a food processor for solid foods, like the pine nuts, cheese, and basil in pesto.

SEASONING: When I say "seasoning," I'm mainly referring to salt—other seasonings, like spices and herbs, are best added in the amounts given in the recipe. Seasoning your food properly with salt really intensifies the flavor of the food. Don't be afraid to taste your food as you cook and add salt when needed. I season my food before, during, and sometimes after cooking. One of the best examples is making homemade stock (see page 26): I flavor the stock with a few aromatics as it simmers, but I add salt only at the end, once it's strained. It goes from tasting like virtually nothing to the most amazing explosion of meaty flavor, all from being properly salted.

Cooking with heat

BRAISING: Searing meat and then simmering it at a low temperature in a flavorful liquid until tender.

BROILING: Cooking with very intense direct heat—basically, you put a dish right under your oven's heat source. In this book there are a few recipes that need to be popped under the broiler for extra browning, melting, or crispiness. Be sure the dish is 3 to 5 inches away from the heat; you don't want it too close or too far away.

DEGLAZING: Scraping up the flavorful brown bits that get stuck to the bottom of a pot or skillet after sautéing meats or veggies. A deglazing liquid is used to help scrape up the pieces; in the recipes in this book, I use either a meat stock or wine.

REDUCING: Cooking a liquid until it thickens and a certain amount of it (often half) has evaporated. This concentrates and intensifies the flavors. It usually takes about 3 to 5 minutes, but it could take longer depending on the volume of the liquid.

SAUTÉING: Quick cooking over moderately high heat while tossing or stirring the ingredients in the pan. For best results, preheat the pan before adding the ingredients.

SEARING: Browning a piece of meat in order to lock in the juices and add deep flavor. Simply preheat a heavy-bottomed pot or skillet over medium-high heat, pour in your fat of choice, add the meat (skin side down, if applicable), and cook without moving it until it's golden brown, then flip to sear the remaining sides.

SHALLOW-FRYING: Frying in oil on the stovetop, but using far less oil than deep-frying does. You'll want to cover the bottom of your pan with about ¼ to ½ inch of oil for shallow-frying. Always be sure your oil is hot before adding anything to the pan. An easy way to test is to sprinkle in a bit of crushed pork rinds—if they sizzle, it's ready!

SIMMERING: Cooking food in liquid just below boiling; when a higher temperature would overcook the foods, simmering keeps it tender. All you have to do to obtain a simmer is bring the liquid to a boil and then turn the heat down to about medium-low. This allows it to gently bubble without coming back to a full boil.

TEMPERING EGGS: Adding hot liquid to beaten eggs to heat the eggs without scrambling them. Simply whisk the eggs in a small bowl and then whisk in a ladle of whatever hot liquid the recipe is using. Then just stir in the tempered eggs into the hot soup or pudding—they won't scramble!

NUTRITIONAL FACTS IN THE RECIPES

Each recipe provides the number of calories and grams of protein, fat, total carbs, net carbs, and fiber. These figures include all the ingredients in the recipe except those marked "optional."

BEFORE YOU START COOKING

Get ready...

Read through the entire recipe first and make sure you have all the necessary ingredients. You don't want to be in the middle of cooking when you realize you don't have a key component of the dish!

Get set...

Set up your mise en place! Prep all your ingredients so everything is ready to use before anything touches the heat. Not only will this ensure that nothing overcooks while you're chopping something else, but it will calm your mind and allow for an even more enjoyable cooking experience.

While you prep the ingredients, preheat your needed tools. Talk about a huge time-saver—with your oven preheating while you chop and slice, everything will be ready at the same time! The same goes for skillets, pots, and even boiling water; start to heat them before they're needed so they are ready when you are.

Go!

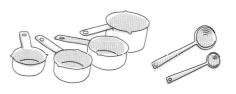

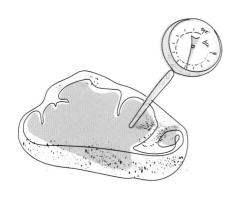

BEEF

Rare, 115°F

Medium-rare. 130°F

Medium, 140°F

Medium-well, 150°F

Well-done, 155°F

GROUND BEEF

160°F

All temperatures are internal and should be read with a meat thermometer.

PORK

Medium, 145°F

Well-done, 160°F

GROUND PORK

165°F

POULTRY (white meat, dark meat, and ground)

165°F

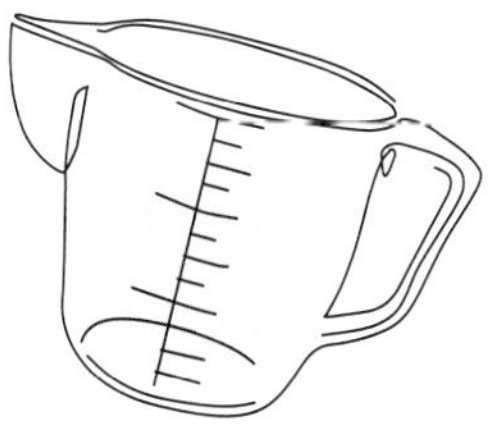

TEASPOONS		TABLESPOONS		FLUID OUNCES
½ tsp.	=	⅙ Tbsp.		
1 tsp.	=	⅓ Tbsp.		
1½ tsp.	=	½ Tbsp.	=	¼ fluid ounce
3 tsp.	=	1 Tbsp.	=	½ fluid ounce
6 tsp.	=	2 Tbsp.	=	1 fluid ounce
9 tsp.	=	3 Tbsp.	=	1½ fluid ounces

CUPS		TABLESPOONS		FLUID OUNCES
¼ cup	=	4 Tbsp.	=	2 fluid ounces
⅓ cup	=	5 Tbsp. + 1 tsp.	=	2⅓ fluid ounces
⅜ cup	=	¼ cup + 2 Tbsp.	=	3 fluid ounces
½ cup	=	8 Tbsp.	=	4 fluid ounces
⅝ cup	=	½ cup + 2 Tbsp.	=	5 fluid ounces
⅔ cup	=	10 Tbsp. + 2 tsp.	=	5⅓ fluid ounces
¾ cup	=	12 Tbsp.	=	6 fluid ounces
⅞ cup	=	¾ cup + 2 Tbsp.	=	7 fluid ounces
1 cup	=	16 Tbsp.	=	8 fluid ounces (½ pint)

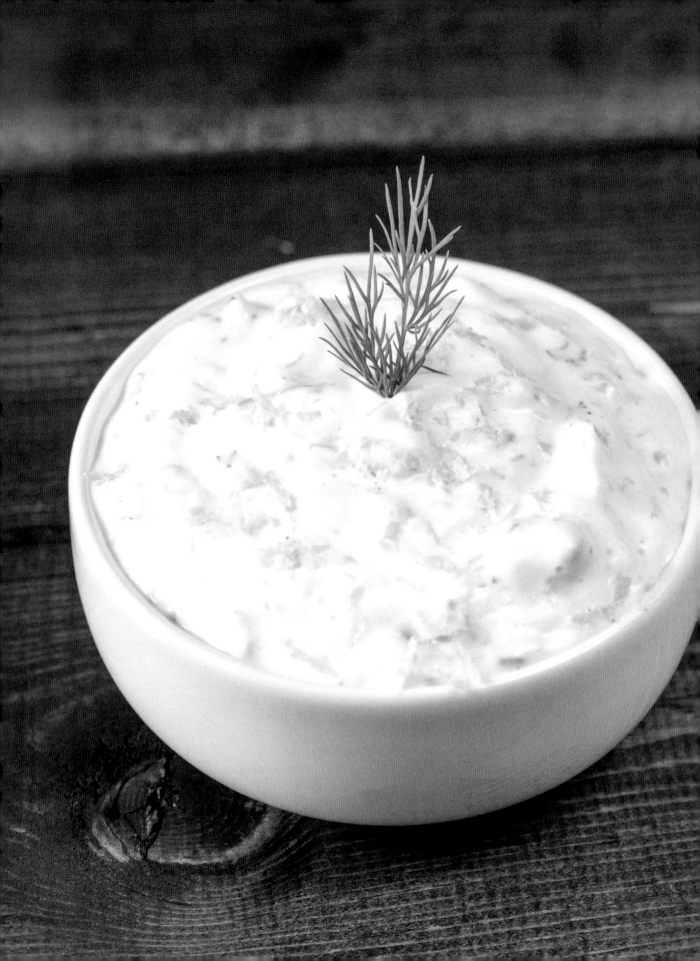

Dressings, Sauces & Seasonings

TACO SEASONING

MINUTES or LESS

MAKES ABOUT 1 CUP
(¼ cup per serving)

The moment I read the ingredients label and saw what was really in my package of taco seasoning—sugar, corn, chemicals, and preservatives—I knew I had to make my own. Turns out, homemade tastes better than any taco seasoning on the market!

¼ cup chili powder

¼ cup dried minced onions

2 tablespoons ground cumin

1 tablespoon plus 1 teaspoon fine sea salt

1 tablespoon plus 1 teaspoon garlic powder

1 tablespoon plus 1 teaspoon onion powder

1 tablespoon plus 1 teaspoon sweet paprika

2 teaspoons cayenne pepper

2 teaspoons ground black pepper

2 teaspoons ground white pepper

1 teaspoon dried oregano leaves

- In a medium-sized bowl, combine all the ingredients and whisk until well mixed.

- Store in an airtight glass jar in the pantry for a few months, or freeze in a resealable bag for up to a year.

Note : To season 1 pound of ground meat, use ¼ cup of this taco seasoning.

PER SERVING
Calories **40** · Fat **1g** · Total Carbs **7g** · Net Carbs **5g** · Fiber **2g** · Protein **1g**

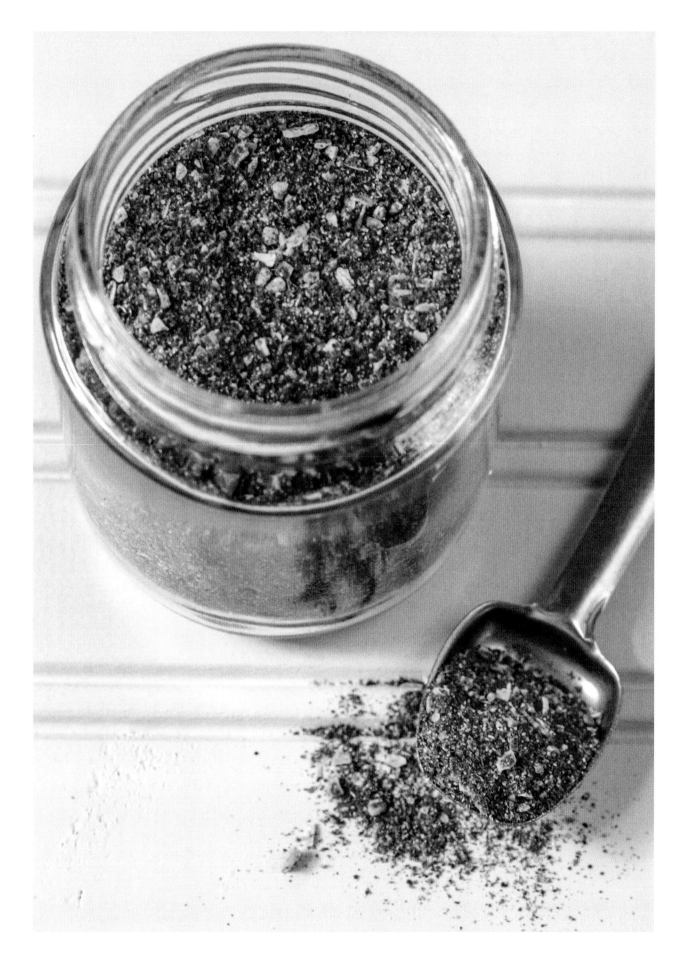

CAJUN SEASONING

This spicy blend of savory flavors works well with just about anything!

MAKES ¼ CUP
(1 teaspoon per
serving)

3 tablespoons sweet paprika

2 tablespoons fine sea salt

2 tablespoons garlic powder

1 tablespoon dried parsley

1 tablespoon dried oregano
leaves

1 tablespoon onion powder

1½ teaspoons cayenne pepper

1½ teaspoons dried thyme leaves

1½ teaspoons ground black
pepper

1½ teaspoons ground white
pepper

• In a medium-sized bowl, combine all the ingredients and whisk until well mixed.

• Store in an airtight glass jar in the pantry for a few months, or freeze in a resealable bag for up to a year.

PER SERVING
Calories **5** · Fat **0g** · Total Carbs **1** · Net Carbs **1** · Fiber **0g** · Protein **0g**

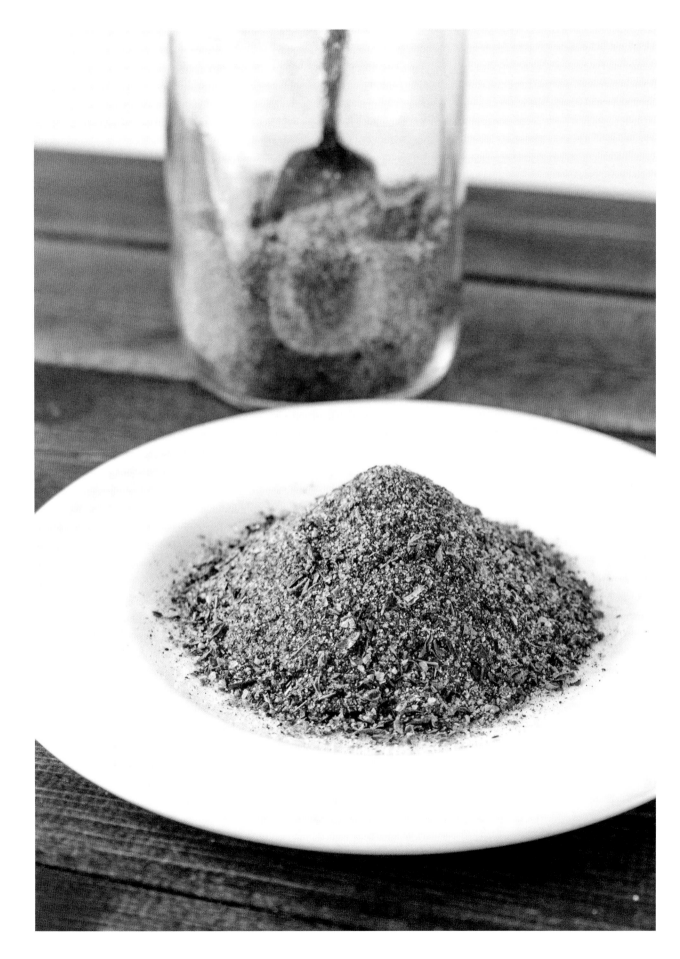

SMOKY BBQ RUB

30 MINUTES or LESS

MAKES ¼ CUP
(1 teaspoon per serving)

Growing up in Memphis, I had my share of amazing barbecue, and it starts with a great-tasting rub. But this rub isn't just for barbecue—I use it on everything from eggs to veggies to fish.

¼ cup granulated erythritol (see page 46)

2 tablespoons smoked paprika

2 tablespoons sweet paprika

1 tablespoon plus 1 teaspoon fine sea salt

2 teaspoons chili powder

2 teaspoons garlic powder

2 teaspoons onion powder

1 teaspoon chipotle powder

1 teaspoon ground black pepper

1 teaspoon ground white pepper

- In a medium-sized bowl, combine all the ingredients and whisk until well mixed.

- Store in an airtight glass jar in the pantry for a few months, or freeze in a resealable bag for up to a year.

PER SERVING

Calories **3** · Fat **0g** · Total Carbs **1g** · Net Carbs **1g** · Fiber **0g** · Protein **0g**

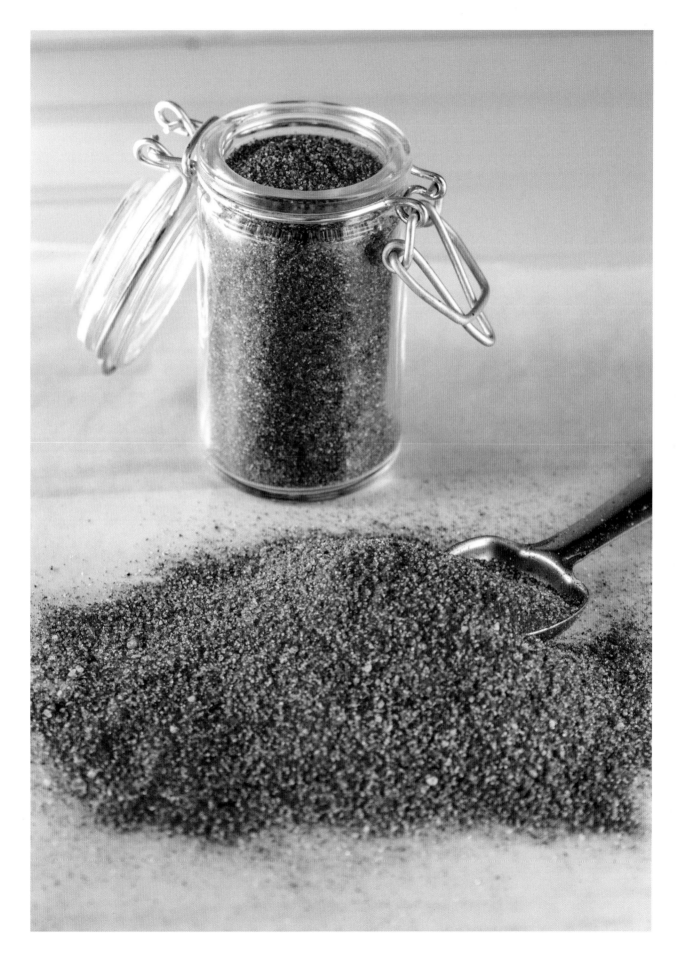

RANCH DRESSING

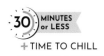

30 MINUTES or LESS

+ TIME TO CHILL

MAKES ABOUT 1 CUP
(2 tablespoons per serving)

Making your own ranch dressing couldn't be simpler, and the difference in flavor between store-bought and homemade is mind-blowing. I always have this in my fridge, and in addition to pouring it on salads, I use it as a dipping sauce for just about everything.

½ cup mayonnaise (see page 43)

¼ cup full-fat sour cream

¼ cup plain, unsweetened almond milk

1 teaspoon lemon juice

1 teaspoon dried dill weed

½ teaspoon dried chives

½ teaspoon dried minced onions

½ teaspoon dried parsley

½ teaspoon garlic powder

½ teaspoon onion powder

¼ teaspoon fine sea salt

⅛ teaspoon ground black pepper

⅛ teaspoon ground white pepper

• In a medium-sized bowl, whisk together the mayonnaise, sour cream, almond milk, and lemon juice until smooth. Add the rest of the ingredients and whisk well to combine.

• Pour the dressing into a 1-pint glass jar and cover tightly. Refrigerate for at least 1 hour before using to allow flavors to blend.

• Store in the fridge for up to 1 week.

Variation: RANCH DIP

Make a thick, delicious ranch dip by omitting the almond milk and increasing the amount of sour cream to ½ cup.

DRESSINGS, SAUCES & SEASONINGS

PER SERVING
Calories **109** · Fat **11g** · Total Carbs **1g** · Net Carbs **1g** · Fiber **0g** · Protein **0g**

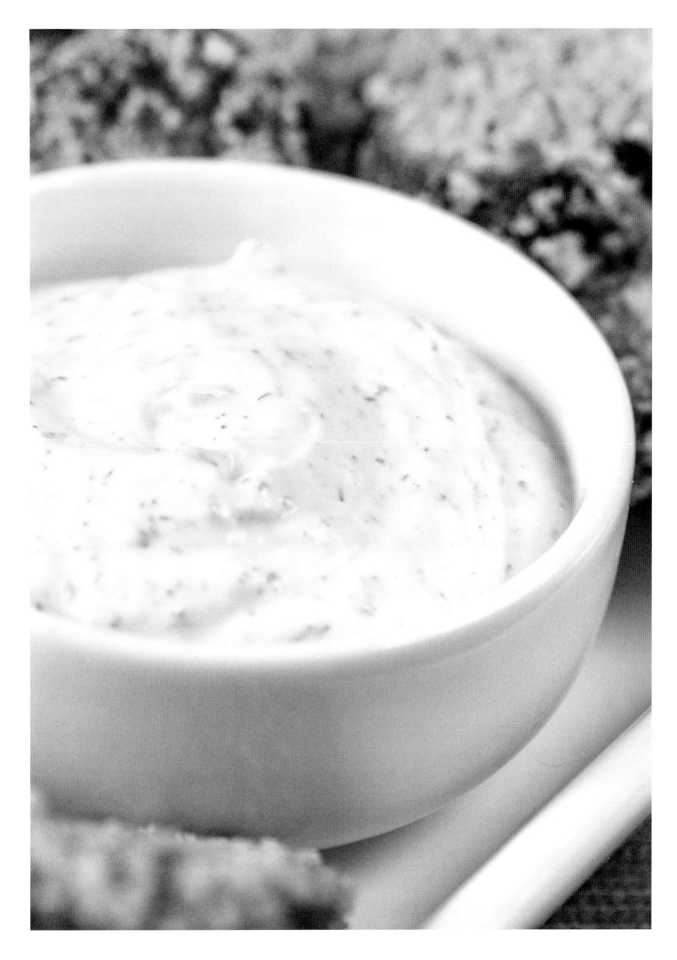

BLUE CHEESE DRESSING

30 MINUTES or LESS

+ TIME TO CHILL

MAKES 1½ CUPS
(3 tablespoons per serving)

This is not your run-of-the-mill bottled blue cheese dressing. This is real deal, chunky and delicious, like a dressing you would find in a fine-dining steakhouse. It needs some time in the fridge before the flavors are perfect, so please plan ahead. Be sure to have a batch on hand for my Blue Cheese Wedge Salad (page 134).

½ cup full-fat sour cream

½ cup mayonnaise (see page 43)

2 tablespoons heavy cream

1 teaspoon lemon juice

1 teaspoon Worcestershire sauce

¼ teaspoon garlic powder

⅛ teaspoon fine sea salt

⅛ teaspoon ground black pepper

⅓ cup crumbled blue cheese, plus more for garnish if desired

- In a medium-sized bowl, combine all the ingredients except the blue cheese and whisk until well combined and smooth. Add the blue cheese and stir while breaking up some of the crumbles with the back of a spoon. The dressing should still be chunky.

- Transfer the dressing to a 1-pint glass jar and cover tightly. Refrigerate for at least 4 hours or overnight to allow the flavors to blend. Garnish with additional blue cheese if desired before serving.

- Store in the fridge for up to 1 week.

Variation: FETA CHEESE DRESSING

Not a fan of blue cheese? Substitute crumbled feta for the blue cheese and double the lemon juice!

PER SERVING
Calories **179** · Fat **18g** · Total Carbs **2g** · Net Carbs **2g** · Fiber **0g** · Protein **2g**

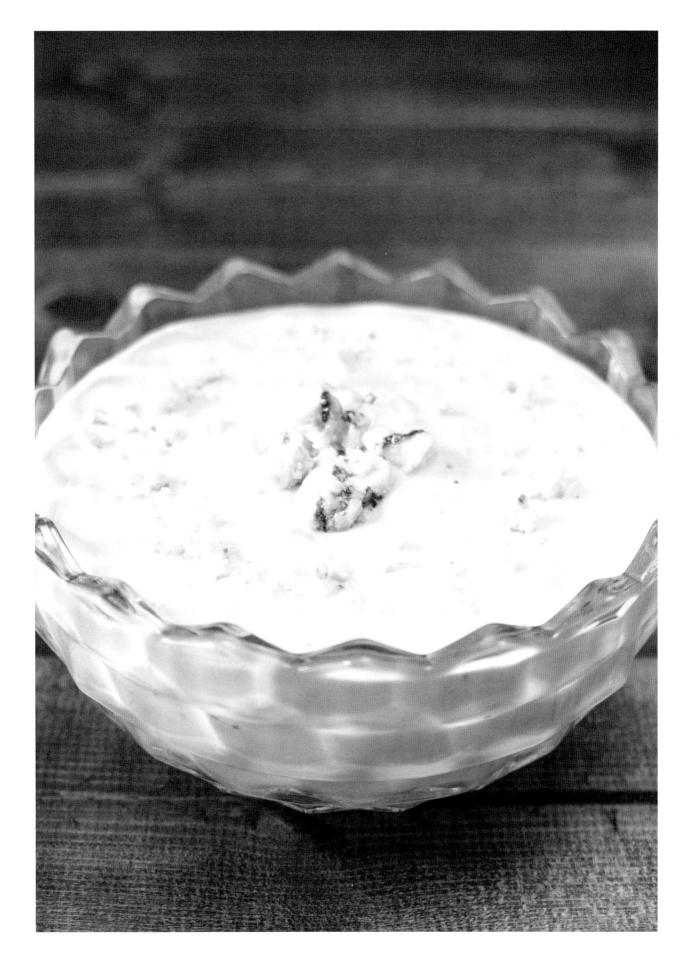

CHIPOTLE BBQ SAUCE

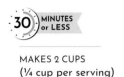

MINUTES
or LESS

MAKES 2 CUPS
(¼ cup per serving)

This tangy, sweet, and spicy barbecue sauce is perfect for slathering on your favorite meats. It's a must for my BBQ Bacon Mini Meatloaves (page 216) and Oven-Roasted Beef Ribs (page 228).

1 tablespoon light olive oil

1 small shallot, minced

1 clove garlic, minced

1½ cups water

⅓ cup tomato paste

2 tablespoons apple cider vinegar

2 tablespoons Dijon mustard

2 tablespoons powdered blended erythritol-stevia sweetener (see page 46)

2 tablespoons Worcestershire sauce

1½ teaspoons liquid smoke

1 teaspoon chipotle powder

¾ teaspoon fine sea salt

½ teaspoon smoked paprika

⅛ teaspoon ground white pepper

• Heat the oil in a medium-sized saucepan over medium-high heat. Add the shallot and garlic to the oil and sauté, stirring continuously, until they soften and become fragrant, about 2 minutes.

• Whisk in the rest of the ingredients. Bring to a light boil, then turn the heat down to medium-low and simmer, stirring occasionally, for 30 minutes, or until thickened. Remove from the heat and allow to cool in the pot.

• Once cool, transfer the sauce to a 1-quart glass jar and cover tightly. This sauce will keep for up to 2 weeks in the fridge.

PER SERVING
Calories **32** · Fat **2g** · Total Carbs **3g** · Net Carbs **3g** · Fiber **0g** · Protein **1g**

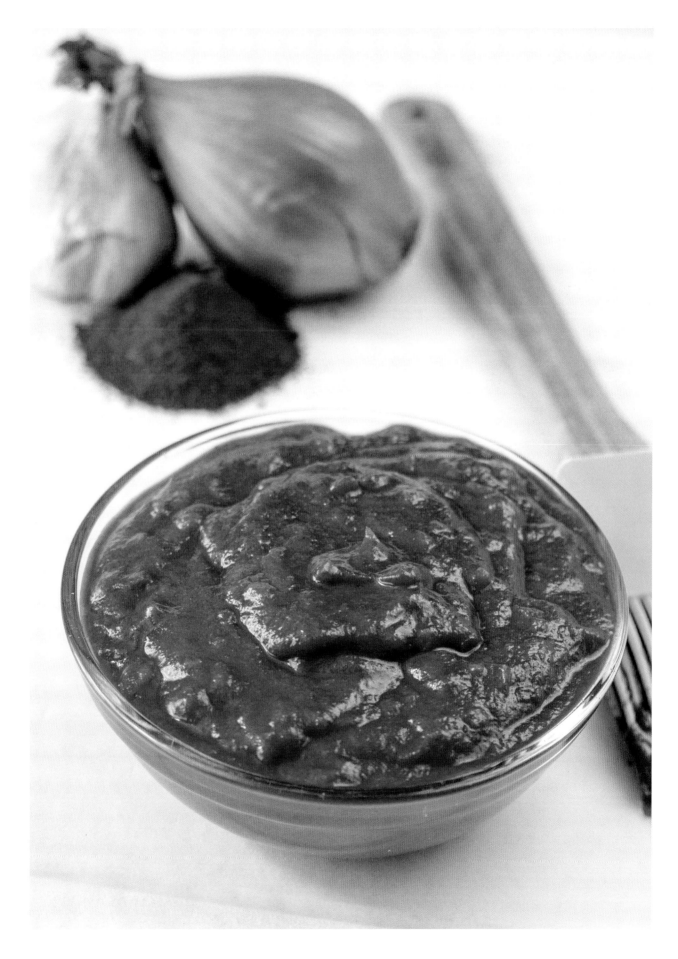

BLOOM SAUCE

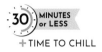

30 MINUTES or LESS

+ TIME TO CHILL

MAKES ¾ CUP
(2 tablespoons per
serving)

You might recognize this as the sauce that accompanies large deep-fried onions at many popular chain restaurants. It has such a zesty flavor that it's a delicious addition to a plethora of meats and veggies. It has become a staple any time I make my Fully Loaded Chicken (page 240).

½ cup mayonnaise (see page 43)

2 tablespoons prepared horseradish

2 tablespoons sugar-free ketchup

¼ teaspoon fine sea salt

¼ teaspoon smoked paprika, plus more for garnish if desired

⅛ teaspoon dried oregano leaves

⅛ teaspoon ground black pepper

Dash of cayenne pepper

• In a small bowl, combine all the ingredients and whisk until well combined.

• Transfer the sauce to a 1-pint glass jar and cover tightly. Refrigerate for at least 1 hour before using to allow the flavors to blend. Garnish with smoked paprika before serving, if desired.

• This sauce will keep for up to 1 week in the fridge.

PER SERVING
Calories **123** · Fat **13g** · Total Carbs **1g** · Net Carbs **1g** · Fiber **0g** · Protein **0g**

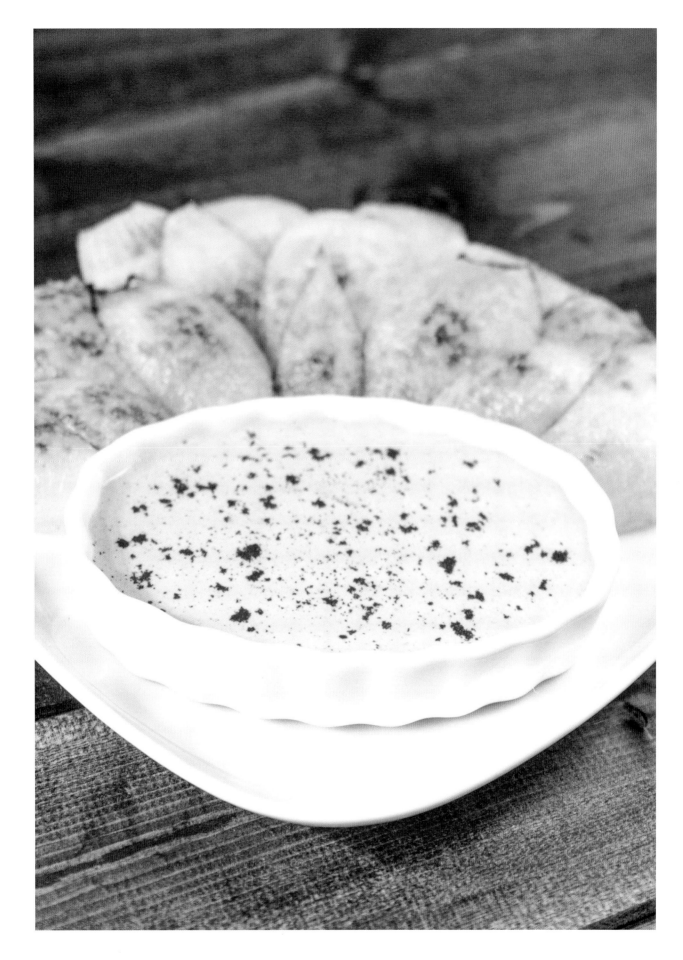

CILANTRO CHIMICHURRI

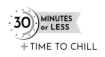

30 MINUTES or LESS

+ TIME TO CHILL

MAKES ½ CUP
(2 tablespoons per
serving)

Cilantro isn't part of traditional chimichurri, but I absolutely love the flavor and brightness it brings to a dish. This fragrant herb condiment is incredible with meat, especially my Barbacoa (page 222) and Carnitas (page 266).

1 bunch fresh cilantro (about 2 ounces)

¼ cup light olive oil

2 tablespoons lemon juice

1 clove garlic, minced

1 teaspoon dried Mexican oregano leaves

¼ teaspoon crushed red pepper

¼ teaspoon fine sea salt

• Rinse the cilantro thoroughly and blot it dry with paper towels. Remove the thick stems, gather the leaves into a bundle, and roughly chop.

• Put the chopped cilantro in a medium-sized bowl and add the rest of the ingredients, then stir everything together until thoroughly combined.

• Transfer the chimichurri to a 1-pint glass jar and cover tightly. Refrigerate for at least 2 hours before using to allow the flavors to develop. Stir before serving.

• Chimichurri will keep for up to 1 week in the fridge, but it will lose its bright green color after a few days. The taste won't be affected, though!

PER SERVING
Calories **126** · Fat **14g** · Total Carbs **1g** · Net Carbs **1g** · Fiber **0g** · Protein **0g**

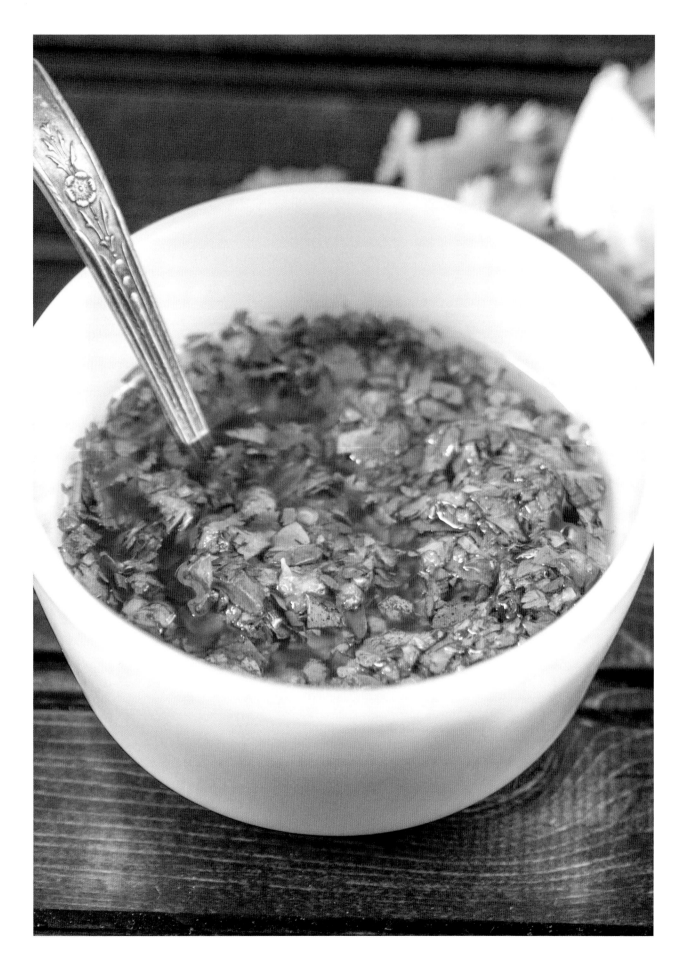

LEMON DILL TARTAR SAUCE

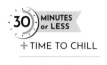

30 MINUTES or LESS

+ TIME TO CHILL

MAKES ¼ CUP
(3 tablespoons per serving)

When I was a kid, I'd only eat fish sticks if they were covered in tartar sauce. Now that I'm an adult, I still have a love for tartar sauce, albeit a grown-up version brimming with salty capers, tangy lemon, and fresh dill. This tartar sauce is perfect for your favorite seafood dishes, and it's especially delicious with my Crispy Pistachio-Crusted Cod (page 278), Crispy Tuna Cakes (page 284), and Sole Grenobloise (page 282).

½ cup mayonnaise (see page 43)

¼ cup minced dill pickles or jarred dill relish

2 teaspoons minced fresh dill

2 teaspoons minced shallots

1 teaspoon capers (reserve the liquid)

½ teaspoon grated lemon zest, plus more for garnish if desired

½ teaspoon lemon juice

⅛ teaspoon capers liquid (from above)

Sprig of dill, for garnish (optional)

• In a medium-sized bowl, combine all of the ingredients and mix thoroughly.

• Transfer the sauce to a 1-pint glass jar and cover tightly. Refrigerate for at least 1 hour to allow the flavors to blend. Garnish with additional lemon zest and a sprig of dill, if desired, before serving.

• Store in the fridge for up to 1 week.

PER SERVING
Calories **186** · Fat **20g** · Total Carbs **2g** · Net Carbs **1g** · Fiber **1g** · Protein **0g**

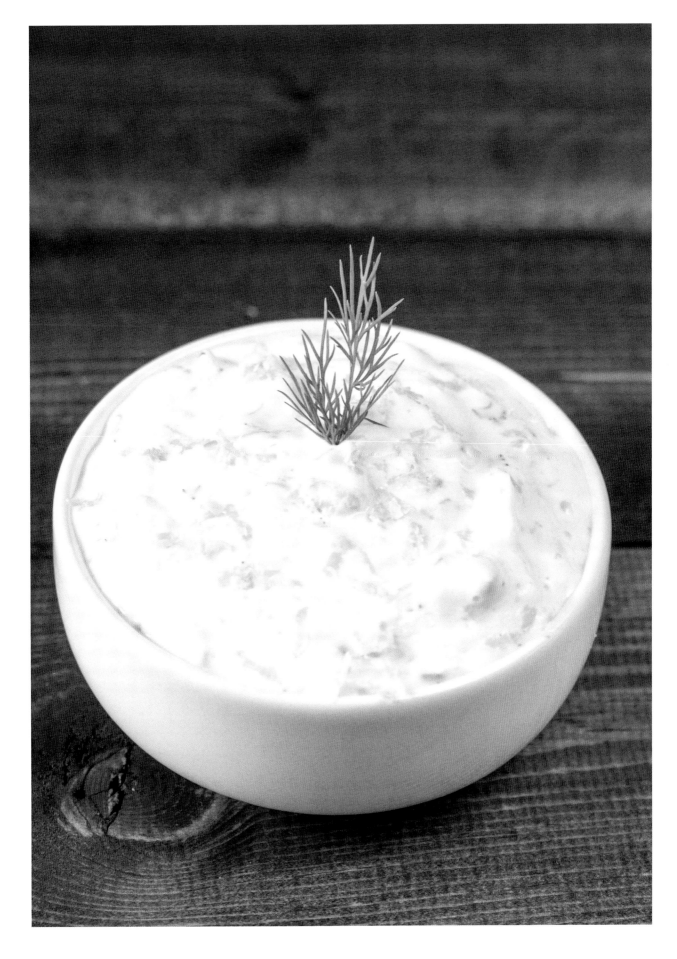

AUTHENTIC ENCHILADA SAUCE

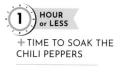

HOUR or LESS

+ TIME TO SOAK THE CHILI PEPPERS

MAKES 2 CUPS
(¼ cup per serving)

If you've ever had authentic enchilada sauce, then you understand that the canned stuff just doesn't cut it. Dried chili peppers are readily available in the international-foods aisle of your supermarket, and they are really what makes this enchilada sauce shine. This rich and flavorful red sauce goes perfectly with my Chile Rellenos (page 176).

1 ounce dried ancho peppers, stems and seeds removed

1 ounce dried pasilla peppers, stems and seeds removed

½ ounce dried guajillo peppers, stems and seeds removed

1 cup water

1 clove garlic, peeled

1 tablespoon light olive oil

2 teaspoons fine sea salt

1 teaspoon powdered blended erythritol-stevia sweetener (see page 46)

1 teaspoon cocoa powder, sifted

½ teaspoon dried Mexican oregano leaves

• Heat a medium-sized skillet over high heat. Add the dried chili peppers to the hot, dry pan and toast until fragrant, 3 to 5 minutes, being careful not to burn them.

• Place the toasted chili peppers in a medium-sized bowl and cover with boiling water. Allow the chili peppers to soften in the water for 30 minutes.

• Once they're softened, put the chili peppers in a blender along with the 1 cup water and garlic. Blend on high speed until smooth. Strain the sauce through a fine-mesh sieve into a medium-sized bowl, pressing as needed to push it through the sieve.

• Heat the oil in a saucepan over medium heat and add the strained sauce, salt, and sweetener, then stir to combine. Simmer, uncovered, for 30 minutes to blend the flavors.

• Remove the pan from the heat and stir in the cocoa powder. Let the sauce cool in the saucepan, then pour it into a 1-quart glass jar and cover tightly.

• Store in the fridge for up to 1 week or in the freezer for up to 2 months. If freezing, be sure to leave an inch of headspace in the jar.

PER SERVING

Calories **41** · Fat **2g** · Total Carbs **4g** · Net Carbs **2g** · Fiber **2g** · Protein **1g**

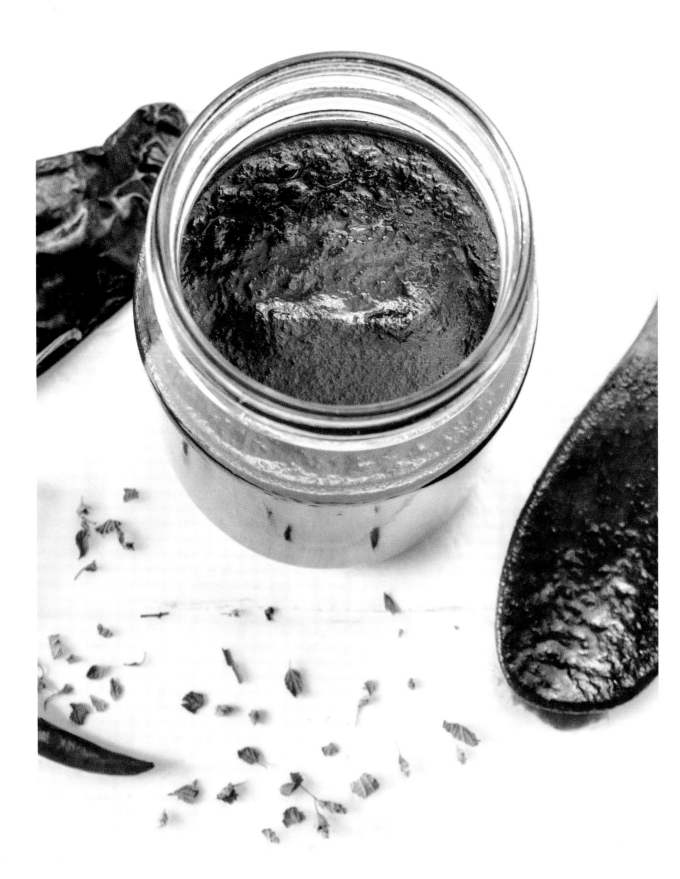

BAJA SAUCE

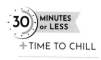

30 MINUTES or LESS

+ TIME TO CHILL

MAKES ¾ CUP
(3 tablespoons per serving)

I came up with this recipe because I wanted a creamy, zesty sauce to add to tacos, but I had no idea how incredible it would turn out! This sauce is so full of flavor, you'll want to put it on everything. It's an absolute must with my Baja Fish Tacos (page 290), and it's amazing on my Shrimp Fajitas (page 280). Plan ahead when you make this, because the longer it sets, the better it gets!

1 large jalapeño pepper, seeded and roughly chopped

⅓ cup full-fat sour cream

⅓ cup mayonnaise (see page 43)

2 tablespoons chopped scallions, both white and green parts

1½ teaspoons white wine vinegar

¼ teaspoon ground black pepper

⅛ teaspoon fine sea salt

⅛ teaspoon garlic powder

⅛ teaspoon ground cumin

Sliced scallions, for garnish (optional)

- Place the jalapeño in a small food processor and pulse until it's very finely minced. Add the rest of the ingredients and pulse until everything is combined. Alternatively, mince the jalapeño and scallions by hand, place them in a large bowl, and stir in the remaining ingredients until well combined. Either way, the sauce should be slightly chunky.

- Pour the sauce into a 1-pint glass jar and cover tightly. Refrigerate for at least 4 hours or overnight to allow the flavors to blend. Garnish with sliced scallions before serving, if desired.

- Store in the fridge for up to 1 week.

PER SERVING
Calories **165** · Fat **17g** · Total Carbs **1g** · Net Carbs **1g** · Fiber **0g** · Protein **1g**

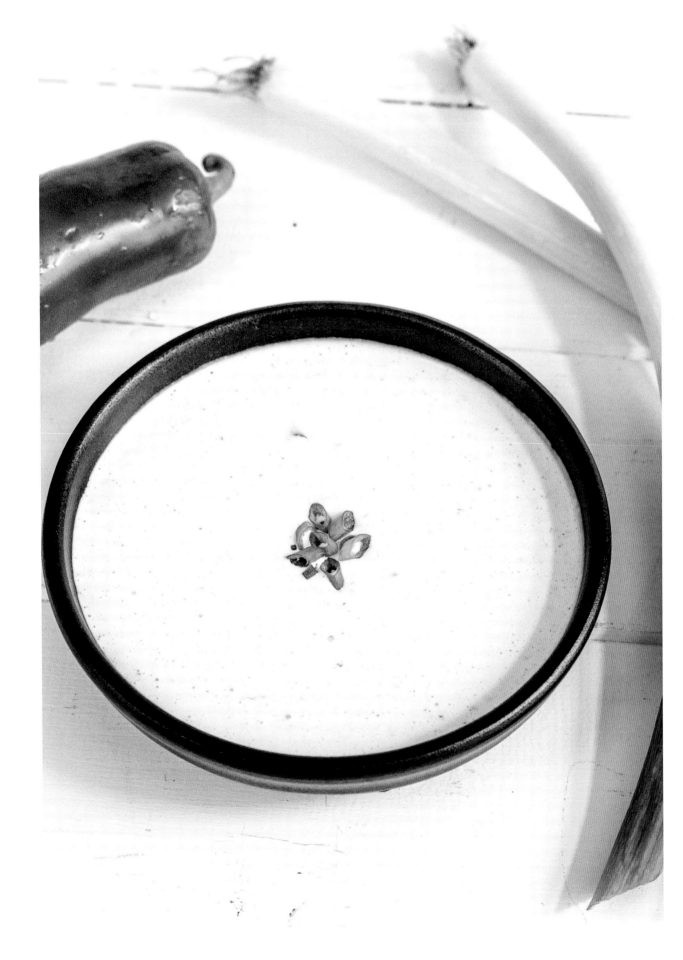

SWEET CHILI SAUCE

MAKES 1 CUP
(2 tablespoons per serving)

I had a mild obsession with the sweet chili sauce from a well-known fast-food restaurant, and I was pretty upset when it was discontinued. Funny enough, though, I never tried to re-create it until long after I had stopped eating sugar—but when I did, it turned out beautifully, savory and sweet, with an Asian zing. It's incredible drizzled over just about any veggie or meat, especially crispy chicken wings!

1 cup water

¼ cup unseasoned rice wine vinegar

2 tablespoons powdered blended erythritol-stevia sweetener (see page 46) (see Notes)

2 tablespoons sambal oelek (see Notes, page 260)

1 tablespoon soy sauce

1 teaspoon garlic powder

⅛ teaspoon crushed red pepper

¼ teaspoon xanthan gum

3 drops toasted sesame oil

· In a medium-sized saucepan over medium-high heat, combine the water, vinegar, and sweetener and whisk until the sweetener is completely dissolved.

· Add the sambal oelek, soy sauce, garlic powder, and crushed red pepper and bring to a light boil. Turn the heat down to medium-low and simmer for 20 minutes, stirring occasionally, until slightly reduced.

· Very slowly add the xanthan gum while whisking to prevent clumps. Simmer for 5 more minutes, until thickened. Remove from the heat and add the toasted sesame oil.

· Let the sauce cool in the saucepan, then pour it into a 1-pint glass jar and cover tightly.

· Store in the fridge for up to 2 weeks.

Notes : For a delicious aioli dipping sauce, combine equal parts mayonnaise (see page 43) and this chili sauce.

I've tried this with other sweeteners, and it never works with anything else—you must use an erythritol-stevia blend for the right balance of flavors.

DRESSINGS, SAUCES
& SEASONINGS

PER SERVING
Calories **4** · Fat **0g** · Total Carbs **3g** · Net Carbs **0g** · Fiber **0g** · Protein **0g**

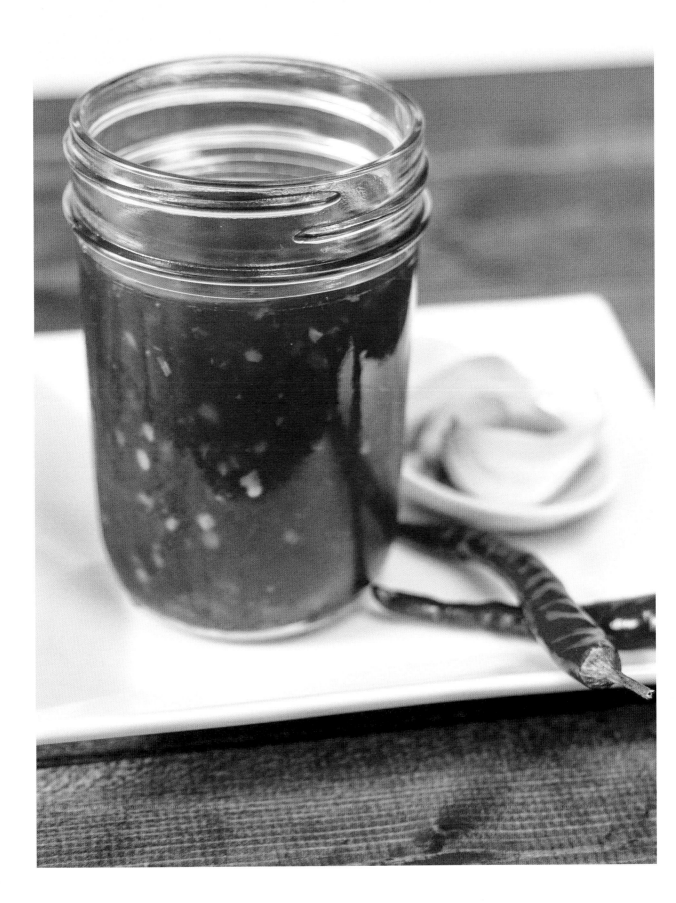

BACON ONION JAM

1 HOUR or LESS

MAKES ABOUT 1 CUP
(2 heaping
tablespoons per
serving)

I originally came up with this jam for my Roast Pork Loin (page 258), but it's so versatile, I use it on any meat or veggie. It's just terrific with eggs or as an addition to an antipasto platter (see page 104).

½ pound thick-cut bacon (about 5 slices)

2 cups diced onions (about 2 medium onions)

½ tablespoon blended erythritol-stevia sweetener (see page 46)

½ teaspoon fine sea salt

¼ teaspoon ground black pepper

2 tablespoons balsamic vinegar

- Stack the bacon slices and halve them lengthwise and then crosswise into ½-inch pieces. Place the bacon in a sauté pan over medium heat and sauté until cooked but still chewy, about 15 minutes. Using a slotted spoon, transfer the bacon to a paper towel–lined plate and set aside.

- Add the onions to the pan and stir to coat them in the bacon drippings. Cook for 10 minutes, stirring occasionally, until softened and lightly browned.

- Turn the heat down to medium-low and stir in the sweetener, salt, and pepper. Continue cooking until the onions have caramelized, about 20 minutes more.

- Turn the heat back up to medium and stir in the balsamic vinegar and reserved bacon pieces. Cook, stirring occasionally, for 5 minutes, or until the consistency is chunky but jam-like. Serve warm or at room temperature.

- Store in an airtight container in the fridge for up to 1 week.

Variation: BACON PEPPER JAM

Swap out the onions for 2 cups diced bell peppers in a variety of colors for a sweeter and more complex flavor.

PER SERVING
Calories **244** · Fat **20g** · Total Carbs **4g** · Net Carbs **3g** · Fiber **1g** · Protein **14g**

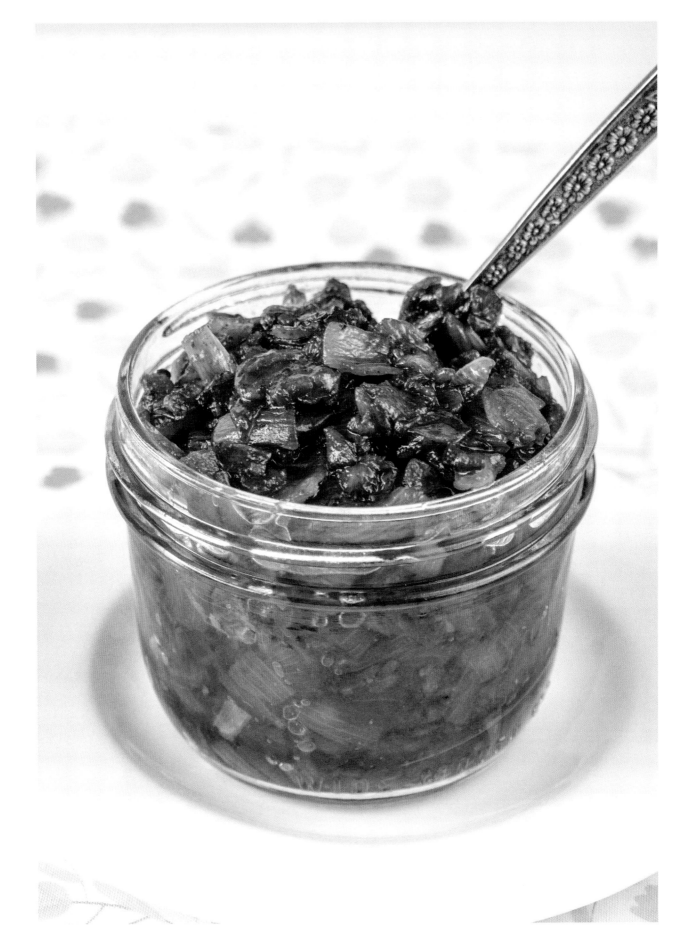

ITALIAN SALSA

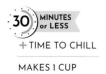

30 MINUTES or LESS

+ TIME TO CHILL

MAKES 1 CUP

I have been making this salsa forever as a topping for grilled chicken, but it's also wonderful with scrambled eggs and my Cheesy Garlic Butter Breadsticks (page 120). It tastes even better after sitting for a day, so I highly recommend making a batch ahead of time to enjoy it in all its glory.

½ cup diced Roma tomatoes

¼ packed cup fresh basil leaves (about 25 leaves), chiffonaded

1 tablespoon balsamic vinegar

1 tablespoon red wine vinegar

½ tablespoon Dijon mustard

1 clove garlic, minced

¼ teaspoon fine sea salt

Sprig of fresh basil, for garnish (optional)

· In a medium-sized bowl, combine all the ingredients and stir to mix well.

· Transfer to a 1-pint glass jar and cover tightly. Refrigerate for at least 2 hours to allow the flavors to blend. Garnish with a sprig of fresh basil before serving, if desired.

· Store this salsa in the fridge for up to 1 week (but it's best consumed within a few days).

PER SERVING

Calories **12** · Fat **0g** · Total Carbs **3g** · Net Carbs **2g** · Fiber **1g** · Protein **0g**

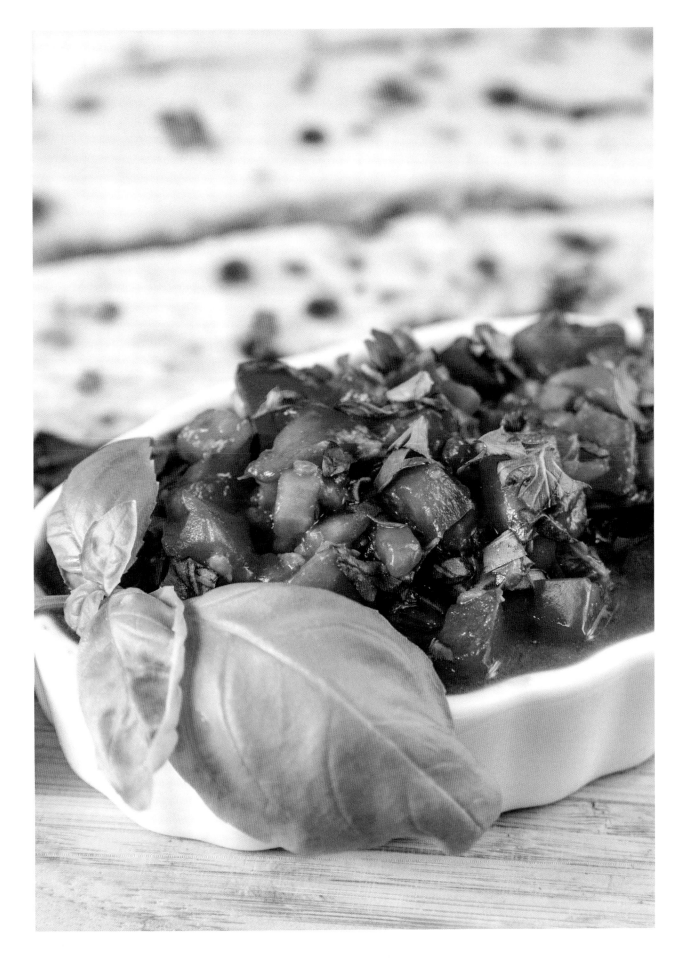

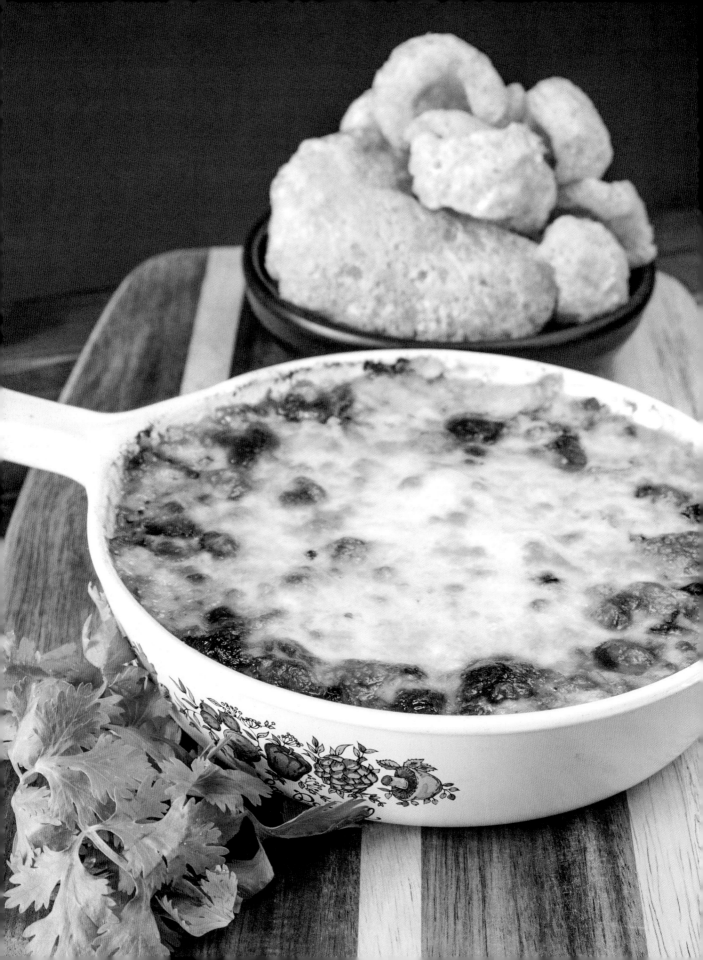

Appetizers & Snacks

ZUCCHINI FRITTE

MINUTES or LESS 30

SERVES 4

I have always loved fried zucchini, and before I started eating keto, I would order it anytime I found it on an appetizer menu. The crushed pork rinds on this low-carb version give these fried zucchini an amazingly crispy exterior. I enjoy them even more than the original!

2 medium zucchini (about 5 ounces each)

1½ cups crushed pork rinds

1 teaspoon Italian seasoning

1 large egg

Fine sea salt

¼ cup light olive oil, for frying

½ cup Ranch Dressing (page 62), for serving

- Cut the zucchini on the bias into slices ½ to ¾ inch thick.

- Mix the crushed pork rinds and Italian seasoning together, then pour onto a large plate.

- Beat the egg in a small bowl with a pinch of salt. Dip both sides of a zucchini slice into the egg, then place it in the crushed pork rinds. Using clean hands, cover the zucchini slice with crushed pork rinds and press down, then flip the zucchini slice over and repeat. Carefully pick up the heavily coated zucchini slice and gently tap one side on the edge of the plate, allowing the excess pork rinds to fall back onto the plate. Set aside. Repeat with remaining zucchini slices.

- Once all the zucchini slices have been coated in crushed pork rinds, heat the oil in a medium skillet over medium-high heat. To test the oil temperature, sprinkle in a pinch of crushed pork rinds; if it sizzles, the oil is ready. Working in batches, shallow-fry the zucchini slices until golden brown, then carefully flip to brown the other side (about 2 minutes per side).

- Transfer to a paper towel–lined plate and lightly sprinkle with salt. Serve with ranch dressing.

- Fried zucchini is best served fresh, but leftovers may be stored in an airtight container for a few days in the fridge. If you have an air fryer, I recommend using it to reheat the zucchini back to its original crunch. Otherwise, reheat in a preheated 400°F oven for 10 minutes. I do not recommend reheating in the microwave because they can become soggy.

PER SERVING

Calories **413** · Fat **37g** · Total Carbs **4g** · Net Carbs **3g** · Fiber **1g** · Protein **16g**

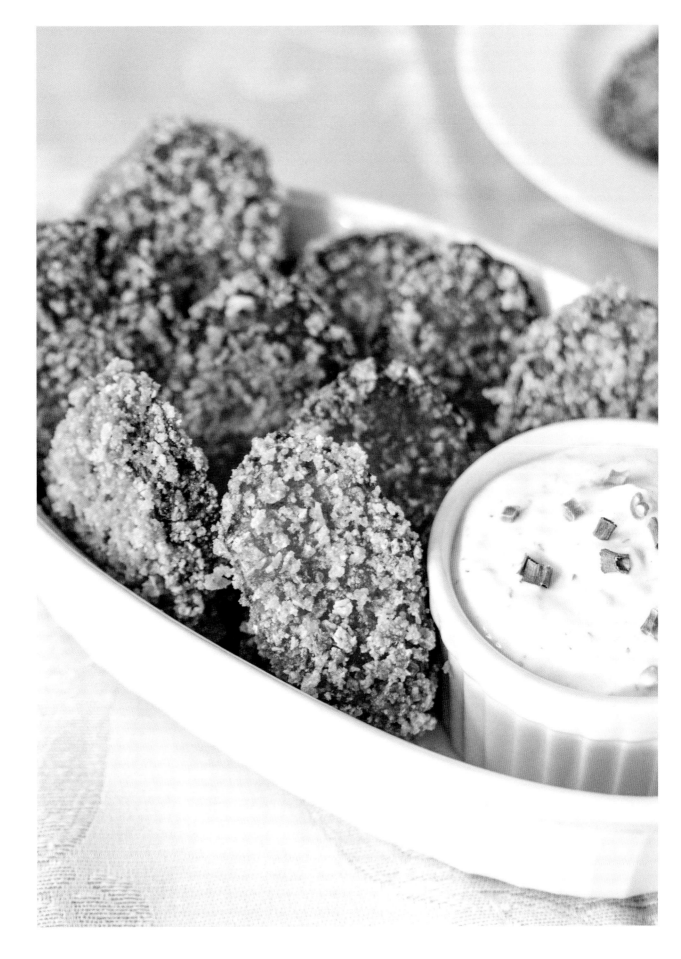

STUFFED MUSHROOMS

30 MINUTES or LESS

MAKES ABOUT 16
MUSHROOMS
(4 per serving)

Stuffed mushrooms are such a wonderful appetizer. Not only are they handheld, so they're easy to snack on while you circulate at a gathering, but they are also filling and delicious. Anytime I have a party, these are the first to go!

2 tablespoons light olive oil, divided

24 ounces large white mushrooms (about 16 mushrooms), cleaned and stemmed

1 tablespoon unsalted butter

2 scallions, minced (both green and white parts)

1 medium shallot, minced

1 clove garlic, minced

1 (8-ounce) package cream cheese, room temperature

¼ cup grated Parmesan cheese

¼ teaspoon onion powder

¼ teaspoon smoked paprika

⅛ teaspoon fine sea salt

⅛ teaspoon ground white pepper

FOR THE TOPPING:

¼ cup crushed pork rinds

1 tablespoon chopped fresh parsley

• Preheat the oven to 400°F.

• Brush a sheet pan with 1 tablespoon of the olive oil. Arrange the mushrooms cup side up on the sheet pan and brush the remaining tablespoon of olive oil over the mushrooms. Bake for 10 minutes.

• While the mushrooms are baking, melt the butter in a small sauté pan over medium-high heat. Add the scallions, shallot, and garlic and cook until everything is light brown, about 5 minutes. Remove from the heat and allow to cool for 5 minutes.

• In a medium-sized bowl, stir together the cream cheese, Parmesan cheese, onion powder, smoked paprika, salt, and pepper until well combined. Add the cooled scallion-shallot mixture and stir until well blended.

• Make the topping: In a small bowl, stir together the crushed pork rinds and parsley until combined.

• Spoon the cream cheese mixture into the baked mushroom cups. Sprinkle the topping evenly over the mushrooms. Return the mushrooms to the oven and bake until the filling is heated through and the topping is browned, about 15 minutes.

• Store leftovers in an airtight container in the fridge for up to 1 week.

PER SERVING
Calories **355** · Fat **31g** · Total Carbs **6g** · Net Carbs **5g** · Fiber **1g** · Protein **13g**

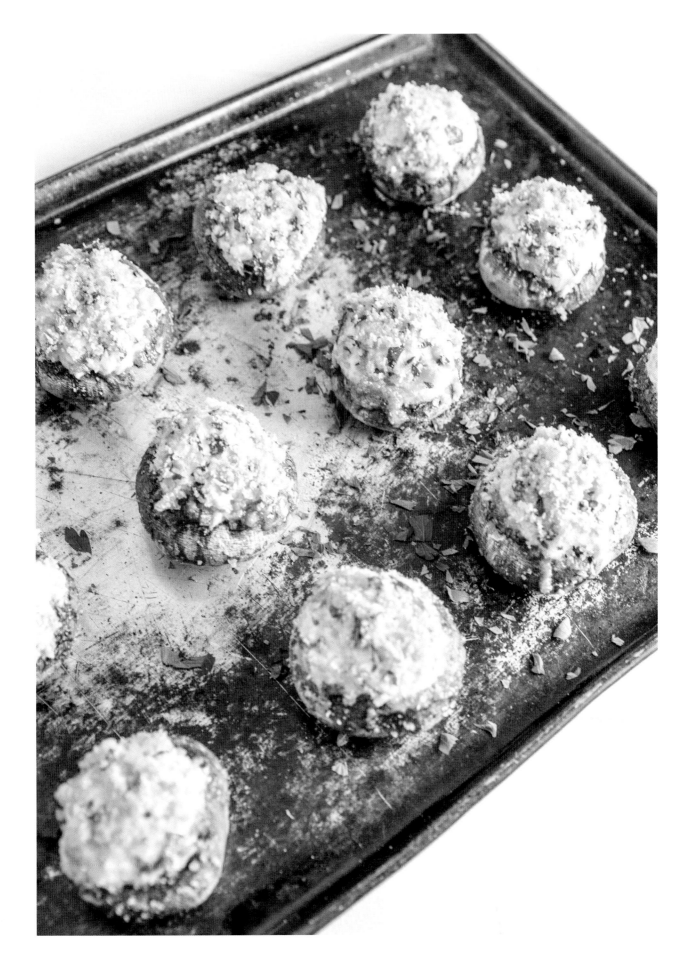

MARINATED MOZZARELLA BITES

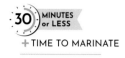

30 MINUTES or LESS

+ TIME TO MARINATE

SERVES 6

I make this anytime I have company; everyone loves it. Fresh mozzarella is great on its own, but once it marinates in this luscious blend, it's truly incredible, with an herby, briny flavor and just a touch of spice. This is a must for an antipasto platter (see page 104).

¼ cup light olive oil

1 teaspoon balsamic vinegar

½ teaspoon fine sea salt

½ teaspoon crushed red pepper

½ teaspoon dried parsley

½ teaspoon dried oregano leaves

½ teaspoon garlic powder

¼ teaspoon ground black pepper

1 pound fresh baby mozzarella balls, drained

• In a medium-sized bowl, whisk together the oil, vinegar, salt, and spices until well blended. Add the mozzarella balls and stir well to coat.

• Cover the bowl tightly with plastic wrap and refrigerate for at least 1 hour before serving for best flavor. Stir once more before serving.

• Store in an airtight container in the refrigerator for up to 1 week.

Variation: **ANTIPASTO SALAD**

For a quick antipasto salad, double the oil, vinegar, salt, and spices and add a 6-ounce can of black olives, drained, and 8 ounces of salami, cubed.

PER SERVING
Calories **273** · Fat **23g** · Total Carbs **1g** · Net Carbs **1g** · Fiber **0g** · Protein **14g**

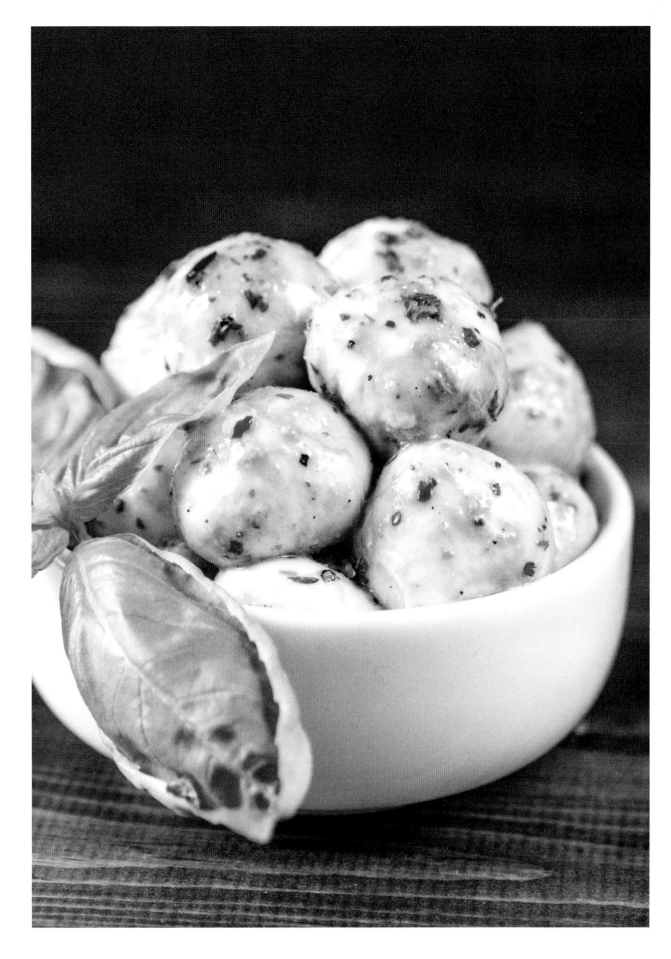

HAM & CHIVES STUFFED EGGS

**MAKES 1 DOZEN
STUFFED EGGS**
(3 per serving)

This is a quick and easy appetizer with a huge flavor payoff! Removing the egg yolks means you can use endless flavor combinations in the stuffing, but this ham-and-chives version continues to be my favorite.

6 large hard-boiled eggs (see page 25), peeled

2 ounces cream cheese (¼ cup), room temperature

¼ cup mayonnaise (see page 43)

½ cup diced no-sugar-added ham (about 2½ ounces)

2 tablespoons sliced chives or scallions, plus more for garnish if desired

⅛ teaspoon fine sea salt

⅛ teaspoon garlic powder

⅛ teaspoon ground white pepper

Note : Instead of discarding the egg yolks, try storing them in an airtight container in the fridge and crumbling them on top of salads for extra flavor and nutrition.

- Slice each egg in half lengthwise. Remove the yolks and discard (see Note).

- In a medium-sized bowl, whisk together the cream cheese and mayo until smooth. Add the remaining ingredients and mix well to combine.

- Fill the egg whites with the cream cheese mixture. Garnish with chives or sliced scallions, if desired, and serve immediately.

- Store in an airtight container in the fridge for up to 1 week.

Variation : TUNA & CELERY STUFFED EGGS

The flavor combinations for the stuffing are limitless. For me, tuna and celery take a close second place to ham and chives! Just swap ½ cup canned tuna, drained, for the ham and 2 tablespoons chopped celery for the chives. Or try different combinations of cooked meats and veggies—just keep the same measurements.

PER SERVING
Calories **298** · Fat **24g** · Total Carbs **2g** · Net Carbs **2g** · Fiber **0g** · Protein **17g**

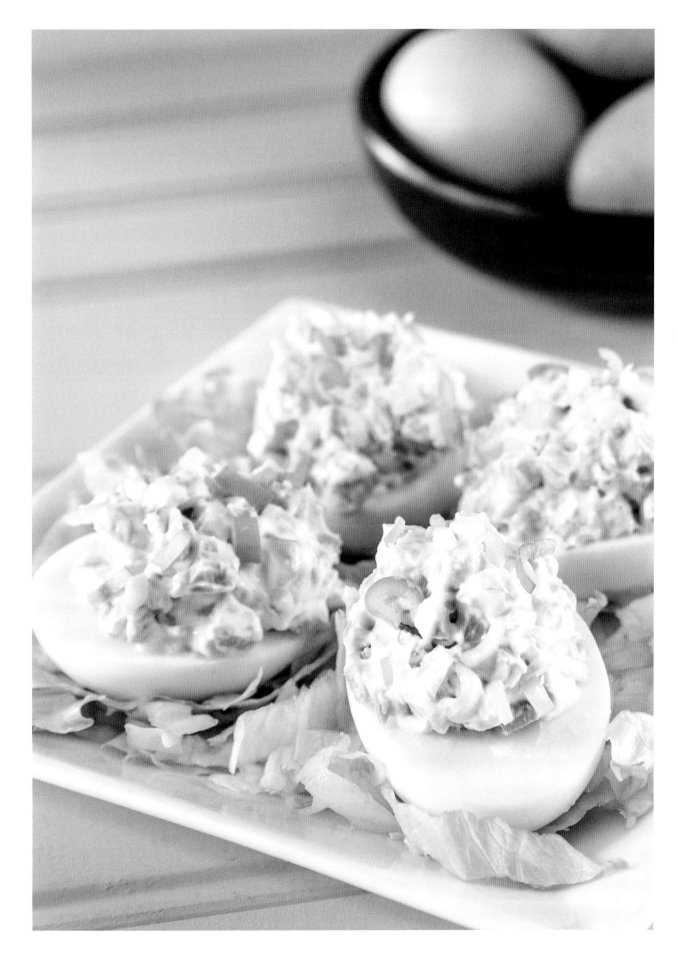

SPINACH DIP

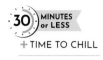

30 MINUTES or LESS

+ TIME TO CHILL

MAKES ABOUT 3½ CUPS
(about ½ cup plus 1 tablespoon per serving)

Spinach dip will forever be my hands-down favorite dip of all time. I'm happy eating it all by itself with a fork, but it is especially delicious served with my Buttery Slider Buns (page 114). Plan ahead to make this dip, as it really needs time in the fridge to become magnificent.

1 (12-ounce) bag frozen chopped spinach

1½ cups full-fat sour cream

½ cup mayonnaise (see page 43)

2 teaspoons dried minced onions

1½ teaspoons dried parsley

1 teaspoon garlic powder

1 teaspoon onion powder

⅛ teaspoon ground white pepper

½ teaspoon fine sea salt

¼ teaspoon blended erythritol-stevia sweetener (see page 46)

1 (8-ounce) can sliced water chestnuts, drained and chopped

4 scallions, sliced

· Cook the spinach as instructed on the package and let cool.

· While the spinach cools, place the sour cream, mayo, spices, salt, and sweetener in a large bowl and whisk until smooth and creamy. Add the chopped water chestnuts and scallions and stir well to combine.

· Once the spinach is cool, squeeze it to remove the excess water, then add it to the bowl with the dip mixture and stir well to combine. Cover the bowl tightly with plastic wrap and refrigerate for at least 2 hours to allow the flavors to blend. Stir well before serving.

· Store in an airtight container in the refrigerator for up to 1 week.

PER SERVING
Calories **251** · Fat **23g** · Total Carbs **6g** · Net Carbs **5g** · Fiber **1g** · Protein **3g**

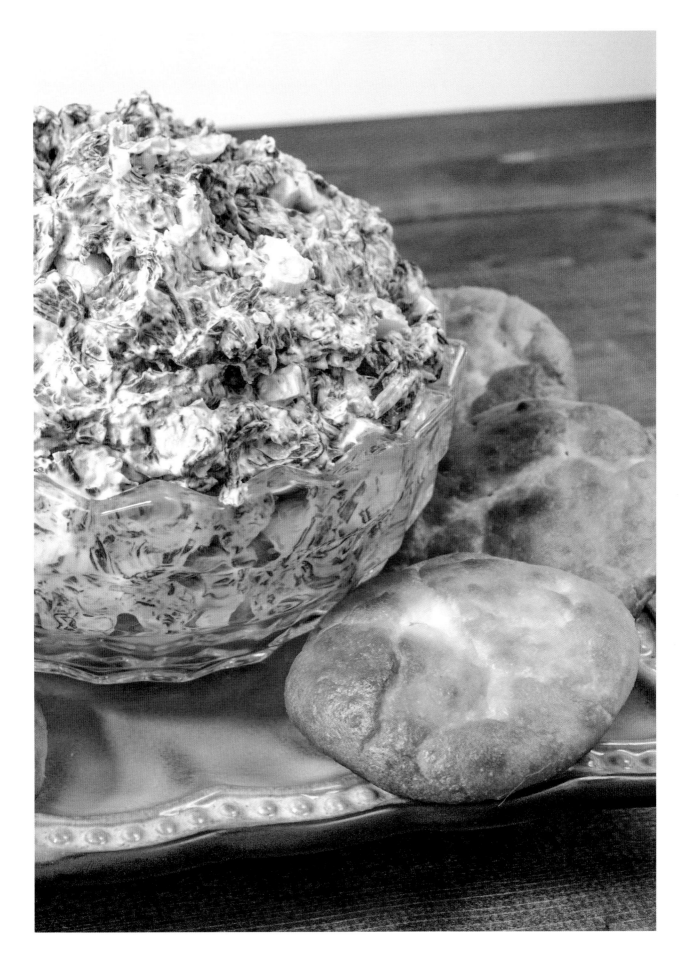

ROASTED NUTS

 MINUTES or LESS

MAKES 2 CUPS
(⅓ cup per serving)

Believe me when I tell you that after making these nuts, you will never buy roasted nuts at the store again. These are fresh and crunchy, and their natural nutty flavor really shines—and bonus, no refined oils! Everyone who tries them can't stop eating them—they're that good!

1½ teaspoons hot water

½ teaspoon fine sea salt

2 cups raw nuts, such as almonds, cashews, pistachios, or a combination

1 tablespoon light olive oil

• Preheat the oven to 375°F. Line a sheet pan with parchment paper.

• In a large heatproof bowl, combine the hot water and salt and stir until the salt is mostly dissolved. Add the nuts to the salt water and toss to coat. Spread the nuts on the lined sheet pan in a single layer.

• Bake until the nuts are lightly browned, about 15 minutes total. Every 5 minutes, remove the nuts from the oven, stir, spread again into a single layer, and then return to the oven.

• When the nuts are done baking, return them to the original large bowl, drizzle with the oil, and toss to coat. Sprinkle with a pinch of sea salt and toss once more. Allow the nuts to cool completely before serving.

• Store in an airtight container at room temperature for up to 3 weeks.

Variation: SEASONED ROASTED NUTS

After tossing the roasted nuts with the olive oil, add your favorite dried herbs or spices, like rosemary and garlic, or my Cajun Seasoning (page 58) for a spicy mix. Start with ½ teaspoon and add more if desired.

PER SERVING
Calories **183** · Fat **16g** · Total Carbs **7g** · Net Carbs **5g** · Fiber **2g** · Protein **6g**

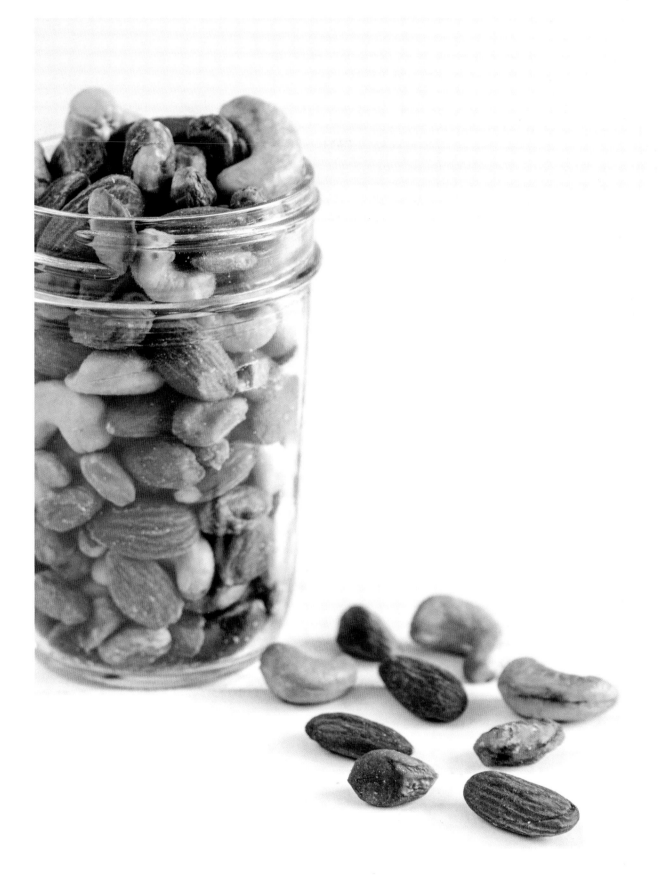

FRIED JALAPEÑO MOZZARELLA BITES

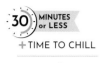

30 MINUTES or LESS

+ TIME TO CHILL

SERVES 4

If you've ever tried to make mozzarella sticks, you know how difficult it can be! This method makes breading much easier, and you can make the bites chock-full of yummy add-ins, like chopped jalapeño. Behold the amazing fried mozzarella bite!

2 cups shredded mozzarella cheese

½ cup chopped jalapeño peppers (about 2 large jalapeños)

1 large egg

1 cup crushed pork rinds

½ cup light olive oil, for frying

- Place the mozzarella in a medium-sized microwave-safe bowl and microwave in 15-second increments until the cheese is completely melted. Stir in the chopped jalapeños. Transfer the mixture to a large serving plate or sheet pan and spread it into an even layer about ½ inch thick. Refrigerate for 30 minutes to harden the cheese, then cut it into the desired shape: sticks, triangles, circles...the choice is yours!

- Set up a "breading" station: Beat the egg in a small bowl and place the crushed pork rinds on a large plate. Dip a cheese bite into the beaten egg and allow the excess egg to drip off. Dredge the cheese bite in the crushed pork rinds, making sure it is well coated. Place the cheese bite on a large plate. Repeat with the remaining cheese bites.

- Heat a heavy-bottomed skillet over medium-high heat and pour in the oil. Test that the oil is hot enough for frying by sprinkling in a few crumbs; if they sizzle, it's ready! Shallow-fry the cheese bites until golden brown on both sides, 3 to 4 minutes per side. Use a slotted spoon to transfer the bites to a paper towel–lined plate.

- Serve immediately with your favorite dipping sauce, such as marinara, ranch, or blue cheese.

- Store in an airtight container in the fridge for up to 1 week. Reheat in a toaster oven or air fryer for best results.

Variation: MEATY MOZZARELLA BITES

Swap out the jalapeños for ½ cup of pepperoni chunks, shredded Buffalo chicken, crumbled bacon, or another cooked meat.

PER SERVING
Calories **420** · Fat **34g** · Total Carbs **2g** · Net Carbs **2g** · Fiber **0g** · Protein **28g**

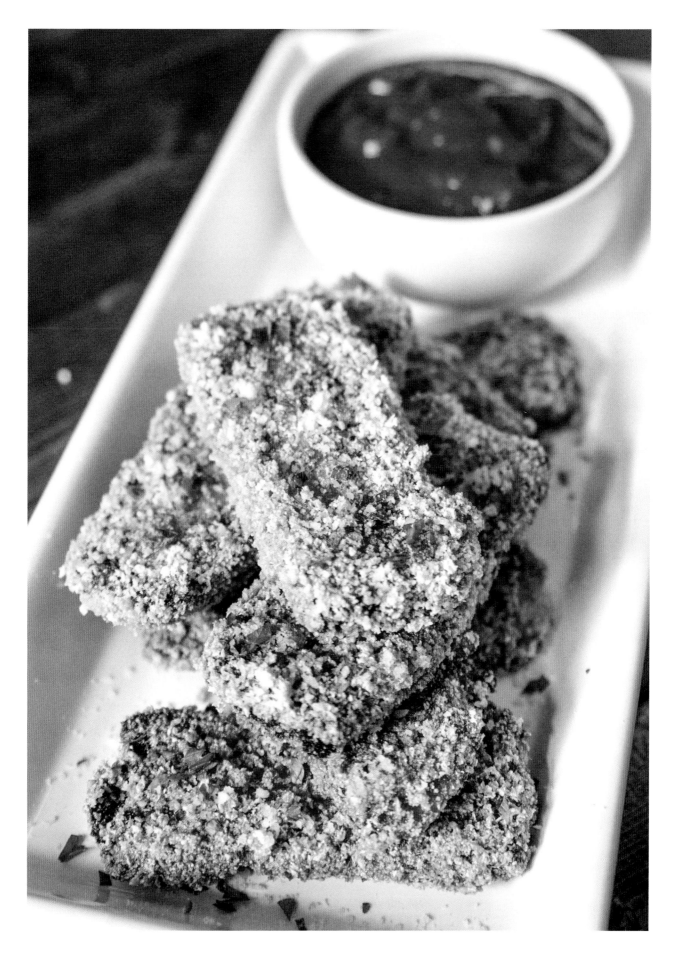

OLIVE DIP

MAKES 3½ CUPS
(about ½ cup plus 1 tablespoon per serving)

If you're an olive lover like me, then this is the dip for you! It's so rich and cheesy, with a delicious salty bite. I've been making this for parties for years and everyone always wants the recipe.

6 ounces pimento-stuffed green olives

6 ounces pitted black olives

2 scallions, minced

1 cup mayonnaise (see page 43)

1 cup shredded sharp cheddar cheese, divided

Chopped fresh parsley, for garnish (optional)

• Preheat the oven to 350°F. Grease an oven-safe au gratin dish or 2-quart casserole dish.

• Chop the olives into small pieces, or place them in a food processor and pulse until chopped into small pieces.

• In a medium-sized bowl, combine the chopped olives, scallions, and mayonnaise and stir until well combined. Add ¾ cup of the shredded cheese and stir to combine.

• Transfer the dip to the prepared baking dish. Top with the remaining ¼ cup of cheddar and bake for 25 minutes, or until the top is browned and bubbly.

• Garnish with chopped fresh parsley if desired. Serve immediately with pork rinds, low-carb crackers, or crudités for dipping. Store in an airtight container in the refrigerator for up to 1 week.

Variation: SWISS OLIVE DIP

Swap Swiss cheese for the cheddar, or even pepper Jack to add a spicy kick!

PER SERVING
Calories **416** · Fat **42g** · Total Carbs **3g** · Net Carbs **3g** · Fiber **0g** · Protein **5g**

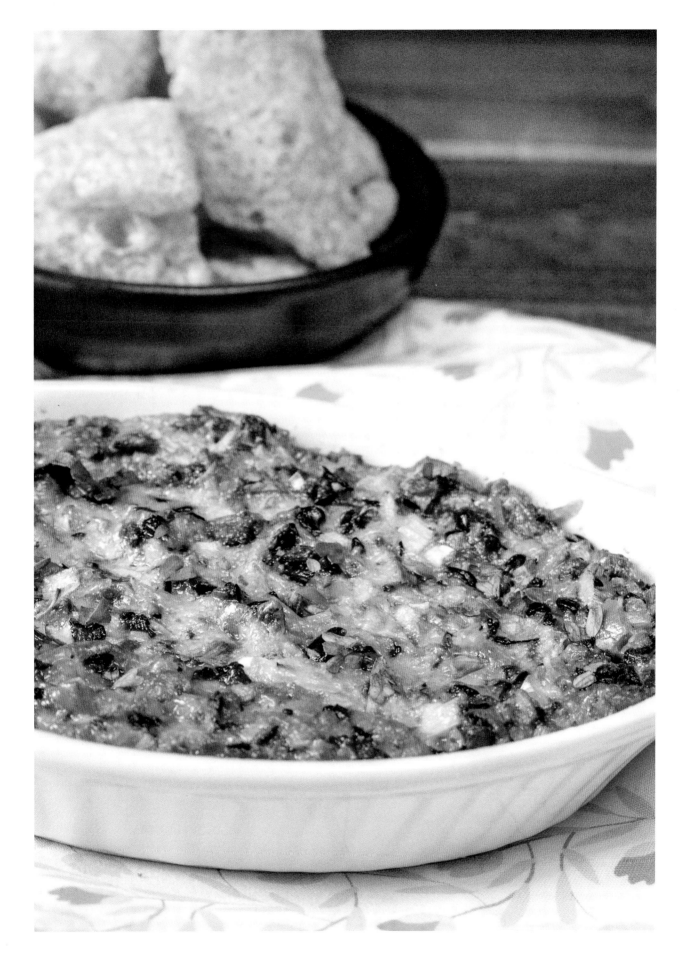

QUESO FUNDIDO

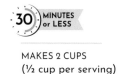

MAKES 2 CUPS
(½ cup per serving)

Queso fundido means "melted cheese," and who doesn't want that?! This ooey-gooey cheesy dip with a subtle spicy and smoky flavor will quickly become a favorite, and it couldn't be easier to make.

2 poblano peppers

1 tablespoon unsalted butter

1 medium onion, diced

1 cup shredded Monterey Jack cheese

1 cup shredded mozzarella cheese

1 cup shredded pepper Jack cheese

• Put an oven rack just under the broiler and turn on the broiler. Line a sheet pan with foil. Grease a 2-quart baking dish.

• Place the poblano peppers on the lined sheet pan and put them directly under the broiler. Broil the peppers until the skin blackens and blisters on all sides, about 10 minutes, flipping as needed to blacken evenly. Remove the peppers from the oven and place in a medium-sized bowl, then cover the bowl with plastic wrap to allow the peppers to steam and their skins to loosen.

• Turn the oven to 375°F.

• While the peppers are steaming, melt the butter in a skillet over medium-high heat. Add the onion and sauté, stirring occasionally, until softened and translucent, about 5 minutes. Remove the pan from the heat and let cool for 15 minutes.

• Once the poblanos have cooled enough to handle, remove and discard their skins, seeds, and stems and chop them into bite-sized pieces. Add the chopped poblanos to the sautéed onion and stir to combine.

• In a medium-sized bowl, combine the three cheeses until well mixed. Spread half the pepper mixture in the bottom of the prepared baking dish and spread half the cheese on top. Repeat with the remaining cheese and pepper mixture; you should have 2 layers of each, 4 layers total. Bake for 20 minutes, or until the cheese is bubbly and golden brown.

• Serve immediately with pork rinds, low-carb crackers, or crudités for dipping. Store in an airtight container in the refrigerator for up to 1 week.

Variation: CHORIZO QUESO FUNDIDO

Add 1 pound of cooked chorizo to the pepper-onion mixture for a more substantial and tasty cheese dip.

PER SERVING
Calories **326** · Fat **25g** · Total Carbs **8g** · Net Carbs **6g** · Fiber **2g** · Protein **19g**

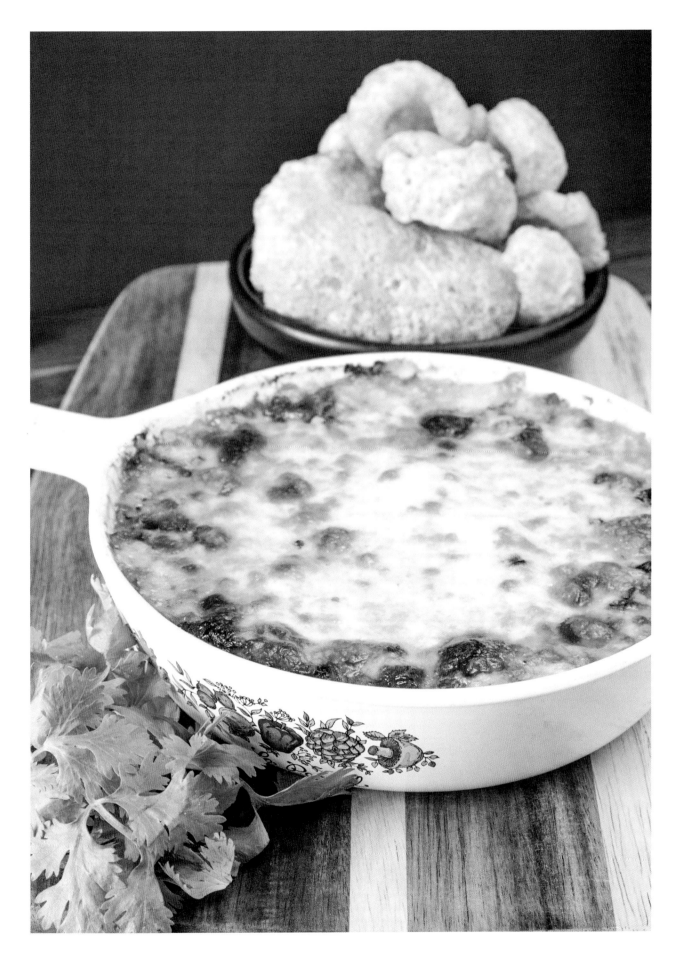

ANTIPASTO PLATTER

30 MINUTES or LESS

Antipasto platters are the ultimate party snack food. There's something for everyone, and they're always a hit! I love that you can be completely creative and make the platters different each time. The list below shows a wide range of options—not all appear in the photo, but they'll all work beautifully on a platter. Be sure to provide plenty of cocktail napkins and toothpicks!

MEATS

Hard chorizo

Mortadella

Pepperoni

Prosciutto

Salami

Soppressata

CHEESES

Hard cheeses

- Cheddar
- Colby
- Gouda
- Manchego
- Monterey Jack
- Parmigiano Reggiano
- Provolone
- Swiss

Soft cheeses

- Blue cheese
- Brie
- Camembert
- Feta
- Garlic Chive Cheese Spread (page 106)
- Havarti
- Mozzarella

VEGGIES & HERBS

Capers

Fresh basil

Giardiniera

Marinated artichoke hearts

Peppers

- Banana peppers
- Hot peppers
- Peperoncini
- Peppadews
- Roasted red peppers

Pickled red onions

Pickles

- Cornichons/gherkins
- Dill slices or spears

Olives

- Black (marinated or plain)
- Green with pimento
- Kalamata
- Stuffed olives (garlic, blue cheese, etc.)

Roasted garlic

Sun-dried tomatoes

FRUITS

Blackberries

Blueberries

Raspberries

Starfruit

Strawberries

BREADS/CRACKERS

Bacon Seed Crackers (page 122)

Best-Ever Flax Buns (page 112)

Buttery Slider Buns (page 114)

Chewy Cheese Bites (page 124)

CONDIMENTS

Blueberry Compote (page 298)

Garlic aioli

Stone-ground mustard

Sugar-free preserves

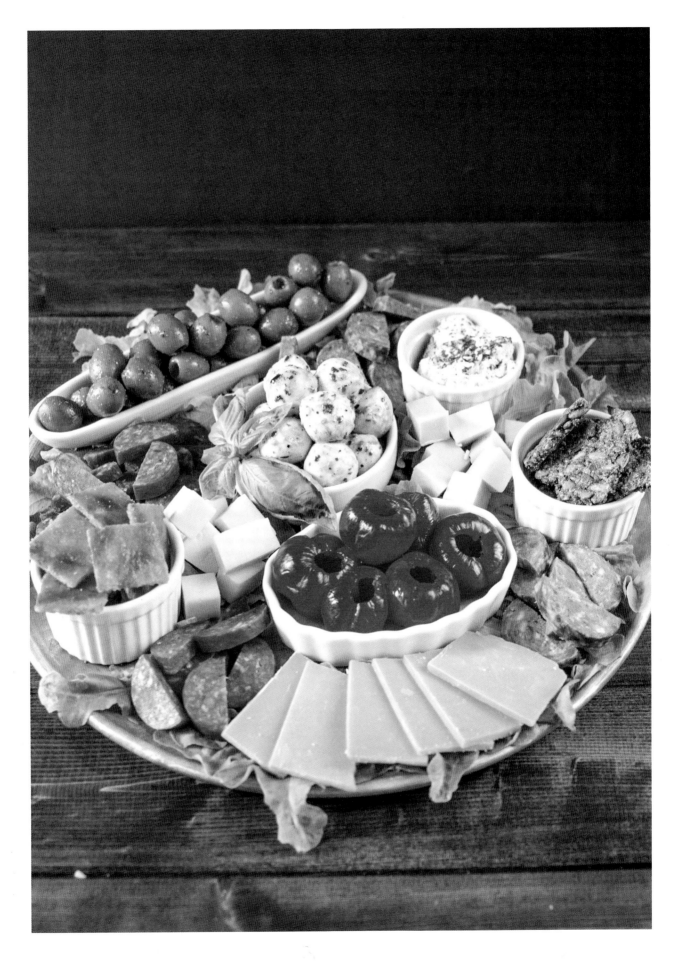

GARLIC CHIVE CHEESE SPREAD

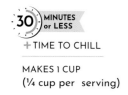

30 MINUTES or LESS

+ TIME TO CHILL

MAKES 1 CUP
(¼ cup per serving)

I've always loved that delicious (and pricey) herbed cheese spread you can find at the store. Now you can save money—and control the flavors—by making it at home! I always include this spread in an antipasto platter (see page 104), and it's really great on my Bacon Seed Crackers (page 122) for a quick and delicious snack. Be sure to allow time for it to chill in the fridge for the best flavor.

1 (8-ounce) package cream cheese, room temperature

2 tablespoons unsalted butter, softened

4 scallions, minced

2 cloves garlic, minced

½ teaspoon chopped fresh dill

¼ teaspoon fine sea salt

⅛ teaspoon ground black pepper

Sliced scallions, for garnish (optional)

• In a medium-sized bowl, mix the cream cheese and butter until smooth and well blended. Add the rest of the ingredients and mix well.

• Cover the bowl tightly with plastic wrap and refrigerate for at least 2 hours for the best flavor. Garnish with sliced scallions, if desired.

• Store in an airtight container in the refrigerator for up to 1 week.

Variation: TOMATO-BASIL SPREAD

Replace the dill with 1 tablespoon minced fresh basil, and replace the scallions with ¼ cup minced sun-dried tomatoes.

Variation: SWEET STRAWBERRY SPREAD

Omit the scallions, garlic, dill, and salt and pepper. Add ¼ cup minced fresh strawberries and ⅛ cup sugar-free strawberry preserves. This is especially wonderful on a toasted Buttery Slider Bun (page 114)!

PER SERVING
Calories **257** · Fat **26g** · Total Carbs **4g** · Net Carbs **4g** · Fiber **0g** · Protein **4g**

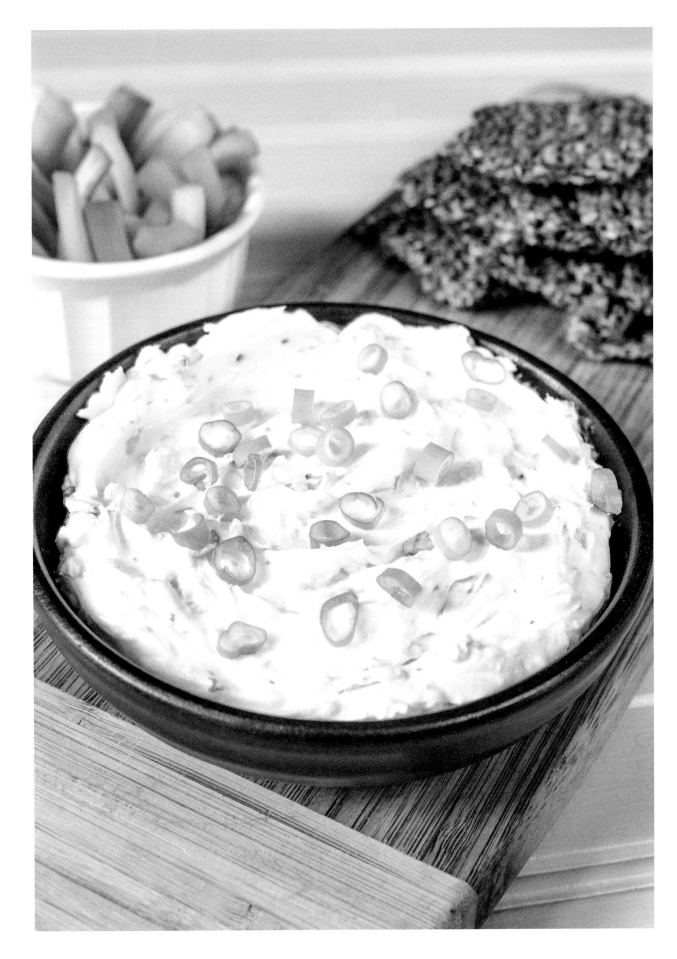

SHRIMP & LOBSTER DIP

Talk about a decadent dip! This is very similar to a dip I used to order at one of my favorite steakhouses, but truth be told, I think mine is better!

MAKES 2 CUPS
(¼ cup per serving)

1 tablespoon unsalted butter

4 ounces peeled and deveined shrimp, chopped

1 lobster tail, shelled and chopped (about 4 ounces after shelling)

1 medium shallot, minced

⅓ cup dry white wine

⅓ cup heavy cream

1 ounce cream cheese (2 tablespoons)

1 tablespoon shredded Parmesan cheese

¼ teaspoon fine sea salt

⅛ teaspoon ground black pepper

1 cup shredded mozzarella cheese, divided

Chopped fresh parsley, for garnish (optional)

- Preheat the oven to 350°F.

- Melt the butter in a skillet over medium heat. Add the shrimp and lobster and gently cook until the shrimp are pink and opaque, about 5 minutes. Use a slotted spoon to transfer the seafood to a plate and set aside.

- Turn the heat up to medium-high and add the shallot to the melted butter. Sauté until softened, about 5 minutes. Deglaze the pan with the wine and simmer until it's reduced by half, 3 to 4 minutes. Add the heavy cream and cream cheese and whisk until smooth. Add the Parmesan cheese, salt, and pepper and whisk to combine.

- Transfer the sauce to a medium-sized bowl and add the cooked seafood. Add ¾ cup of the mozzarella and stir to combine.

- Grease an ovenproof 1-quart serving dish, such as an au gratin dish, and fill it with the dip. Top with the remaining ¼ cup of mozzarella.

- Bake for 15 minutes to heat through, then turn the oven to broil and move the dish directly under the broiler. Broil until the cheese is brown and bubbly, 2 to 3 minutes.

- Garnish with chopped fresh parsley if desired. Serve immediately with pork rinds, low-carb crackers, or crudités for dipping. Store in an airtight container in the refrigerator for up to 1 week.

Variation : SHRIMP & CRAB DIP

Try using 4 ounces crabmeat in place of the lobster for a delicious variation. You can also omit the shrimp and the lobster and use 8 ounces crabmeat instead!

PER SERVING
Calories **316** · Fat **20g** · Total Carbs **4g** · Net Carbs **4g** · Fiber **0g** · Protein **26g**

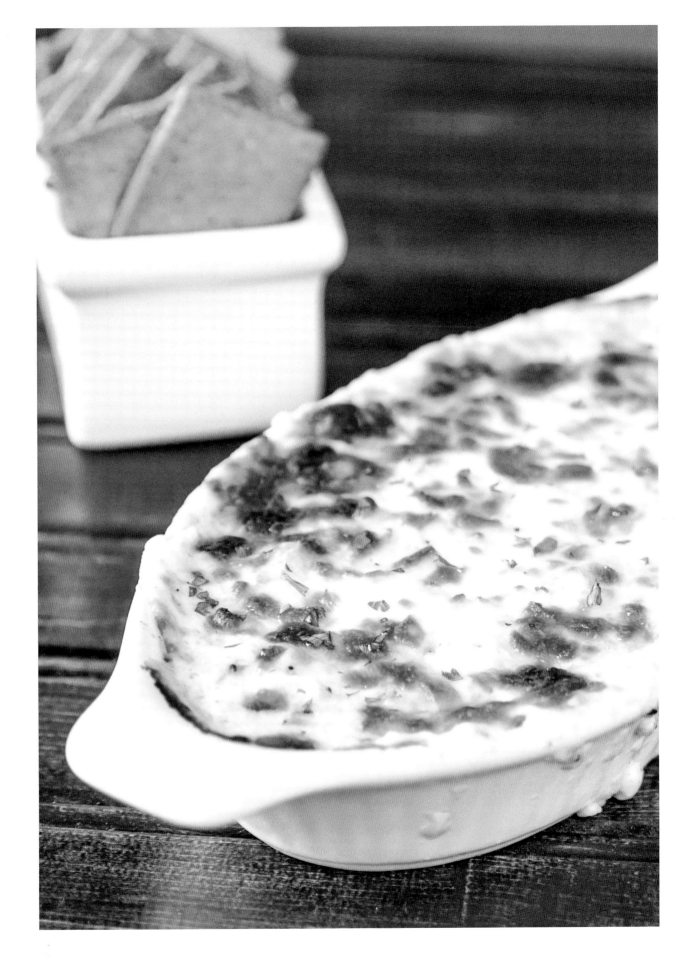

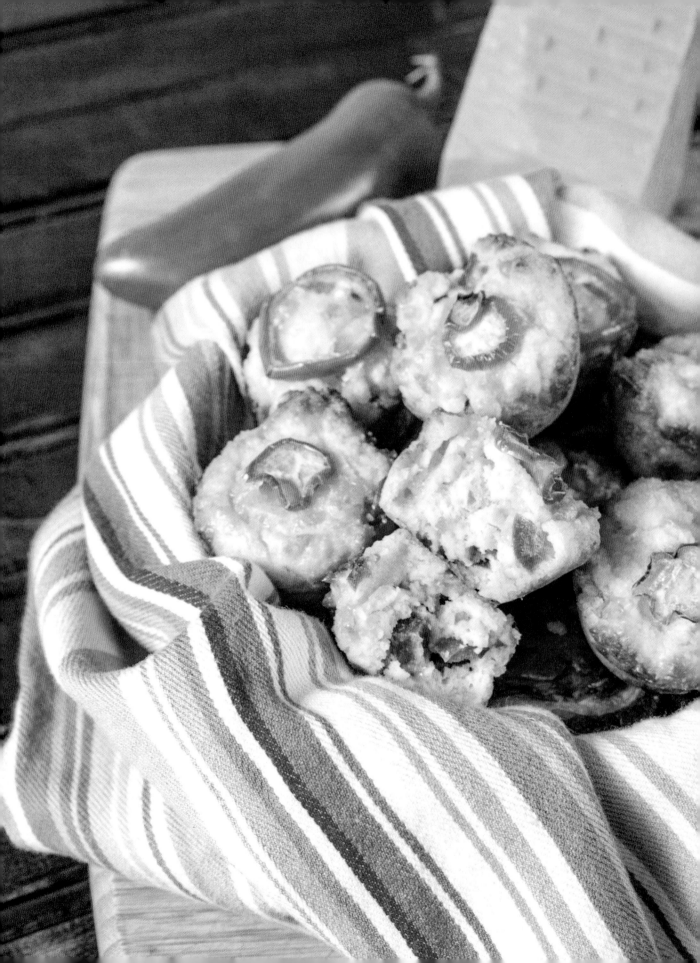

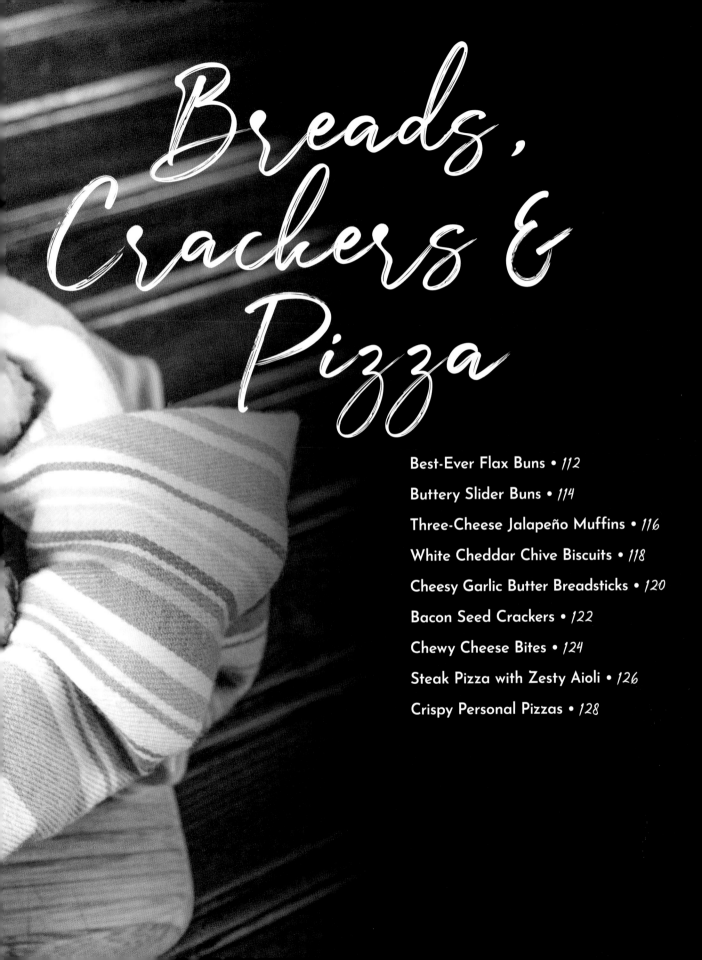

Breads, Crackers & Pizza

BEST-EVER FLAX BUNS

MAKES 8 BUNS
(1 per serving)

I've always preferred whole-wheat bread, and when I started keto, there weren't really any good wheat bread substitutes available. So I created these buns, and they came out beautifully! These are my go-to for most sandwiches, and they are a must for my Cuban Sandwiches (page 270).

¾ cup flaxseed meal

½ cup shredded mozzarella cheese

3 large eggs

3 tablespoons unsalted butter, melted

1 teaspoon baking powder

½ teaspoon blended erythritol-stevia sweetener (see page 46)

⅛ teaspoon fine sea salt

⅛ teaspoon ground black pepper

- Preheat the oven to 350°F. Line a sheet pan with parchment paper.

- Combine all the ingredients in a large bowl and stir to mix well. Wet your hands, then divide the dough into 8 equal pieces. Place the sections in mounds on the prepared sheet pan, 3 inches apart, and form into rounded bun shapes.

- Bake for 10 minutes, or until crusty and lightly browned. Transfer the buns to a baking rack to cool completely.

- Store in an airtight container in the fridge for up to 1 week.

Variation: BEST-EVER FLAX LOAVES

Making the buns as directed will result in the perfect sandwich thin when sliced in half. For a thicker bun or loaf, divide the dough into 4 equal sections and place them in 4 greased 8-ounce ramekins or 4 mini loaf pans. Bake in a preheated 350°F oven for 15 minutes, or until crusty and lightly browned. Allow to cool before removing and slicing.

PER SERVING
Calories **89** · Fat **11g** · Total Carbs **3g** · Net Carbs **1g** · Fiber **2g** · Protein **6g**

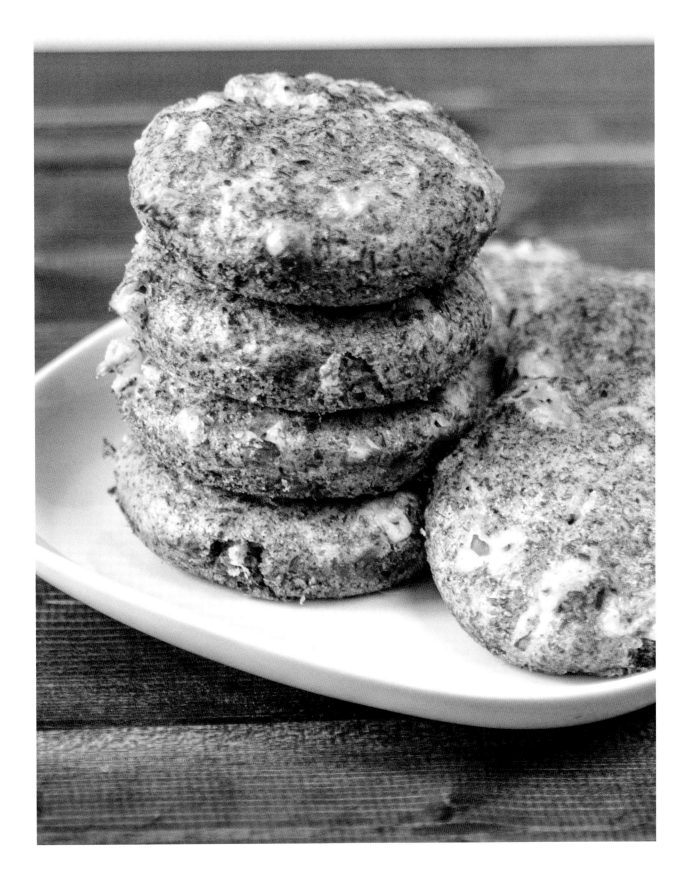

BUTTERY SLIDER BUNS

MAKES 14 BUNS
(1 per serving)

These delicious buttery buns came about when my daughter asked me to make white bread for her sandwiches. This is one of the most popular recipes on my website, not only because they are so delicious but also because they're so versatile. I love using this dough to make pizza crust; it works wonderfully for my Steak Pizza with Zesty Aioli (page 126).

3 large eggs

⅓ cup coconut flour, sifted

½ teaspoon baking powder

½ teaspoon onion powder

¼ teaspoon garlic powder

Pinch of fine sea salt

¾ cup shredded mozzarella cheese

3 ounces cream cheese (¼ cup plus 2 tablespoons)

2 tablespoons unsalted butter

- Preheat the oven to 400°F. Line a baking sheet with parchment paper.

- Crack the eggs into a small bowl and whisk until frothy. In a separate small bowl, whisk together the coconut flour, baking powder, onion powder, garlic powder, and salt until well combined. Set both bowls aside.

- Put the mozzarella, cream cheese, and butter in a large microwave-safe bowl and microwave in 20-second intervals, stirring after each interval, until the mixture is smooth and completely combined.

- Quickly dump the flour mixture and beaten eggs into the cheese mixture and stir with a fork until completely combined.

- To make 14 small slider buns, each about 2 inches in diameter, use a 2-tablespoon cookie scoop to scoop up some of the bun mixture and place it on the prepared baking sheet. Repeat with the rest of the dough, leaving 2 inches between the buns.

- Bake the buns for 10 to 12 minutes, until lightly browned. Remove from the oven and allow to cool on the baking sheet before serving.

- Wrap leftover buns in plastic wrap and store in the refrigerator for up to 1 week. To freeze, wrap in plastic wrap, then in foil and store in the freezer for up to 1 month. Let frozen buns thaw in fridge overnight.

Variation: **BUTTERY SANDWICH BUNS**

Follow the recipe as written, but when forming the buns, use a large 4-tablespoon cookie scoop to scoop up the dough for each bun. If you don't have a 4-tablespoon cookie scoop, simply use two smaller scoops of dough, using the 2-tablespoon cookie scoop, for each bun. (Makes 7 large buns, about 4 inches in diameter)

PER SERVING
Calories **81** · Fat **7g** · Total Carbs **2g** · Net Carbs **1g** · Fiber **1g** · Protein **3g**

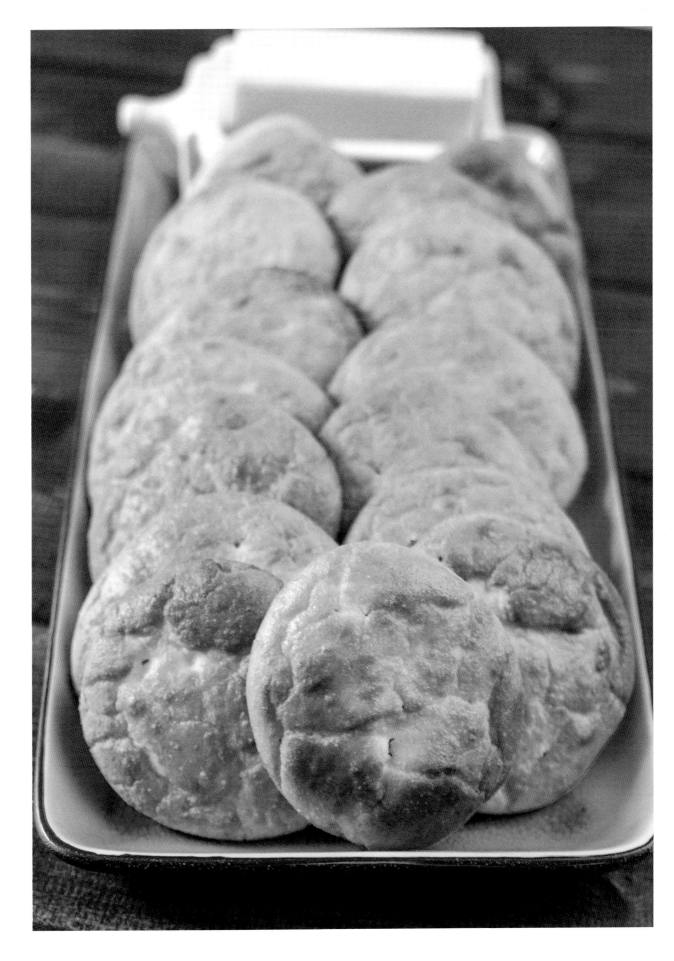

THREE-CHEESE JALAPEÑO MUFFINS

MAKES 6 STANDARD-
SIZE MUFFINS
(1 per serving)
or 1 DOZEN MINI
MUFFINS
(2 per serving)

You really can't go wrong with cheesy muffins, and these are such a nice accompaniment for many soups. I especially love serving them with Albondigas Soup (page 152).

1¼ cups blanched almond flour

1 teaspoon baking powder

½ teaspoon fine sea salt

1 large egg

¼ cup shredded Monterey Jack cheese

¼ cup shredded pepper Jack cheese

¼ cup shredded sharp cheddar cheese

2 tablespoons unsalted butter, melted

2 tablespoons full-fat sour cream

1 large jalapeño pepper, finely diced (about ¼ cup)

6 or 12 pickled jalapeño slices, for garnish (optional)

SPECIAL EQUIPMENT: *24-well mini muffin tin (optional)*

- Preheat the oven to 350°F and grease 6 wells of a standard-sized 12-well muffin tin or 12 wells of a 24-well mini muffin tin.

- In a small bowl, mix together the almond flour, baking powder, and salt.

- In a medium-sized bowl, beat the egg, then stir in the remaining ingredients. Stir the dry ingredients into the wet ingredients and combine thoroughly.

- Drop ¼ cup of the mixture into each greased well of the standard-sized muffin tin. If you're using a mini muffin tin, drop 2 tablespoons into each greased well. Top each muffin with a pickled jalapeño slice, if desired, and bake for 12 to 15 minutes, until golden brown and a toothpick inserted in the middle comes out clean. Serve warm.

- Store leftovers in an airtight container in the fridge for up to 1 week.

Variation : CHEESY BREAKFAST MUFFINS

These muffins are a great side for breakfast if you swap ¼ cup crumbled cooked bacon for the diced jalapeños.

PER SERVING
Calories **252** · Fat **23g** · Total Carbs **5g** · Net Carbs **2g** · Fiber **3g** · Protein **10g**

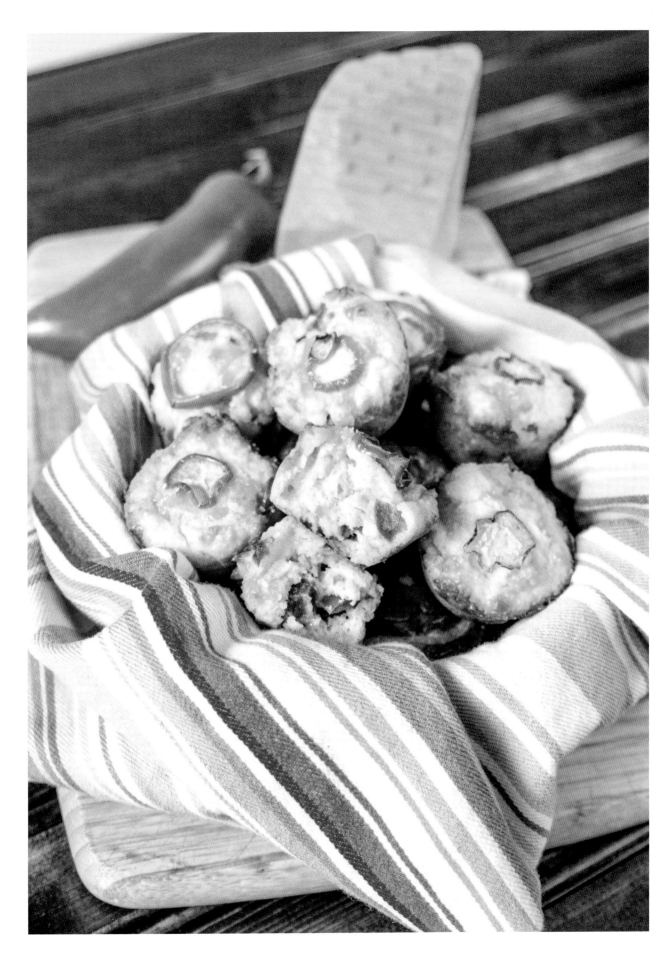

WHITE CHEDDAR CHIVE BISCUITS

MAKES 6 BISCUITS
(1 per serving)

These biscuits are so tender and delicious. I love topping them with sausage gravy, filling them with eggs and bacon for delicious breakfast sandwiches, and dunking them into soup, like Bacon Clam Chowder (page 160).

1¼ cups blanched almond flour

1 teaspoon baking powder

½ teaspoon fine sea salt

½ teaspoon onion powder

¼ teaspoon ground white pepper

3 tablespoons cold unsalted butter, diced

1 large egg

½ cup shredded white cheddar cheese

¼ cup full-fat sour cream

2 tablespoons sliced chives or scallions

• Preheat the oven to 350°F and line a baking sheet with parchment paper.

• In a small bowl, mix together the almond flour, baking powder, salt, onion powder, and white pepper. Add the cold diced butter and use a fork or pastry cutter to work it into the dry mixture until the mixture resembles wet sand.

• In a medium-sized bowl, beat the egg, then stir in the cheddar, sour cream, and chives. Stir the dry ingredients into the wet ingredients and mix thoroughly.

• Using a ¼-cup measuring cup, scoop some of the mixture onto the prepared baking sheet and round it into a biscuit shape. Repeat with the remaining mixture, spacing the biscuits 3 inches apart.

• Bake for 20 minutes, or until golden brown and a toothpick inserted in the middle comes out clean. Serve warm.

• Store leftovers in an airtight container in the fridge for up to 1 week.

PER SERVING
Calories **258** · Fat **23g** · Total Carbs **6g** · Net Carbs **3g** · Fiber **3g** · Protein **9g**

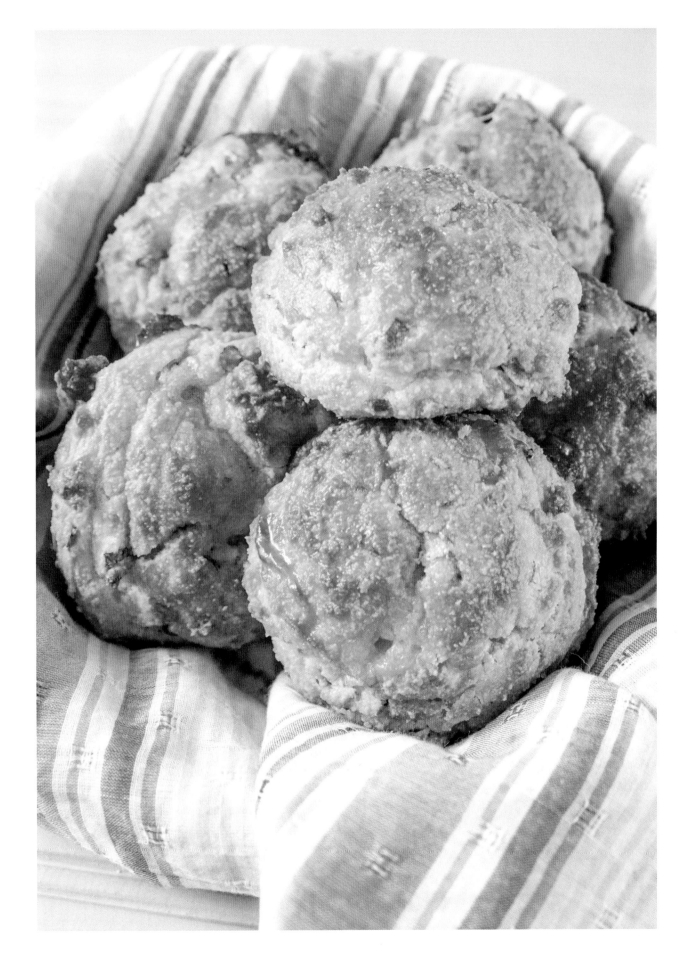

CHEESY GARLIC BUTTER BREADSTICKS

30 MINUTES or LESS

MAKES 16
BREADSTICKS
(2 per serving)

I have always loved cheesy bread, especially when it's dripping with garlic butter. When I created these delicious breadsticks of gooey cheese, I thought they would be incredible with any Italian dish, like my Bolognese Zucchini Lasagna (page 226), which they are, but it turns out, they're just as good dipped in my Italian Salsa (page 82). Cheesy Garlic Butter Bruschetta, anyone?

⅓ cup coconut flour, sifted

½ teaspoon baking powder

½ teaspoon onion powder

¼ teaspoon crushed red pepper (optional)

¼ teaspoon garlic powder

¼ teaspoon fine sea salt

⅛ teaspoon ground black pepper

3 large eggs

¾ cup shredded mozzarella cheese

3 ounces cream cheese (¼ cup plus 2 tablespoons)

3 tablespoons unsalted butter

FOR THE GARLIC BUTTER:

2 tablespoons unsalted butter

1 clove garlic, minced

Pinch of fine sea salt

1½ cups shredded mozzarella, for topping

Chopped fresh parsley, for garnish

- Preheat the oven to 400°F. Line a sheet pan with parchment paper.

- In a small bowl, combine the coconut flour, baking powder, onion powder, crushed red pepper, garlic powder, salt, and pepper. Mix together until well combined, then set aside.

- In a small bowl, beat the eggs until frothy. Set aside.

- Put the mozzarella, cream cheese, and butter in a medium-sized microwave-safe bowl. Microwave on high in 30-second increments, stirring after each round, until the cheese has melted and the mixture is smooth.

- Quickly dump the coconut flour mixture and the beaten eggs into the cheese mixture and stir well to combine. It will seem at first like the components won't mix together, but they will!

- Using a rubber spatula, spread the mixture onto the prepared sheet pan in a 9 by 13-inch rectangle that's about ⅛ inch thick. Bake for 10 minutes, or until the crust is just starting to brown.

- While the breadsticks bake, make the garlic butter: Melt the butter in a small saucepan over medium heat. Add the garlic and salt. Simmer until the garlic is fragrant and just starting to brown, about 3 minutes, then remove the pan from the heat.

- Remove the breadsticks from the oven and brush with half of the garlic butter. Top with the shredded mozzarella.

- Place an oven rack directly under the broiler and turn the oven to the broil setting. Return the breadsticks to the oven and broil until the crust is crispy and the cheese is bubbly, about 3 minutes.

- Remove the breadsticks from the oven and brush with the remaining garlic butter. Slice into 16 breadsticks, garnish with fresh parsley, and serve immediately.

- Store in an airtight container in the fridge for up to 1 week.

PER SERVING
Calories **216** · Fat **16g** · Total Carbs **5g** · Net Carbs **3g** · Fiber **2g** · Protein **13g**

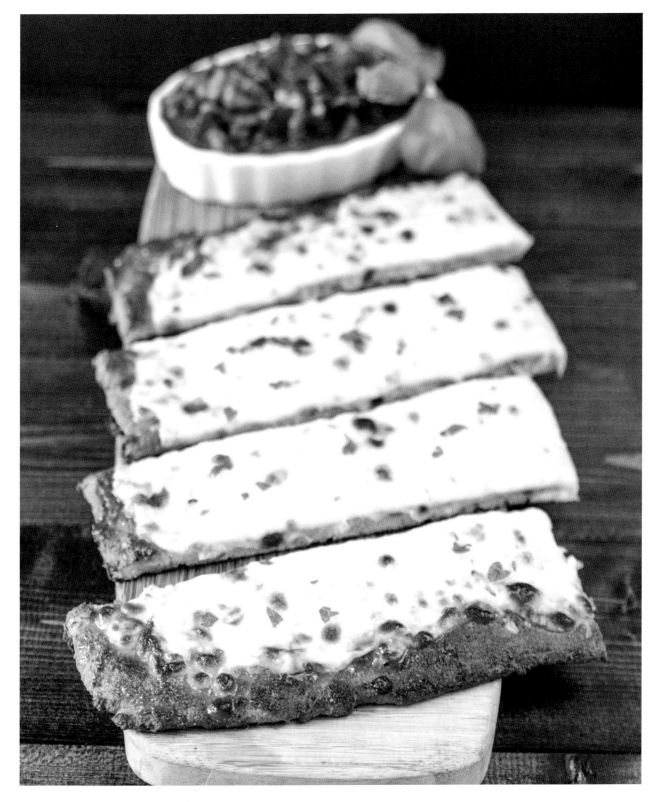

Variation: PIZZA BREADSTICKS

Turn these cheesy breadsticks into pizza breadsticks by adding 32 pepperoni slices on top of the shredded mozzarella before broiling. Dip the breadsticks in your favorite warmed sugar-free pizza sauce.

121

BACON SEED CRACKERS

HOUR or LESS

SERVES 6

One day I was cleaning out my pantry and decided to use up a bunch of odds and ends by throwing them together in what I hoped would be an edible cracker. It turned out to be one of the best things I ever did—everyone who has tried these absolutely loves them! These delicate little morsels are prone to crumbling, but the good news is, the crumbles are fabulous on top of a salad and add a nice crunch! I really enjoy the smoky bacon flavor that the bacon grease brings, but butter is equally delicious.

½ cup chicken stock (see page 26)

⅓ cup blanched almond flour

⅓ cup shelled roasted sunflower seeds

⅓ cup roasted pumpkin seeds

⅓ cup toasted hemp seeds (see Note)

¼ cup bacon grease or salted butter, melted

1 tablespoon flaxseed meal

1 tablespoon psyllium husk powder

½ teaspoon fine sea salt

Note : Make sure you use hemp seeds, not hemp hearts! Hemp hearts are hulled hemp seeds, and we want the added crunch of that shell.

- Place an oven rack in the lowest position and preheat the oven to 300°F. Line a large baking sheet with parchment paper.

- Combine all the ingredients in a large bowl and stir well to thoroughly combine. Place the dough on the prepared baking sheet.

- Using a silicone spatula, spread the dough out and push it down until it becomes an even sheet about ⅛ to ¼ inch thick. Bake for 1 hour, or until the dough starts to lightly brown and smell amazing.

- Remove from the oven and let cool completely, then break into pieces.

- Store in an airtight container in the fridge for up to 2 weeks.

PER SERVING
Calories **237** · Fat **22g** · Total Carbs **5g** · Net Carbs **3g** · Fiber **2g** · Protein **7g**

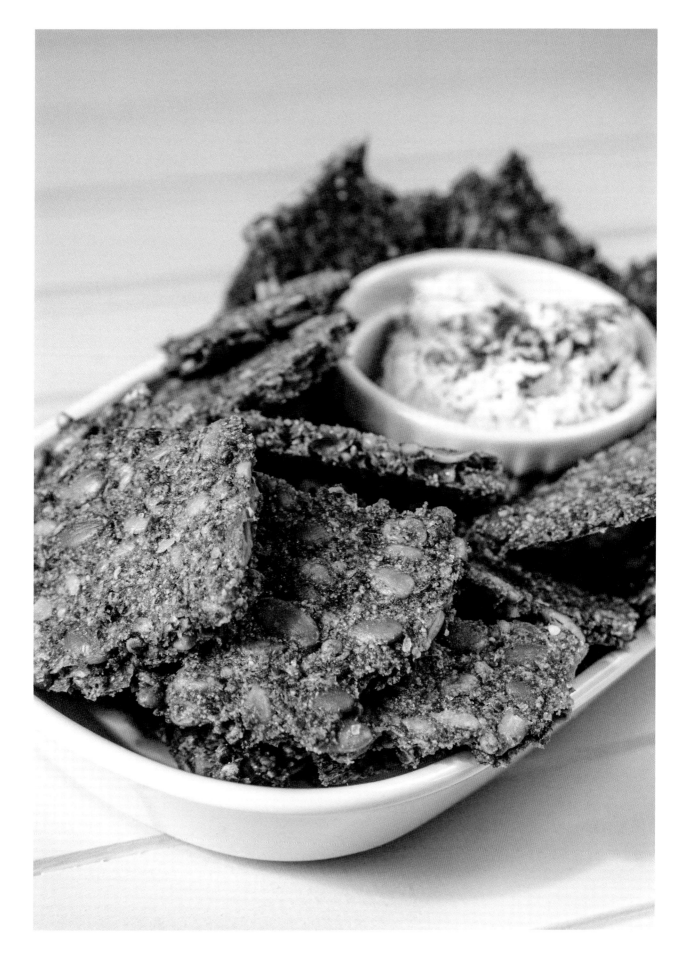

CHEWY CHEESE BITES

30 MINUTES or LESS

MAKES 60 BITES
(10 per serving)

My kids asked for cheese crackers, so I went to work putting together something crispy and cheesy for them. Well, one out of two isn't bad, right? I told them I'd have to try again to make them crunchy, but they said they loved the chewiness as much as the tangy flavor! I hope you enjoy these cheesy chews as much as my kids do.

¾ cup shredded mozzarella cheese

½ cup shredded sharp cheddar cheese

½ cup blanched almond flour

¼ cup crumbled feta cheese

1 large egg

2 tablespoons full-fat sour cream

2 teaspoons coconut flour, sifted

¼ teaspoon fine sea salt

¼ teaspoon smoked paprika

· Preheat the oven to 400°F.

· Combine all the ingredients in a large bowl and stir to mix well.

· Place a large piece of parchment paper, about 11 by 17 inches, on the countertop, place the dough on the parchment, and cover it with another piece of parchment paper. Use a rolling pin to roll the dough out as thin as possible without tearing, into a rectangle about 9 by 13 inches. Remove the top piece of parchment and use a pizza cutter to score the dough to create 60 squares. Slide the bottom piece of parchment and the dough onto a large baking sheet.

· Bake for 7 minutes, then flip the dough with a spatula and bake for 3 to 5 minutes more, until the bites start to lightly brown. Remove from the oven and let cool completely. Run the pizza cutter over the scored lines once more to separate the bites.

· Store in an airtight container in the fridge for up to 1 week.

PER SERVING
Calories **174** · Fat **14g** · Total Carbs **3g** · Net Carbs **2g** · Fiber **1g** · Protein **9g**

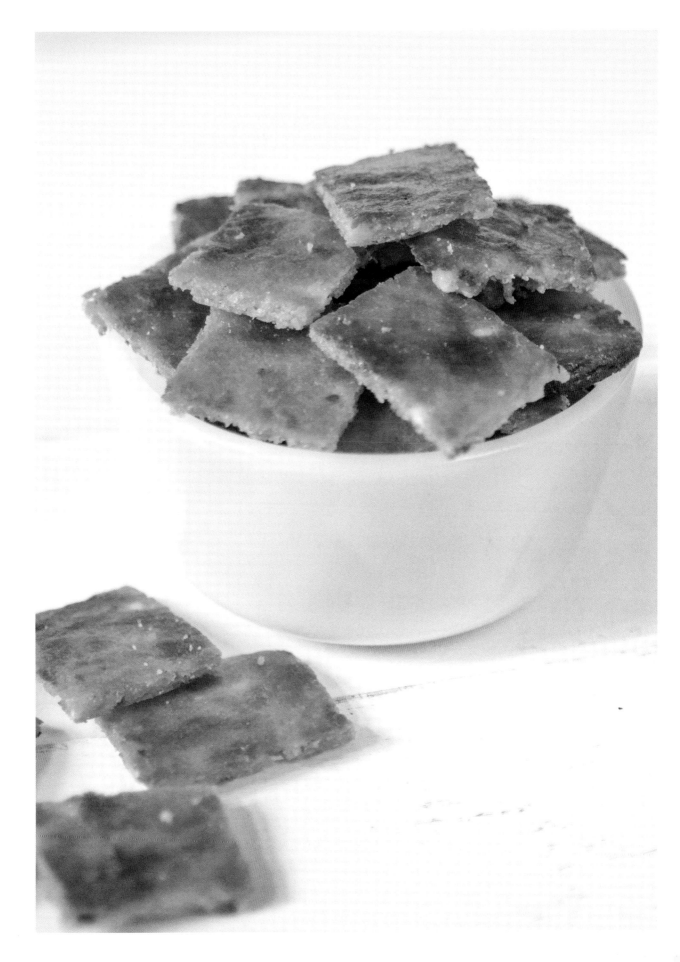

STEAK PIZZA *with* ZESTY AIOLI

MAKES ONE 9 BY
13-INCH PIZZA
(4 servings)

I really love this crust for its versatility and texture. It's more of a bready crust than traditional pizza crust—in fact, it's the same dough that I use for my Cheesy Garlic Butter Breadsticks (page 120)—and it pairs really well with virtually all toppings and flavors. In this version, the juicy steak, peppery arugula, and zesty aioli create an amazing taste experience.

FOR THE CRUST:

⅓ cup coconut flour, sifted

½ teaspoon baking powder

½ teaspoon onion powder

¼ teaspoon crushed red pepper (optional)

¼ teaspoon garlic powder

¼ teaspoon fine sea salt

⅛ teaspoon ground black pepper

3 large eggs

¾ cup shredded mozzarella cheese

3 ounces cream cheese (¼ cup plus 2 tablespoons)

3 tablespoons unsalted butter

FOR THE AIOLI:

¼ cup mayonnaise (see page 43)

1 clove garlic, minced

1 teaspoon lemon juice

½ teaspoon grated lemon zest

⅛ teaspoon fine sea salt

⅛ teaspoon ground black pepper

FOR TOPPING:

1 lightly packed cup arugula

1 tablespoon lemon juice

Pinch of fine sea salt

Pinch of ground black pepper

1 pound flank steak, cooked and sliced on the bias

½ small red onion, thinly sliced

- Preheat the oven to 400°F. Line a sheet pan with parchment paper.

- Make the crust: In a small bowl, combine the coconut flour, baking powder, onion powder, crushed red pepper, garlic powder, salt, and pepper. Mix together until well combined, then set aside.

- In a small bowl, beat the eggs until frothy. Set aside.

- In medium-sized microwave-safe bowl, combine the mozzarella, cream cheese, and butter. Microwave on high in 30-second increments, stirring after each round, until the cheese has melted and the mixture is smooth.

- Quickly dump the coconut flour mixture and the beaten eggs into the cheese mixture and stir well to combine. It will seem at first like the components won't mix together, but they will!

- Using a rubber spatula, spread the mixture onto the prepared sheet pan in a 9 by 13-inch rectangle that's about ⅛ inch thick. Bake for 13 minutes, or until golden. When the crust is done, remove it from the oven and let cool.

- While the crust bakes, make the aioli: Put all the aioli ingredients in a small bowl and mix until well combined. Set aside.

- Dress the arugula for the topping: In a medium-sized bowl, toss together the arugula, lemon juice, salt, and pepper.

- To assemble the pizza, spread the aioli on the crust and add the sliced flank steak, dressed arugula, and red onion slices.

- Store in an airtight container in the fridge for up to 1 week.

PER SERVING
Calories **558** · Fat **42g** · Total Carbs **9g** · Net Carbs **5g** · Fiber **4g** · Protein **37g**

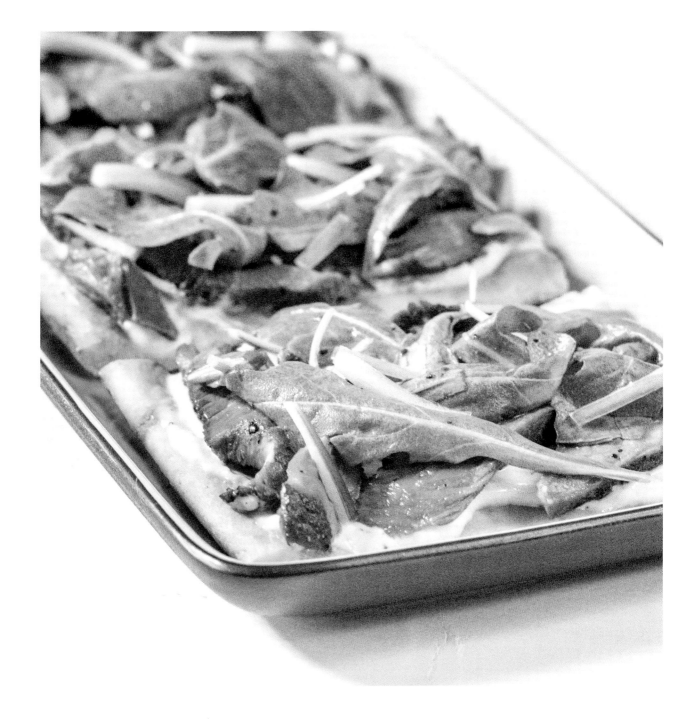

Variation: HAM AND CHEDDAR GRINDER PIZZA

I love to top this pizza crust with cheddar cheese and ham. It's like a pizza sandwich! Follow the instructions for making the crust, then add slices of sharp cheddar cheese and ham. Place an oven rack directly under the broiler and turn the oven to the broil setting, then broil the pizza until the cheese is bubbly and the ham is lightly browned, about 3 minutes. Meanwhile, in a large bowl, combine ¼ cup mayo, 1½ teaspoons apple cider vinegar, ⅛ teaspoon dried oregano leaves, a pinch of fine sea salt, and a pinch of ground black pepper. Stir together until smooth. Toss the mixture with 2 cups shredded lettuce and ½ cup thinly sliced onions. After the pizza has cooled slightly, top it with zigzags of mustard, then add the dressed lettuce and onions. It tastes incredible!

CRISPY PERSONAL PIZZAS

MAKES TWO 6-INCH
PIZZAS
(4 servings)

This is the pizza my family asks me to make the most. It's nice and crispy without being heavy, like some low-carb crusts can be. Here, I've suggested topping it with pepperoni and olives, but any and all toppings are welcome on this pizza—sky's the limit!

FOR THE CRUST:

1 boneless, skinless chicken breast (6 to 8 ounces), cooked (see Notes)

1 cup crushed pork rinds

¼ cup mayonnaise (see page 43)

¼ cup shredded mozzarella

2 large eggs

1 teaspoon Italian seasoning

FOR TOPPING:

½ cup no-sugar-added pizza sauce

2 cups shredded mozzarella

20 slices pepperoni

10 green olives, sliced

Notes : I've found that poaching is the quickest and easiest method of cooking chicken—see page 28 for instructions.

You can use this pizza crust to make other sizes as well:

Large pizza: Use all of the crust mixture; makes one 12-inch pizza.

Small pizzas: Use ¼ cup of the crust mixture for each; makes four 3-inch pizzas.

Mini pizzas: Use ⅛ cup of the crust mixture for each; makes eight 1½-inch pizzas.

- Preheat the oven to 400°F. Line 2 medium-sized sheet pans with parchment paper.

- Make the crust: If the chicken breast was just cooked, allow it to cool. Place the chicken breast in a food processor and pulse until it forms a fine crumb. Alternatively, mince the chicken by hand with a sharp knife.

- In a medium-sized bowl, combine the chicken and the remaining crust ingredients and mix well. Using wet hands, split the chicken mixture in half. Form one half into a ⅛-inch-thick circle on the prepared baking sheet. Repeat with the other half of the mixture.

- Bake until the crusts are crispy and golden, about 10 minutes.

- Spread half of the pizza sauce in a thin layer on each baked crust. Top each pizza with half of the mozzarella, pepperoni, and olives. Return the pizzas to the oven and bake until the cheese is melted and bubbly, about 5 minutes. Slice and serve immediately.

- Store leftovers in an airtight container in the fridge for up to 1 week.

*Variation : *BBQ CHICKEN PIZZA

Replace the pizza sauce with sugar-free BBQ sauce, the pepperoni with 1 cup shredded poached chicken, and the olives with jalapeños, and you have delicious BBQ chicken pizza.

PER SERVING
Calories **511** · Fat **38g** · Total Carbs **4g** · Net Carbs **4g** · Fiber **0g** · Protein **39g**

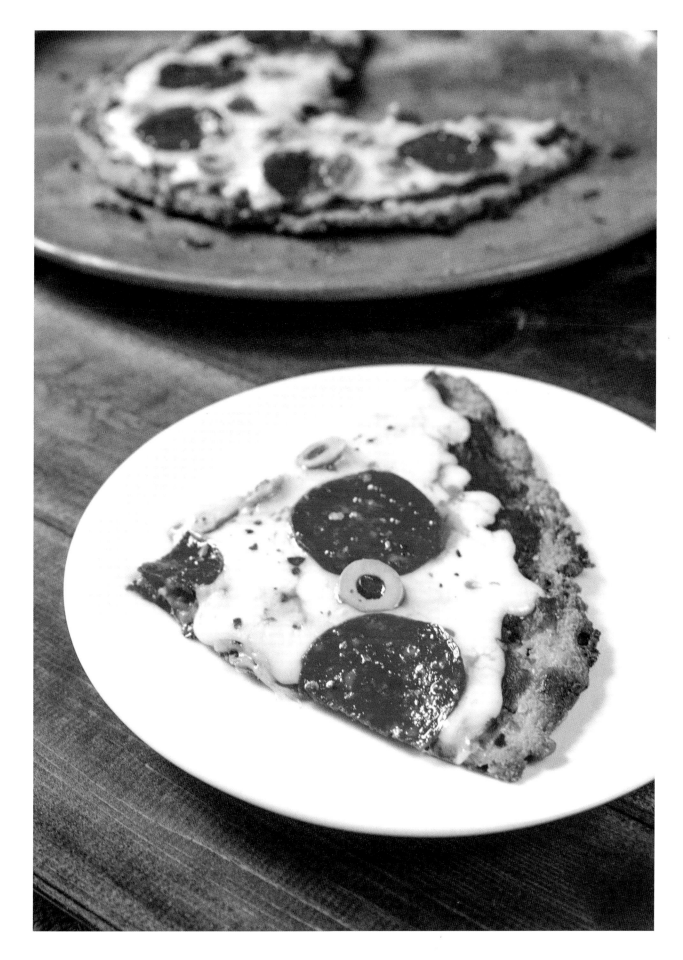

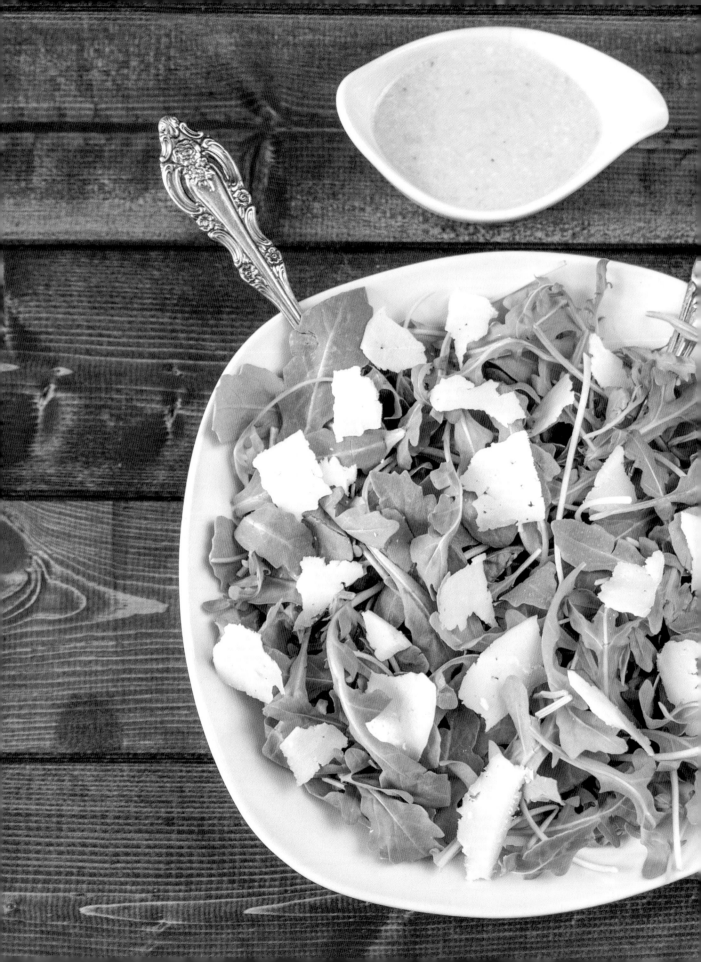

Salads

HEIRLOOM CAPRESE SALAD

 30 MINUTES or LESS

I think everyone loves caprese salad! Using heirloom tomatoes lets you make this classic in a bright variety of colors and turns the flavor up to eleven.

SERVES 4

3 heirloom tomatoes, any variety, any color

6 ounces fresh mozzarella cheese

12 fresh basil leaves, plus extra for garnish

Fine sea salt

Cracked black pepper

• Cut each tomato into 4 thick slices and set aside. Slice the mozzarella into 12 slices, each about ¼ inch thick.

• On a serving plate, layer a slice of mozzarella and a basil leaf on top of a tomato slice. Repeat in a circle around the serving plate until all the tomato, mozzarella, and basil are used; you should end up with 12 stacks. Sprinkle with salt and pepper, then garnish with additional basil leaves. Serve immediately.

• Store leftovers in an airtight container in the fridge for 2 to 3 days.

Variation: BALSAMIC CAPRESE SALAD

Make your own balsamic reduction: In a small saucepan, bring ¼ cup balsamic vinegar to a boil, then turn the heat down to medium-low and simmer for about 15 minutes, until it reduces by half. Allow the reduction to cool, then drizzle it over the caprese salad for a stunning presentation and burst of flavor.

PER SERVING
Calories **119** · Fat **8g** · Total Carbs **4g** · Net Carbs **3g** · Fiber **1g** · Protein **8g**

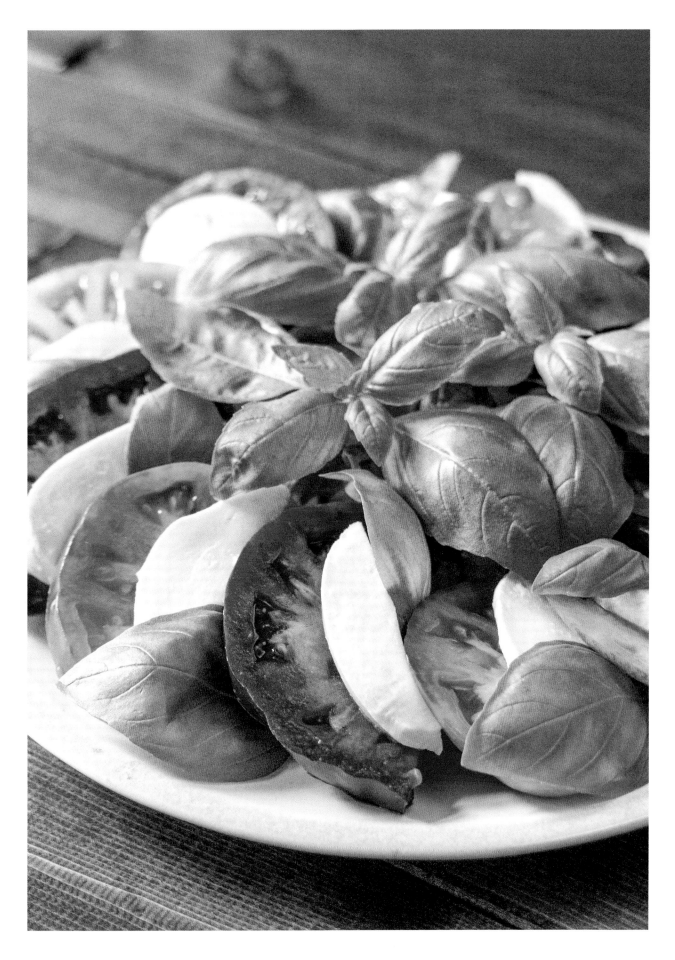

BLUE CHEESE WEDGE SALAD

SERVES 4

Wedge salads are so visually appealing, and they are super quick and easy to make. I love the crunch of the iceberg mixed with the indulgent blue cheese and bacon—absolute perfection.

8 slices bacon, cut into 1-inch pieces

1 head iceberg lettuce (see Note)

¾ cup Blue Cheese Dressing (page 64)

⅓ cup crumbled blue cheese

2 Roma tomatoes, diced

Cracked black pepper (optional)

Note : Wedge salads are best when the lettuce is straight from the fridge and ice-cold.

• Heat a skillet over medium-high heat and drop in the bacon. Cook until brown and crispy, about 10 minutes. Using a slotted spoon, transfer the bacon to a paper towel–lined plate and set aside to cool.

• Cut the head of lettuce into 4 equal wedges and set each wedge on a separate plate. Pour 3 tablespoons of blue cheese dressing over each wedge. Sprinkle equal amounts of blue cheese, tomatoes, and bacon over the wedges. Top each with a few grinds of fresh cracked black pepper, if desired, and serve immediately.

PER SERVING
Calories **326** · Fat **26g** · Total Carbs **8g** · Net Carbs **5g** · Fiber **3g** · Protein **12g**

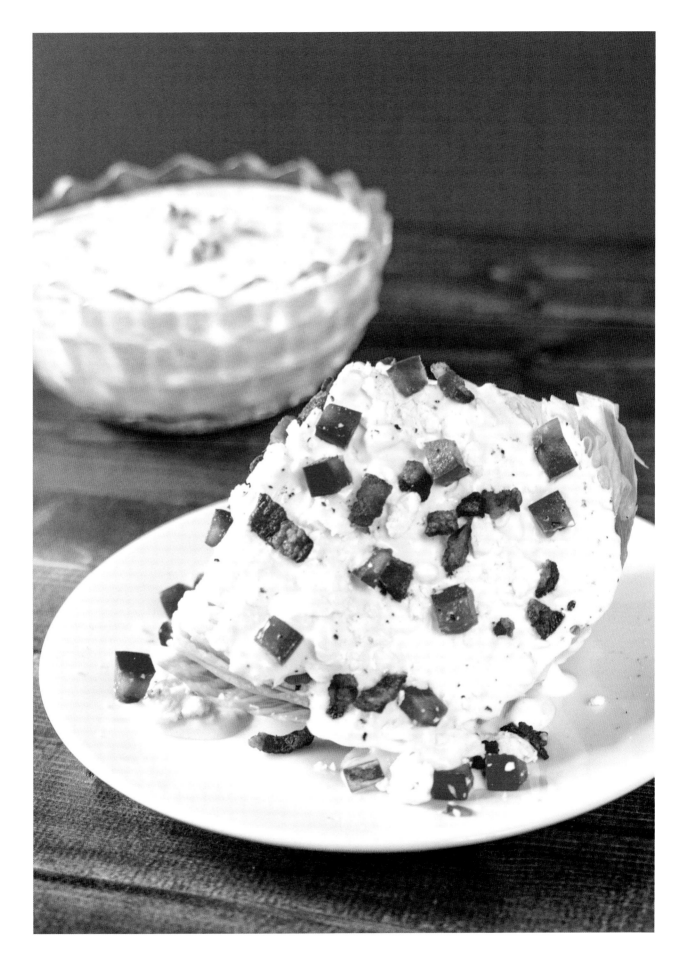

SPINACH SALAD *with* WARM BACON DRESSING

 MINUTES or LESS

SERVES 4

Spinach is one of my favorite vegetables, and this salad does it right. It has a nice smokiness from the bacon, and a touch of sweetness in the dressing balances its acidity.

8 slices bacon, cut into 1-inch pieces

8 large button mushrooms, sliced

½ pound baby spinach

2 large hard-boiled eggs (see page 25), sliced

½ small red onion, thinly sliced

FOR THE DRESSING:

3 tablespoons bacon drippings (reserved from above)

2 tablespoons red wine vinegar

2 teaspoons blended erythritol-stevia sweetener (see page 46)

1 teaspoon Dijon mustard

Pinch of fine sea salt

Pinch of ground black pepper

Note : Check out page 25 for how to make perfect hard-boiled eggs.

• Heat a skillet over medium-high heat and drop in the bacon. Cook until brown and crispy, about 10 minutes. Using a slotted spoon, transfer the bacon to a paper towel–lined plate and set aside. Transfer 3 tablespoons of bacon drippings from the pan to a small bowl and set aside.

• Add the mushrooms to the bacon drippings in the pan and sauté until tender and lightly browned, about 5 minutes. Transfer the mushrooms to a plate to cool.

• Divide the spinach between 4 plates and top each plate with equal amounts of mushrooms, egg slices, bacon, and red onion slices.

• In a small skillet over medium-low heat, whisk together the reserved bacon drippings and remaining dressing ingredients until well combined. Drizzle the warm dressing evenly over each salad and serve immediately.

PER SERVING
Calories **146** · Fat **9g** · Total Carbs **5g** · Net Carbs **3g** · Fiber **2g** · Protein **12g**

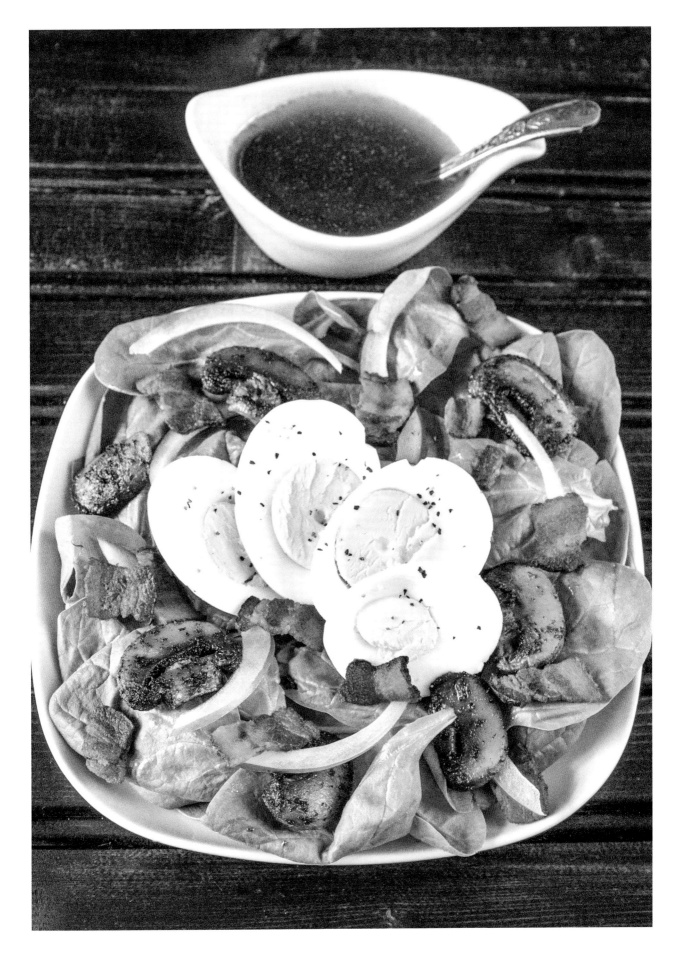

BACON BROC-CAULI SALAD

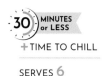

30 MINUTES or LESS

+ TIME TO CHILL

SERVES **6**

"Broc-Cauli"—see what I did there? I've been making this salad for years and it's always a huge hit. I love the combination of broccoli and cauliflower with smoky bacon and the sweet and tangy dressing. This goes really well with my Cuban Sandwiches on page 270. Plan ahead to give this time to chill in the fridge for best flavor.

6 slices bacon, cut into 1-inch pieces

2½ cups riced broccoli (about 8 ounces whole) (see Notes)

2½ cups riced cauliflower (about 8 ounces whole) (see Notes)

2 scallions, both green and white parts, minced

FOR THE DRESSING:

⅔ cup mayonnaise (see page 43)

⅔ cup full-fat sour cream

2 teaspoons apple cider vinegar

1 teaspoon blended erythritol-stevia sweetener (see page 46)

¾ teaspoon fine sea salt

¼ teaspoon ground black pepper

• Heat a skillet over medium-high heat and drop in the bacon. Cook until brown and crispy, about 10 minutes. Using a slotted spoon, transfer the bacon to a paper towel–lined plate and set aside to cool.

• In a large bowl, combine the broccoli, cauliflower, and scallions.

• In a medium-sized bowl, whisk together the dressing ingredients until smooth. Pour the dressing over the salad and stir well to combine. Stir in the bacon pieces.

• Cover the bowl tightly with plastic wrap and refrigerate for at least 1 hour to allow the flavors to develop. Stir well before serving.

• Store leftovers in an airtight container in the fridge for up to 1 week.

Notes : This salad is wonderful using all broccoli or all cauliflower as well.

To rice the broccoli and cauliflower, chop the heads into large pieces and, working in batches, pulse them in a food processor or blender until the pieces are about the size of a grain of rice. You can also rice them by hand with a hand grater.

PER SERVING
Calories **259** · Fat **24g** · Total Carbs **6g** · Net Carbs **4g** · Fiber **2g** · Protein **6g**

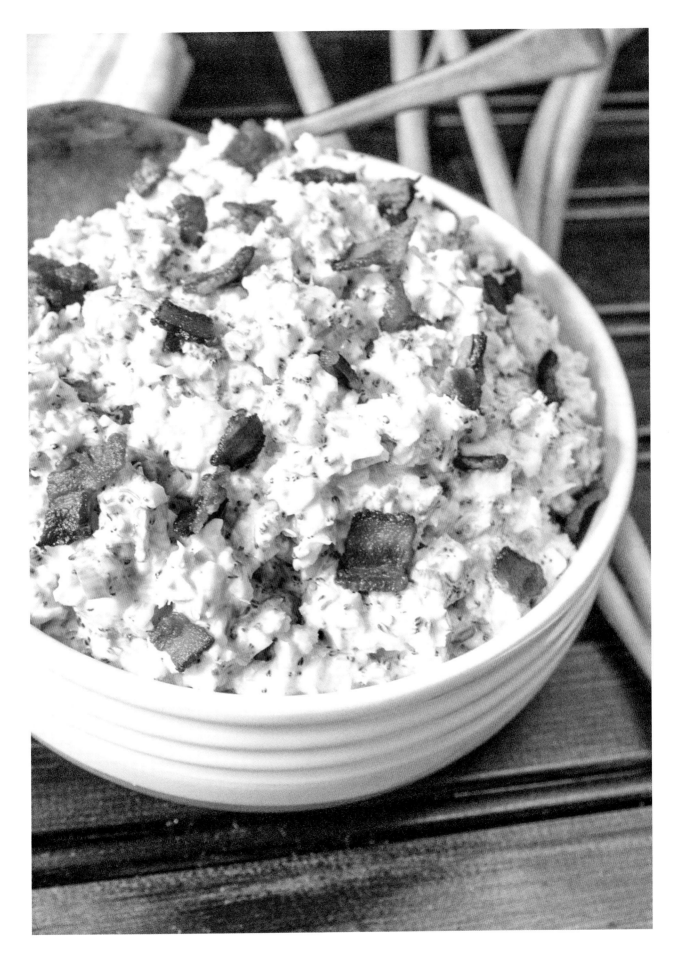

GRAPE TOMATO SALAD
with FETA & PISTACHIOS

SERVES 4

This salad is the result of a spur-of-the-moment decision to throw together a few things that I had on hand. Serendipity! The crunchy roasted pistachios mixed with the sweet, juicy tomatoes and tangy feta is such a delicious combination.

10 ounces grape tomatoes, halved lengthwise

1 teaspoon lemon juice

Pinch of fine sea salt

½ cup crumbled feta cheese

¼ cup unsalted roasted pistachios

6 fresh basil leaves, chiffonaded

Note: Do not toss or stir this salad—the tomato juice will turn the feta pink, which takes away from the presentation.

• Put the grape tomatoes on a serving plate and season with the lemon juice and salt. Sprinkle the feta cheese and pistachios on top of the tomatoes and top with the basil. Serve immediately.

• Store leftovers in an airtight container in the fridge for 2 to 3 days.

PER SERVING
Calories **95** · Fat **6g** · Total Carbs **7g** · Net Carbs **6g** · Fiber **1g** · Protein **4g**

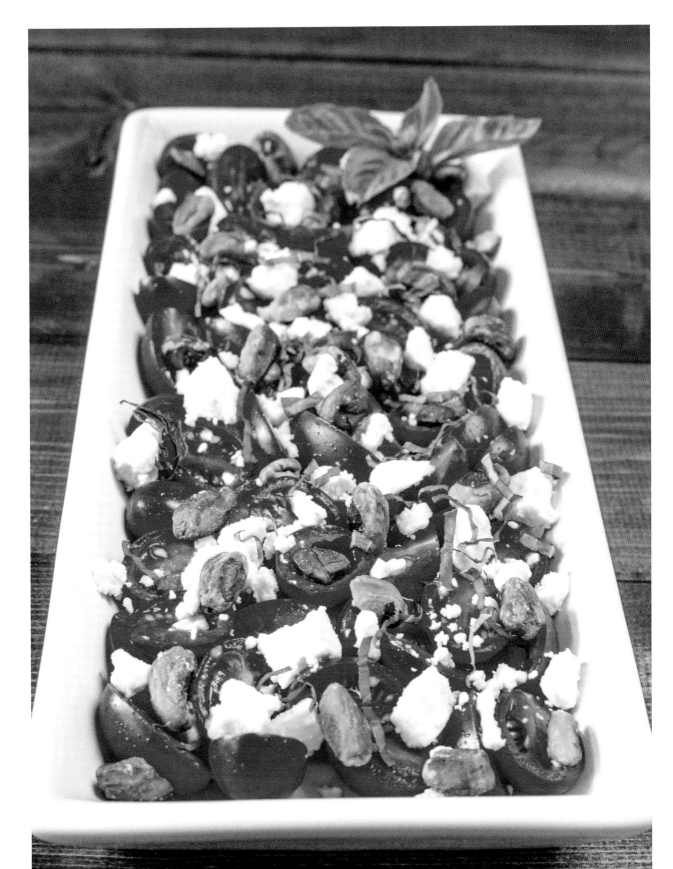

CLASSIC SHRIMP SALAD

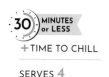

30 MINUTES or LESS

+ TIME TO CHILL

SERVES 4

I absolutely love shrimp any way I can get it, but this salad is one of my favorite preparations. The fresh flavor of the shrimp mixed with the creamy, tangy dressing is truly spectacular. I enjoy eating this as is, but it's also fabulous wrapped in butter lettuce.

1 tablespoon light olive oil

1 pound raw medium shrimp, peeled and deveined (see Note)

½ teaspoon fine sea salt

¼ teaspoon ground white pepper

FOR THE DRESSING:

¼ cup mayonnaise (see page 43)

2 stalks celery, finely diced

2 tablespoons full-fat sour cream

2 tablespoons minced shallots (about 1 small shallot)

1 teaspoon minced fresh dill

½ teaspoon grated lemon zest

½ teaspoon lemon juice

⅛ teaspoon fine sea salt

Note : I opt for medium shrimp (36/40) for this recipe, but any size will work.

• Heat the oil in a skillet over medium-high heat. While it heats, season the shrimp with the salt and pepper. Place the shrimp in the hot pan and sauté until pink and opaque, about 5 minutes. Transfer the shrimp to a plate and set aside to cool.

• In a medium-sized bowl, combine all of the dressing ingredients and toss with the cooled shrimp. Cover and chill in the fridge for at least 30 minutes before serving.

• Store leftovers in an airtight container in the fridge for up to 1 week.

Variation : MEXICAN SHRIMP SALAD

Swap out the lemon zest and lemon juice for equal amounts of lime zest and lime juice, substitute 1 tablespoon chopped fresh cilantro for the dill, and use 2 tablespoons seeded and chopped jalapeño instead of the shallot.

PER SERVING
Calories **222** · Fat **16g** · Total Carbs **3g** · Net Carbs **2g** · Fiber **1g** · Protein **16g**

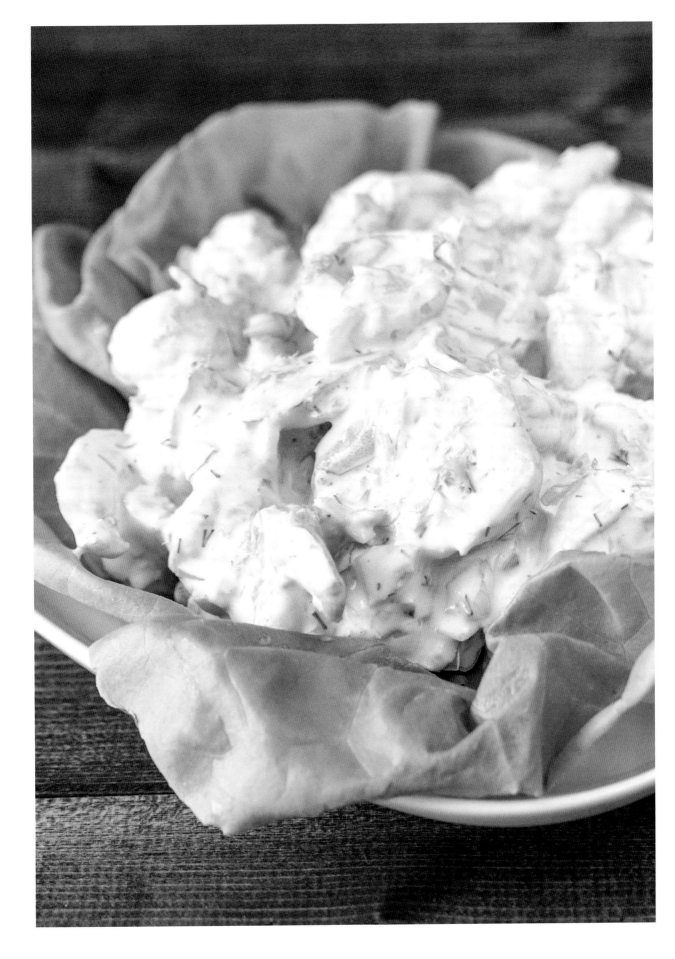

LEMON TARRAGON CHICKEN SALAD

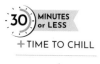

MINUTES or LESS

+ TIME TO CHILL

SERVES 4

I adore chicken salad in any flavor combination, but this one might just be my favorite. With the bright acidic tang of the lemon and the flavorful and aromatic tarragon, this chicken salad is truly special. This is best served after at least two hours in the fridge, so plan ahead.

1 pound boneless, skinless chicken breast, cooked and shredded

2 stalks celery, diced

2 scallions, both green and white parts, minced

½ cup mayonnaise (see page 43)

½ cup full-fat sour cream

2 teaspoons minced fresh tarragon

1 teaspoon lemon juice

¼ teaspoon fine sea salt

Note: For some crunch, add ¼ cup chopped roasted pecans, pistachios, or almonds.

• Place the chicken in a large bowl along with the celery and scallions, then stir to mix well.

• In a medium-sized bowl, whisk together the mayonnaise, sour cream, tarragon, lemon juice, and salt until smooth. Add the mixture to the chicken and vegetables and mix well to combine.

• Cover the bowl tightly with plastic wrap and refrigerate for at least 2 hours to allow the flavors to blend. Stir well before serving.

• Store leftovers in an airtight container in the fridge for up to 1 week.

PER SERVING
Calories **354** · Fat **29g** · Total Carbs **2g** · Net Carbs **1g** · Fiber **1g** · Protein **23g**

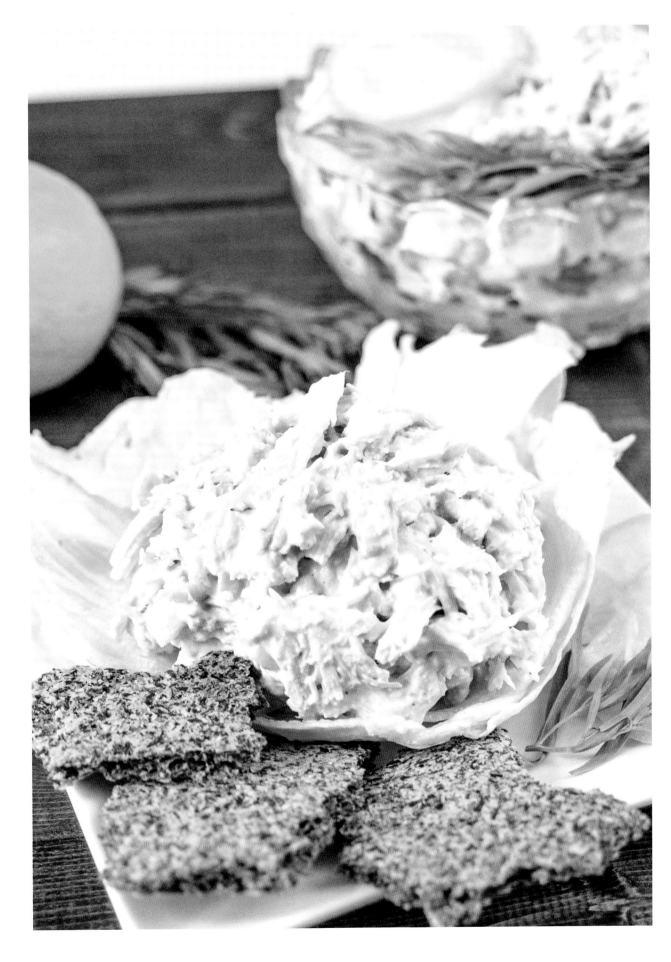

SWEET DIJON COLESLAW

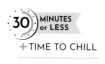

30 MINUTES or LESS

+ TIME TO CHILL

SERVES 4

I never really liked coleslaw until I made this version—I can eat bowls of this stuff! I highly recommend serving this alongside my Oven-Roasted Beef Ribs (page 228). This coleslaw needs some time to chill in the fridge before serving, so plan ahead.

1 cup mayonnaise (see page 43)

2 tablespoons Dijon mustard

1 teaspoon blended erythritol-stevia sweetener (see page 46)

1 teaspoon dried dill weed

1 teaspoon garlic powder

½ teaspoon apple cider vinegar

¼ teaspoon ground white pepper

⅛ teaspoon fine sea salt

5 cups shredded green cabbage (about 1 medium head)

Chopped fresh dill, for garnish (optional)

- In a medium-sized bowl, whisk together the mayo, mustard, and sweetener until smooth. Add the dill weed, garlic powder, vinegar, pepper, and salt and whisk to combine.

- Place the cabbage in an extra-large bowl. Add the mayo mixture to the cabbage and toss well to coat. Transfer the salad to a smaller container and cover tightly with plastic wrap. Refrigerate for at least 1 hour to allow the flavors to blend. Stir well before serving. Garnish with chopped fresh dill, if desired.

- Store leftovers in an airtight container in the fridge for up to 1 week.

Switch It Up:

Try using a mixture of purple and green cabbage for a vibrant pop of color and substitute yellow mustard for the Dijon for a bit more tang.

PER SERVING
Calories **259** · Fat **26g** · Total Carbs **5g** · Net Carbs **3g** · Fiber **2g** · Protein **1g**

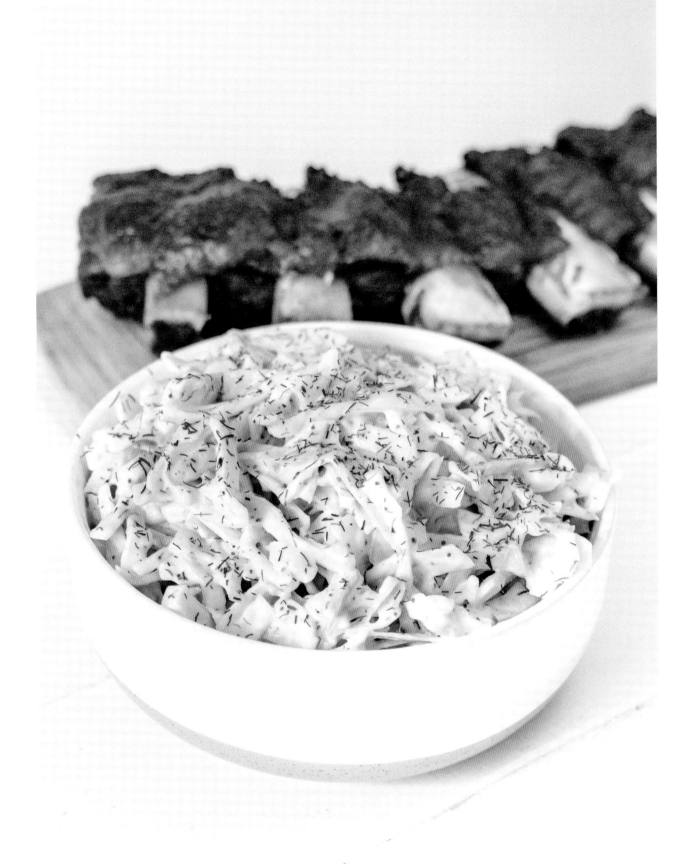

PARMESAN ARUGULA SALAD

 MINUTES or LESS

SERVES 4

This is a great light salad, combining the peppery bite of the arugula and the salty Parmesan. It goes well with just about anything, but I especially love it piled onto my Crispy Personal Pizzas (page 128).

FOR THE SALAD:

5 ounces arugula (about 5 cups)

⅓ cup shaved Parmesan cheese

FOR THE DRESSING:

⅓ cup light olive oil

¼ cup white wine vinegar

¼ cup grated Parmesan cheese

2 tablespoons minced shallots (about 1 small shallot)

Pinch of fine sea salt

Cracked black pepper

- In a large bowl, combine the arugula and shaved Parmesan.

- In a medium-sized bowl, mix together all of the dressing ingredients until well combined.

- Dress the salad and toss just before serving.

Variation: **PARMESAN CHICKEN SALAD**

Add 1 pound of chopped grilled chicken for a quick and easy meal.

PER SERVING
Calories **221** · Fat **21g** · Total Carbs **2g** · Net Carbs **1g** · Fiber **1g** · Protein **6g**

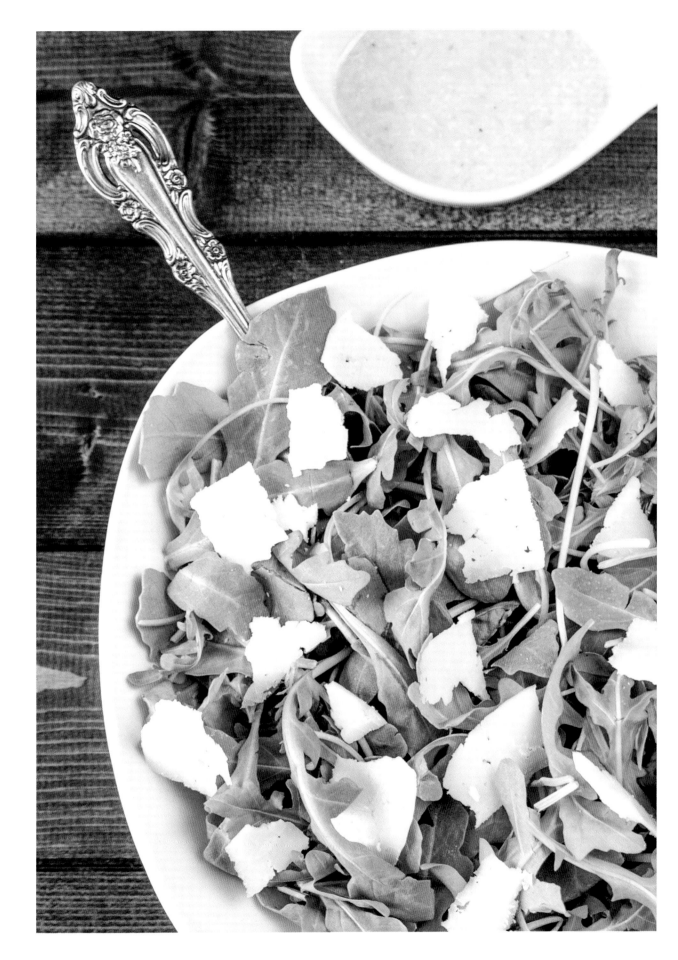

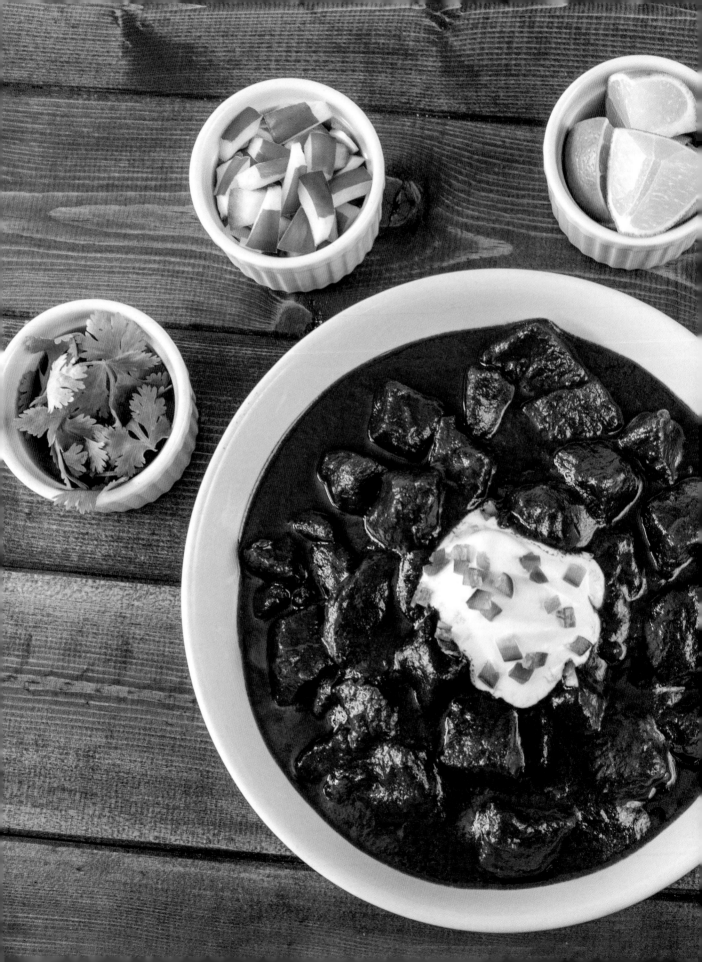

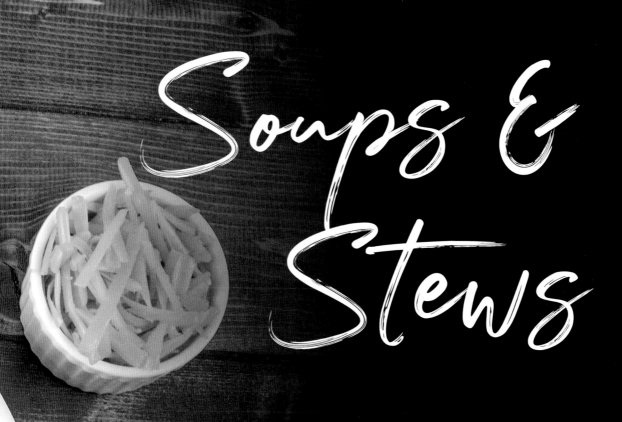

Soups & Stews

ALBONDIGAS SOUP

 1 HOUR or LESS

This Mexican meatball soup is bursting with southwestern flavor. I really enjoy serving this with my Three-Cheese Jalapeño Muffins (page 116).

SERVES **6**

1 pound ground beef, 80% lean

2 jalapeño peppers, seeded and diced

1 small onion, diced

1 large egg

2 cloves garlic, minced, divided

2 tablespoons minced cilantro

1 teaspoon fine sea salt

½ teaspoon ground black pepper

3 tablespoons bacon grease, divided

1 bunch fresh kale (about 6 ounces), stemmed and roughly chopped (about 2 cups)

2 stalks celery, diced

1 medium carrot, peeled and diced

1 tablespoon chili powder

6 cups chicken stock (see page 26)

1 (10-ounce) can diced tomatoes with green chili peppers (see Notes)

1 medium zucchini or yellow squash, cut into ½-inch dice

FOR GARNISH (OPTIONAL):

Cilantro leaves

Sliced jalapeños

Sliced scallions

• In a large bowl, combine the ground beef, jalapeños, onion, egg, garlic, cilantro, salt, and pepper and mix well with your hands. Form the mixture into meatballs, any size you like. I prefer using a 2-tablespoon cookie scoop, both for its size and how easy it makes forming the meatballs.

• Heat 1 tablespoon of the bacon grease in a small pot over medium-high heat. Working in batches if necessary to avoid overcrowding the pan, fry the meatballs, rolling them around in the pot occasionally, until completely browned, about 10 minutes. Using a slotted spoon, transfer the meatballs to a plate.

• To the drippings in the pot, add the kale and a pinch of salt. Sauté, stirring occasionally, until wilted, then transfer the kale to a cutting board. Chop and set aside.

• Melt the remaining 2 tablespoons of bacon grease in the pot and add the celery, carrot, and a pinch of salt. Sauté, stirring frequently, until the veggies begin to soften, about 5 minutes. Stir in the chili powder and cook for 2 minutes more to blend the flavors. Pour in the chicken stock and tomatoes, then stir to combine. Add the kale and meatballs, along with any juices. Taste to check the seasoning and add salt if needed.

• Bring the soup to a boil, then turn the heat down to medium-low and simmer for 5 minutes, then add the zucchini. Simmer until tender, about 20 minutes.

• Garnish with the cilantro, jalapeños, and scallions before serving.

• Store leftovers in an airtight container in the fridge for up to 1 week or in the freezer for up to 2 months.

PER SERVING
Calories **313** · Fat **22g** · Total Carbs **9g** · Net Carbs **6g** · Fiber **3g** · Protein **18g**

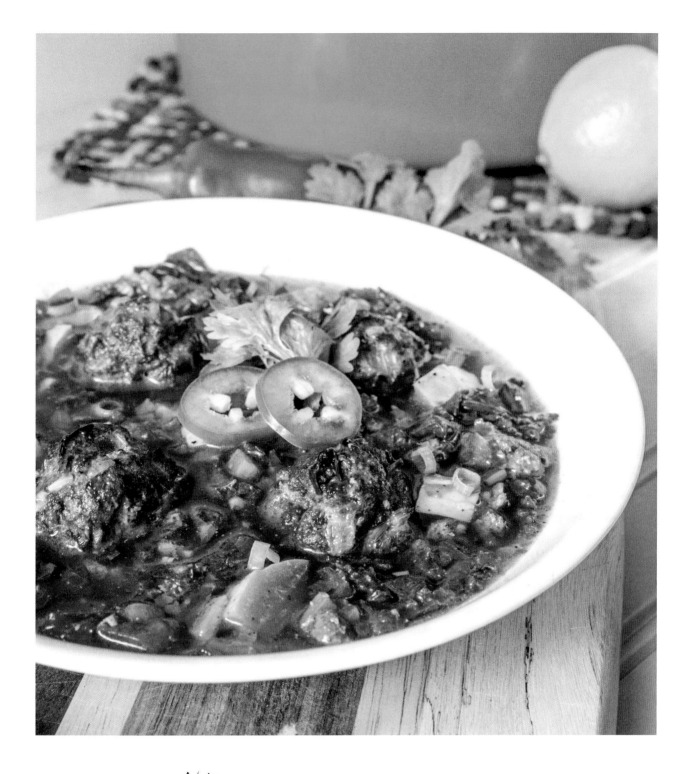

Note : If you prefer less heat, replace the canned tomatoes and green chili peppers with 1 (14-ounce) can diced tomatoes.

Instead of forming the meat mixture into meatballs, here's a super-quick workaround:

Preheat the oven to 350°F. After combining the ingredients for the meatball mixture as described above, press the mixture onto a sheet pan, about 1 inch thick, and bake for 20 minutes. Remove from the oven and use a spatula to divide the meat into 1-inch squares. Set aside to cool. Add the meat squares to the soup in place of the meatballs.

LOADED CAULI LEEK SOUP

1 HOUR or LESS

This low-carb twist on potato leek soup and loaded potato soup is so creamy and satisfying, you won't miss the carbs.

SERVES 6

½ pound bacon, cut into 1-inch pieces

1 leek, cleaned (see page 41), trimmed, and cut into ½-inch slices

1 clove garlic, minced

1 medium head cauliflower, chopped into 2-inch chunks

1½ teaspoons fine sea salt

½ teaspoon ground black pepper

3 cups chicken stock (see page 26) (see Note)

½ cup heavy cream

2 ounces cream cheese (¼ cup), room temperature

1 tablespoon unsalted butter

FOR GARNISH:

1 cup shredded cheddar cheese

2 scallions, sliced

Reserved bacon pieces (from above)

¼ cup plus 2 tablespoons full-fat sour cream

Note : If you're using store-bought chicken stock instead of my homemade chicken stock from page 26, you may need to use more salt. Taste after pureeing and add more salt if necessary.

• Heat a large pot over medium-high heat and drop in the bacon. Cook, stirring occasionally, until brown and crispy, about 10 minutes. Using a slotted spoon, transfer the bacon to a paper towel–lined plate. Set aside.

• Pour most of the bacon drippings from the pot into a 1-pint glass jar, leaving 2 tablespoons in the pot. Add the leek and stir to coat it in the drippings. Cook until softened, about 5 minutes. Add the garlic and cook for 3 minutes more, until fragrant, then add the cauliflower, salt, and pepper. Pour in the chicken stock and bring to a boil. Turn the heat down to medium, cover, and cook until the cauliflower is tender, about 15 minutes.

• Remove the pot from the heat. Carefully puree the soup until smooth using an immersion blender. Alternatively, puree it in a regular blender in batches, then return it to the pot. Be careful not to overfill the blender to avoid any burning-hot accidents.

• Return the pot to the stovetop over medium heat. To the soup, add the cream, cream cheese, and butter and stir well. Cook until the butter and cream cheese have melted.

• Spoon the soup into serving bowls and garnish each bowl with equal amounts of the cheese, scallions, reserved bacon, and sour cream.

• Store leftovers in an airtight container in the fridge for up to 1 week.

Variation : CHICKEN CAULI LEEK SOUP

Add shredded cooked chicken—or another meat, such as steak or sausage—to each serving bowl to make this a complete meal.

PER SERVING
Calories **417** · Fat **32g** · Total Carbs **10g** · Net Carbs **7g** · Fiber **3g** · Protein **22g**

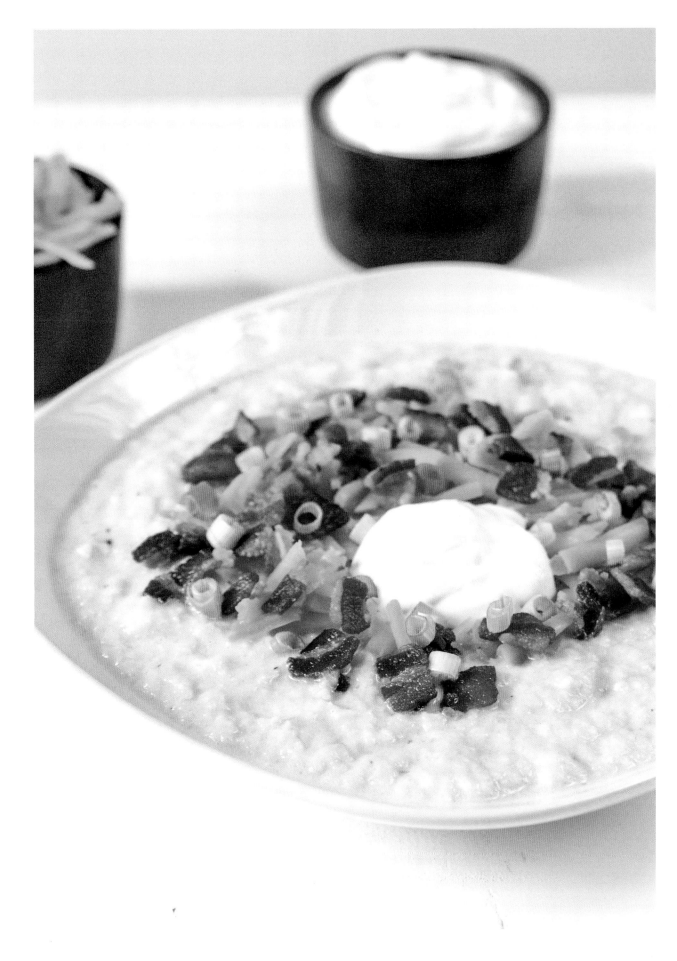

LOBSTER BISQUE

HOUR or LESS

SERVES 4

Lobster bisque is a decadent classic that will impress just about anyone, and they never have to know just how easy it really is! I recommend using lobster juice, which can be found in just about any gourmet supermarket, but feel free to substitute clam juice.

3 cups water

4 lobster tails, about 4 ounces each

1 tablespoon unsalted butter

1 medium shallot, minced

1 medium carrot, peeled and diced

2 stalks celery, diced

1 tablespoon tomato paste

¾ cup dry white wine

¾ teaspoon fine sea salt

¼ teaspoon ground black pepper

⅛ teaspoon blended erythritol-stevia sweetener (see page 46)

8 ounces lobster juice or clam juice

1 cup heavy cream

Minced fresh parsley, for garnish

Variation:
SHRIMP BISQUE

Substitute 1 pound of shrimp for the lobster to make shrimp bisque.

· Bring the water to a boil in a medium-sized saucepan. Add the lobster tails, turn the heat down to low, and simmer until the tails turn bright red, about 10 minutes. Remove the pot from the heat, then use tongs to carefully move the tails to a plate to cool. Keep the cooking water in the pot.

· Once the tails have cooled enough to handle, remove the lobster meat from the shells, chop it into bite-sized pieces, and set aside. Return all the emptied shells back to the pot and bring to a boil. Turn the heat down to low and simmer until the broth has reduced by more than half, about 25 minutes.

· While the shells simmer, melt the butter in a large pot over medium-high heat. Add the shallot, carrot, and celery. Sauté, stirring often, until the veggies have softened and are starting to brown, about 10 minutes. Stir in the tomato paste, then add the wine and deglaze the pan, scraping the browned bits off the bottom. Turn the heat down to low and simmer until the liquid has reduced by half, about 5 minutes.

· Add the salt, pepper, and sweetener and stir to combine. Add the lobster juice.

· Strain the broth with the shells through a fine-mesh sieve into the pot with the veggies. Discard the shells. Using an immersion blender, puree the soup until silky-smooth. Alternatively, puree the soup in a regular blender in batches and then return all the soup to the pot.

· Simmer over low heat for 10 minutes to blend the flavors. Pour in the heavy cream and simmer for 5 minutes. Taste and add more salt if needed.

· Divide the chopped lobster meat into 4 bowls. Ladle the hot soup over the lobster meat and serve garnished with the parsley.

· Store leftovers in an airtight container in the fridge for up to 1 week.

PER SERVING
Calories **290** · Fat **25g** · Total Carbs **7g** · Net Carbs **6g** · Fiber **1g** · Protein **2g**

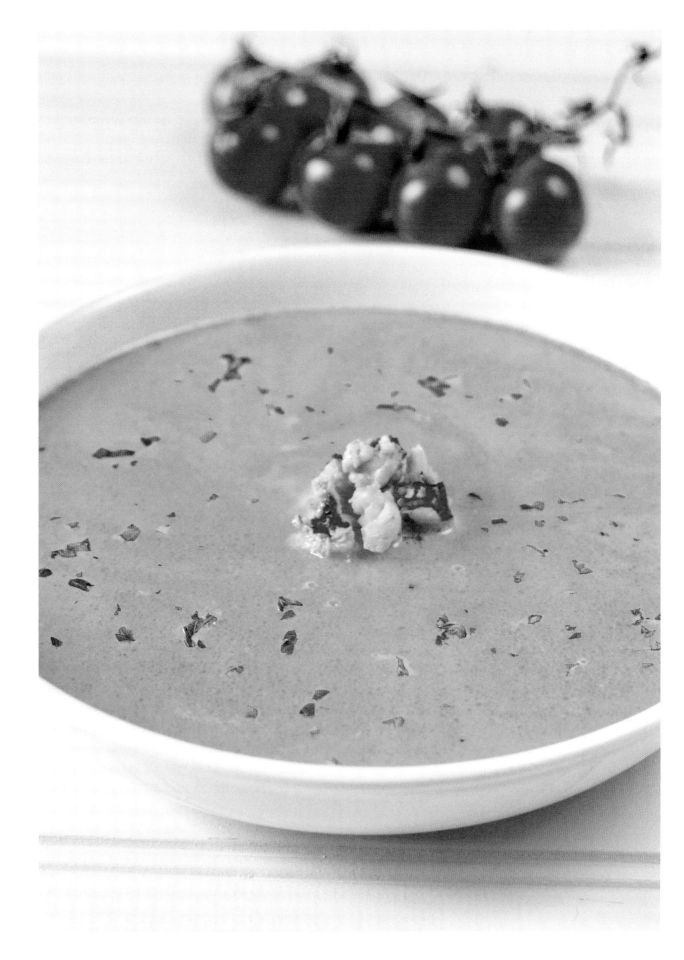

FRENCH ONION SOUP

 1 HOUR or LESS

SERVES 4

I've always been a huge soup lover, but French onion is probably my absolute favorite. It has such a rich and decadent broth, and the cheese—oh, the cheese! Crispy and bubbly Gruyère just begging you to dive in and take a bite.

3 tablespoons unsalted butter

2 medium onions, thinly sliced

1½ teaspoons fine sea salt

½ teaspoon ground black pepper

½ teaspoon blended stevia-erythritol sweetener (see page 46)

½ cup chardonnay

3 cups beef stock

8 slices provolone cheese

1 ⅓ cups shredded Gruyère cheese

• Melt the butter in a large pot over medium heat. Add the onions, salt, pepper, and sweetener and cook until the onions are softened and caramelized, about 30 minutes. Add the chardonnay, turn the heat down to low, and simmer until the wine has evaporated, about 5 minutes. Pour in the beef stock and simmer for 10 minutes to blend the flavors.

• Position an oven rack directly under the broiler and turn the oven on to broil.

• Ladle the broth into soup crocks or ovenproof bowls. Top each bowl with 2 slices of provolone and ⅓ cup Gruyère. Broil until the cheese is browned and bubbly. Serve immediately.

• Store leftovers in an airtight container in the fridge for up to 1 week.

Variation: BEEFY FRENCH ONION SOUP

Add ⅓ cup of braised shredded beef to each bowl of soup before topping the bowls with cheese to make this a complete meal.

PER SERVING
Calories **493** · Fat **35g** · Total Carbs **10g** · Net Carbs **8g** · Fiber **2g** · Protein **28g**

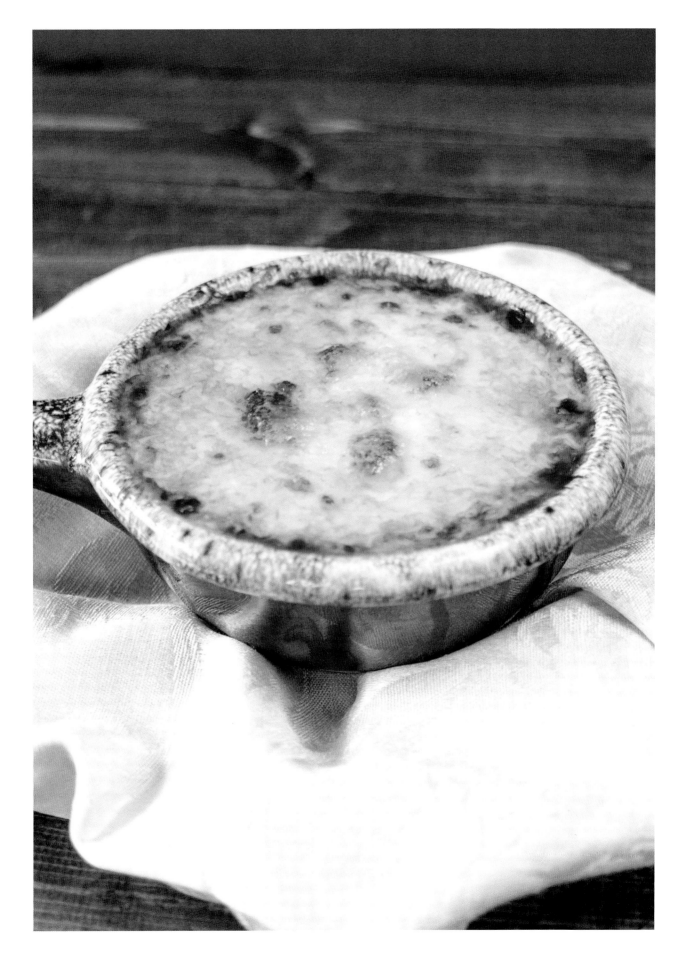

BACON CLAM CHOWDER

HOUR or LESS

SERVES 4

I grew up outside Boston, where clam chowder was on every menu of every restaurant. I have probably had more clam chowder than anyone I know! This recipe is one of my favorites. I highly recommend using higher-quality canned clams and clam juice because they don't contain any added sugar.

4 slices bacon, cut into 1-inch pieces

1 tablespoon unsalted butter

½ medium onion, diced

2 stalks celery, diced

1 clove garlic, minced

½ teaspoon fine sea salt

¼ teaspoon ground black pepper

2 (6.5-ounce) cans chopped clams with juices

8 ounces clam juice

2 ounces cream cheese (¼ cup), room temperature

½ cup heavy cream

Chopped fresh parsley, for garnish (optional)

• Heat a large pot over medium-high heat and drop in the bacon pieces. Sauté, stirring occasionally, until the bacon is browned and crispy, about 10 minutes. Using a slotted spoon, transfer the bacon to a paper towel–lined plate, leaving the drippings in the pot. Set aside.

• Add the butter to the bacon drippings in the pot and stir in the onion and celery. Sauté until the veggies are softened, about 5 minutes. Add the garlic, salt, and pepper and stir to combine. Add the clams with their juices; do not drain. Pour in the clam juice and bring to a boil, then turn the heat down to low and simmer for 5 minutes to blend the flavors.

• Stir in the cream cheese and heavy cream. Simmer for 10 minutes, or until the soup starts to thicken. Taste and add more salt if needed. Top with the reserved bacon and chopped fresh parsley, if desired, before serving.

• Store leftovers in an airtight container in the fridge for up to 1 week.

Variation: SEAFOOD CHOWDER

Try adding ½ pound of shrimp and ½ pound of cod along with the clams and an additional bottle of clam juice for a hearty seafood chowder.

PER SERVING
Calories **282** · Fat **22g** · Total Carbs **4g** · Net Carbs **3g** · Fiber **1g** · Protein **17g**

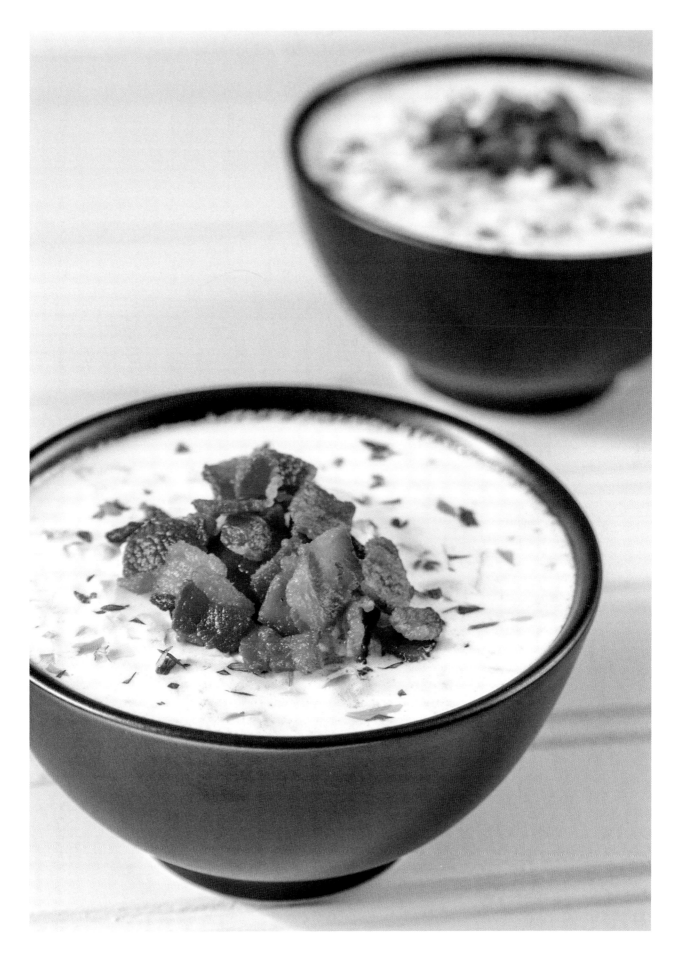

GOLDEN MUSHROOM SOUP

SERVES 4

This recipe couldn't be easier, and it's absolutely delicious. Smooth and creamy, with an incredible mushroom flavor, it's perfect for just about any occasion. I love to serve this alongside my Garlic Roast Beef with Horseradish Cream (page 212).

1 pound button or baby bella mushrooms

2 tablespoons unsalted butter, divided

1 cup diced onion

¼ cup dry white wine

4 cups chicken stock (see page 26)

1 cup heavy cream

½ teaspoon fine sea salt

⅛ teaspoon ground white pepper

Chopped fresh parsley, for garnish (option al)

Note: If you're using store-bought chicken stock instead of my homemade chicken stock from page 26, you may need to use more salt. Taste before serving and add more salt if necessary.

• Slice one mushroom. Stem and chop the rest of the mushrooms.

• Melt 1 tablespoon of the butter in a large pot over medium-high heat. Add the chopped mushrooms to one side of the pot and the sliced mushroom to the other side. Sauté, stirring occasionally but keeping the sliced and chopped mushrooms separate, until golden brown, about 5 minutes. Sprinkle the chopped mushrooms with a pinch of salt, transfer to a bowl, and set aside. Transfer the mushroom slices to a plate and set aside to use as a garnish.

• Melt the remaining tablespoon of butter in the pot and add the onion and a pinch of salt. Sauté until the onion is soft and translucent, about 3 minutes. Add the wine and deglaze the pot, scraping the browned bits off the bottom. Cook until the wine has reduced by half, about 5 minutes.

• Return the chopped mushrooms to the pot and add the chicken stock, cream, salt, and pepper. Simmer for 15 minutes to blend the flavors. Divide the soup among 4 bowls and garnish with the reserved mushroom slices and chopped fresh parsley, if desired.

• Store leftovers in an airtight container in the fridge for up to 1 week.

Variation: BEEF AND MUSHROOM SOUP

For a complete meal, add 1 pound of cooked shredded beef when you return the mushrooms to the pot.

PER SERVING
Calories **331** · Fat **28g** · Total Carbs **10g** · Net Carbs **8g** · Fiber **2g** · Protein **9g**

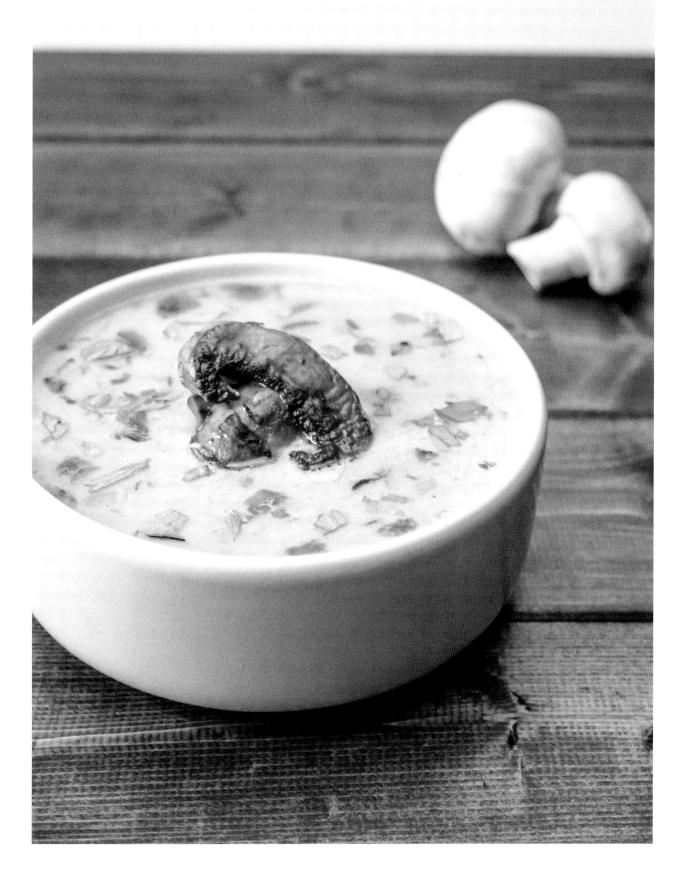

CREAMY STEAK SOUP

2 HOURS or LESS

SERVES 4

This soup came about when I threw together odds and ends I found in the fridge and freezer. It turned out marvelous! I make it all the time and everyone loves it. This is a meal in a bowl and oh so comforting.

1 pound sirloin tips, cut into bite-sized pieces

1 teaspoon salt

½ teaspoon ground black pepper

½ teaspoon garlic powder

1 tablespoon unsalted butter

4 cups beef stock

⅔ cup frozen pearl onions

6 ounces frozen spinach

2 ounces cream cheese (¼ cup)

⅓ cup heavy cream

⅓ cup no-sugar-added salsa

• Season the steak with the salt, pepper, and garlic powder.

• Melt the butter in a heavy-bottomed large pot over medium-high heat. Working in batches to avoid overcrowding the pot, add the steak and sear until browned on all sides, about 5 minutes. Return all the steak to the pot, add the beef stock, and bring to a boil. Turn the heat down to low and simmer until the meat is tender, about 30 to 45 minutes.

• Add the frozen pearl onions and frozen spinach and cook until heated through, about 5 minutes. Stir in the cream cheese, cream, and salsa and stir until well combined. Taste and add salt if needed.

• Simmer for 10 minutes, then serve.

• Store leftovers in an airtight container in the fridge for up to 1 week.

Variation: CREAMY CHICKEN SOUP

For an even quicker meal, replace the steak with cooked chicken and the beef stock with chicken stock (see page 26)—no need to brown the chicken, since it's already cooked; just simmer it in the stock for about 30 minutes and continue with the rest of the recipe.

PER SERVING
Calories **342** · Fat **22g** · Total Carbs **6g** · Net Carbs **5g** · Fiber **1g** · Protein **27g**

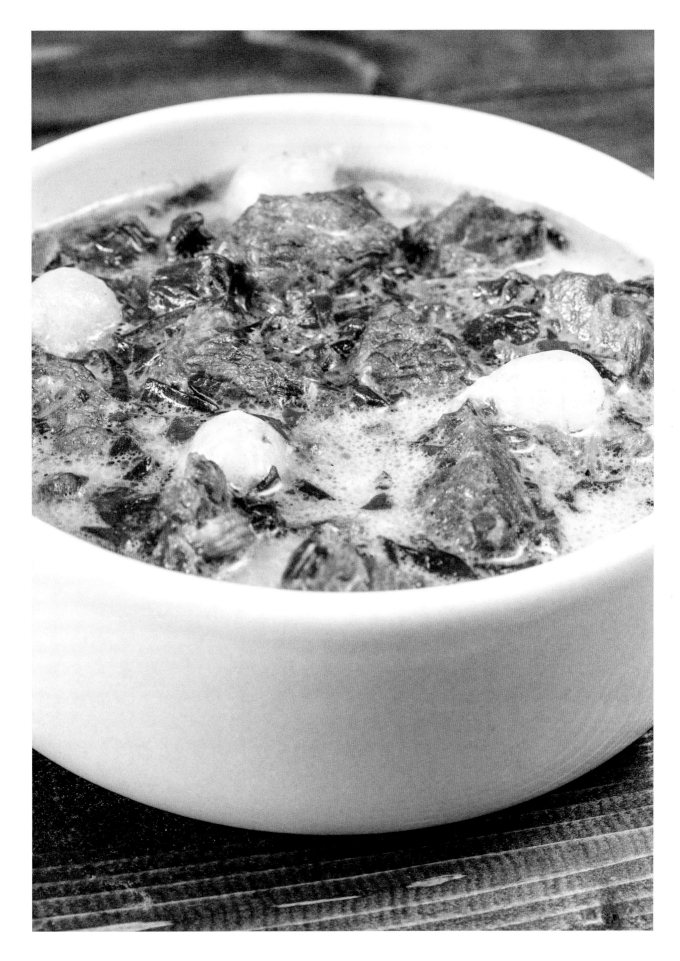

CHICKEN BACON POBLANO SOUP

 1 HOUR or LESS

This soup is so filling, and it has the most delicious smokiness from the roasted poblanos and jalapeños.

SERVES 4

2 poblano peppers

1 jalapeño pepper

5 slices bacon, cut into 1-inch pieces

½ cup diced white onion

1½ teaspoons fine sea salt

½ teaspoon ground black pepper

1 pound cooked boneless, skinless chicken breast, cut into bite-sized pieces

2 cups chicken stock (see page 26)

¾ cup heavy cream

4 ounces cream cheese (½ cup), room temperature

- Position an oven rack directly under the broiler, turn the oven to the broil setting, and line a sheet pan with foil.

- Place the poblanos and jalapeños on the lined sheet pan and set it directly under the broiler. Broil the peppers until the skins blacken and blister on all sides, about 10 minutes, flipping the peppers as needed. Remove the peppers from the oven and place them in a medium-sized bowl, then cover the bowl tightly with plastic wrap. The peppers will steam in the bowl, causing the skins to loosen. After 15 minutes, remove and discard the outer skin and seeds. Mince the jalapeño and chop the poblanos into bite-sized pieces. Set aside.

- Heat a large pot over medium-high heat and drop in the bacon pieces. Cook the bacon, stirring occasionally, until it's brown and crispy, about 10 minutes. Using a slotted spoon, transfer the bacon to a paper towel–lined plate and set aside.

- Add the onion to the bacon drippings in the pot and cook until soft and starting to brown, about 5 minutes. Add the roasted peppers, salt, and pepper to the pot, then stir to combine. Transfer about 2 tablespoons of the onion-pepper mixture to a bowl and set aside to use as a garnish.

- Add the chicken to the pot and stir to combine. Pour in the chicken stock and bring to a boil, then turn the heat down to medium-low and simmer for 5 minutes to blend the flavors. Add the cream and cream cheese and simmer for 5 minutes more, until the cream cheese has melted.

- Garnish with the bacon pieces and top with the reserved onion-peppers mixture before serving.

- Store leftovers in an airtight container in the fridge for up to 1 week.

Variation: PORK BACON POBLANO SOUP

Replace the chicken with 1 pound shredded cooked pork for an even more savory soup.

PER SERVING
Calories **441** · Fat **33g** · Total Carbs **7g** · Net Carbs **6g** · Fiber **1g** · Protein **31g**

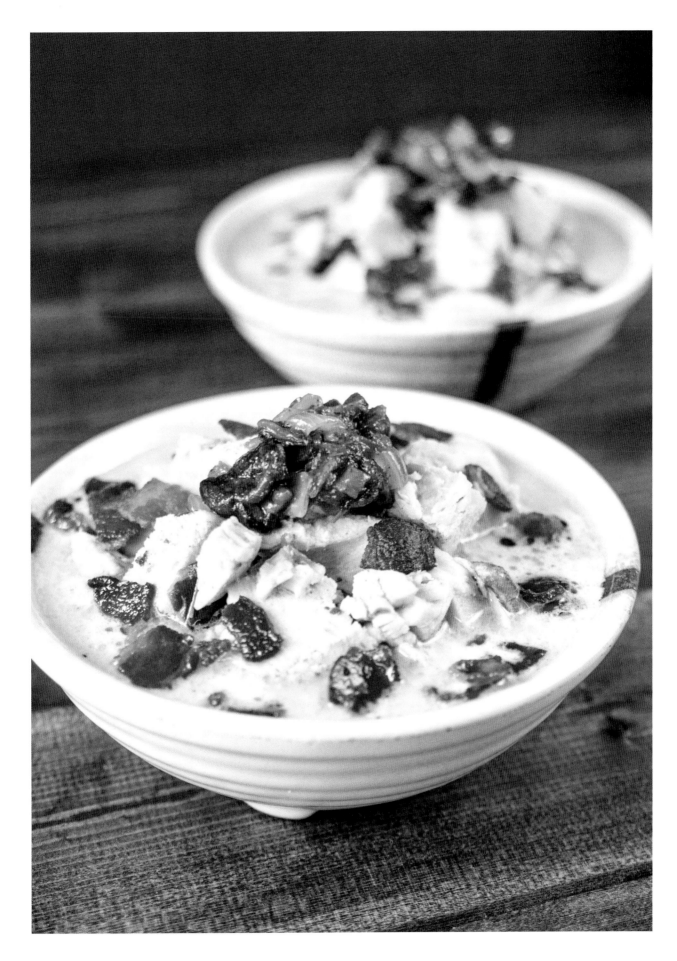

CHILI CON CARNE

IDEAL FOR MEAL PREP

SERVES 4

This chili con carne is extremely rich and smoky, with a punch of heat. (Don't worry, it's easily cooled down with some sour cream.) The longer cook time is well worth it to end up with melt-in-your-mouth beef.

2 dried ancho peppers

2 dried pasilla peppers

2 dried guajillo peppers

1 tablespoon light olive oil

1½ pounds beef chuck, cut into 1-inch cubes

1 tablespoon unsalted butter

½ medium onion, diced

3 cloves garlic, minced

¼ cup water

1 teaspoon fine sea salt

1 teaspoon ground cumin

½ teaspoon dried Mexican oregano leaves

½ teaspoon ground black pepper

3 cups beef stock

1 tablespoon white vinegar

1 teaspoon blended erythritol-stevia sweetener (see page 46)

FOR TOPPINGS (OPTIONAL):
Chopped fresh cilantro

Diced jalapeño

Diced red onion

Full-fat sour cream

Lime wedges

Shredded cheddar cheese

Note: This dish freezes really well, so I generally make a double or triple batch for quick and easy meals later.

• Heat a medium-sized skillet over high heat. Add the dried chili peppers to the hot dry pan and toast until fragrant, about 3 to 4 minutes. Be careful not to burn them.

• Place the toasted chili peppers in a medium-sized bowl and cover with boiling water. Allow the chili peppers to soften in the water for 20 minutes.

• While the chili peppers are softening, heat the oil in a heavy-bottomed sauté pan over medium-high heat. Lightly season the beef with salt and pepper and, working in batches to avoid overcrowding the pan, sear until browned on all sides. Using a slotted spoon, transfer the beef to a plate, leaving the drippings in the pan. Set aside.

• Melt the butter in the beef drippings and add the onion. Sauté for 5 minutes, until softened. Add the garlic and sauté for 3 minutes more, or until the garlic is fragrant.

• While the onion and garlic are cooking, put the chili peppers in a blender along with the water, salt, cumin, oregano, and pepper. Blend on high speed until smooth. Strain the sauce through a fine-mesh sieve into the pot with the onion and garlic, pressing as needed to push it through the sieve. Stir to combine and cook, still over medium-high heat, just for a moment, then return the beef chunks to the pan and add the beef stock.

• Bring to a boil, then turn the heat down to medium-low and simmer until the meat is fall-apart tender, about 3 hours.

• Stir in the vinegar and sweetener, then taste and add salt if needed. Add your choice of toppings before serving.

• Store leftovers in an airtight container in the fridge for up to 1 week, or freeze in an airtight container, leaving an inch of headspace, for up to 2 months. Allow to thaw overnight in the fridge and reheat in the microwave on 50 percent power until warmed through, about 5 minutes, stirring occasionally.

168   SOUPS & STEWS

PER SERVING
Calories **514** · Fat **36g** · Total Carbs **12g** · Net Carbs **9g** · Fiber **3g** · Protein **35g**

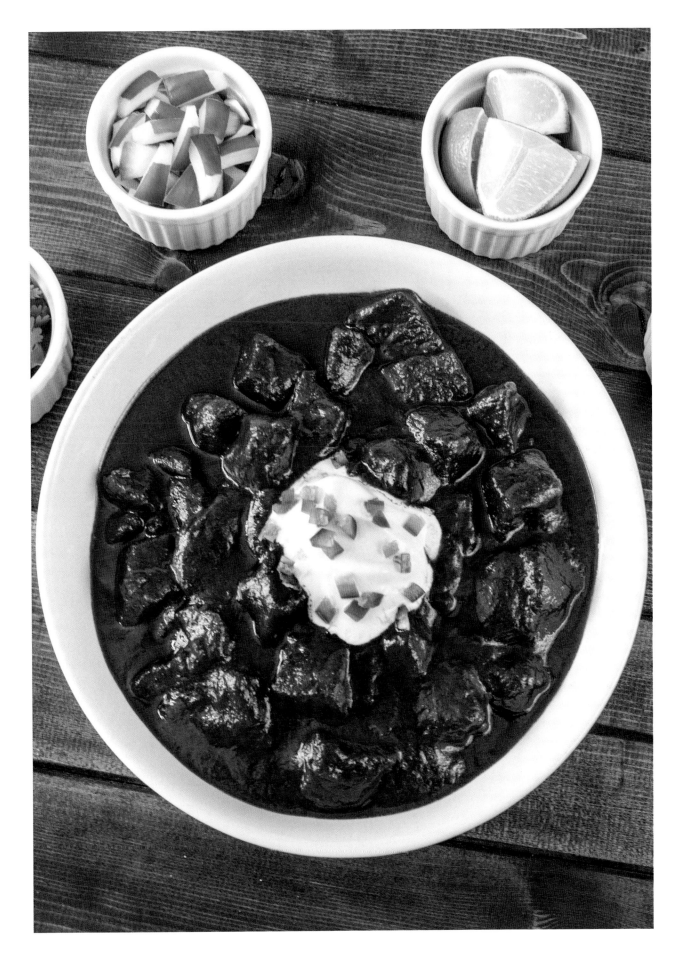

AVGOLEMONO

SERVES 4

This is the Greek version of chicken soup, and it is bursting with bright lemon flavor. If you've never tried this, you must!

1 tablespoon unsalted butter

3 scallions, sliced

2 stalks celery, diced

1 medium carrot, peeled and diced

1 pound cooked boneless, skinless chicken breast, shredded

1½ teaspoons fine sea salt

3 cups chicken stock (see page 26)

¼ cup lemon juice

2 large eggs, separated

½ cup heavy cream

2 teaspoons chopped fresh parsley

• Melt the butter in a large pot over medium-high heat and add the scallions, celery, and carrot. Sauté, stirring often, until the veggies just start to soften, about 5 minutes. Add the chicken and salt, then stir to combine. Pour in the chicken stock and bring to a boil, then turn the heat down to low and simmer for 10 minutes to blend the flavors.

• While the soup is simmering, temper the eggs: Whisk the lemon juice into the egg yolks until well blended. Whisking continuously, slowly stream a ladle of chicken stock from the pot on the stove into the egg-and-lemon-juice mixture.

• Pour the tempered egg mixture into the soup and stir in the heavy cream. Simmer for 5 minutes, or until the soup starts to thicken. Taste and add more salt if needed, then remove from the heat, stir in the parsley, and serve.

• Store leftovers in an airtight container in the fridge for up to 1 week.

Variation: AVGOLEMONO AND CAULI RICE SOUP
For a hearty and low-carb Greek-style chicken and rice soup, add 2 cups of cooked cauliflower rice (see page 202) with the parsley.

PER SERVING
Calories **230** · Fat **17g** · Total Carbs **6g** · Net Carbs **5g** · Fiber **1g** · Protein **14g**

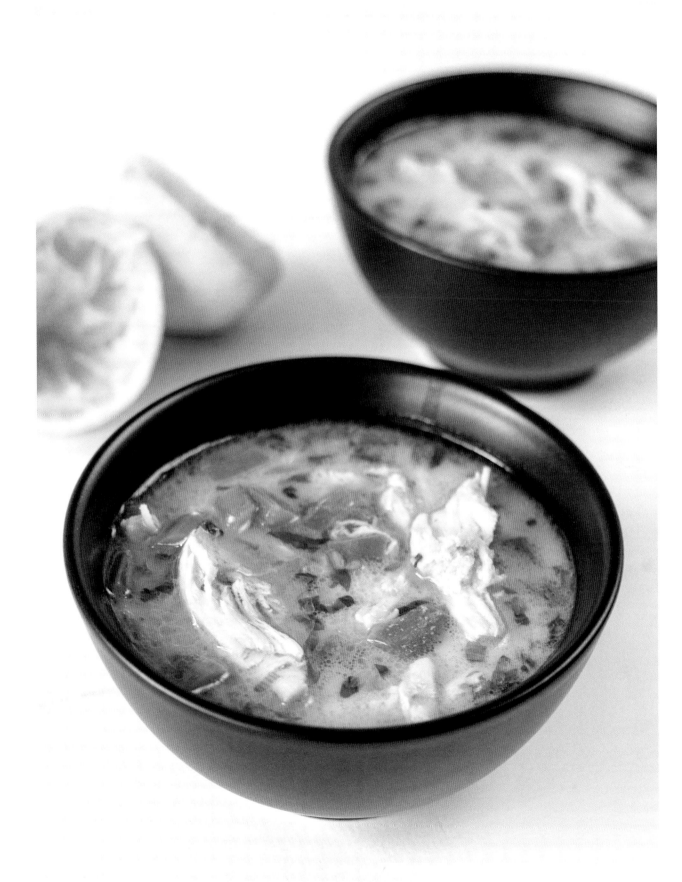

GUMBO

 30 MINUTES or LESS

SERVES 4

I've been making this for years and years, and to make it keto-friendly, all I had to do was omit the roux. Luckily, a bit of heavy cream instead gives it the perfect richness. This is absolute perfection on top of my Cauli Risotto (page 184).

1 tablespoon unsalted butter

1 pound no-sugar-added kielbasa, sliced

3 stalks celery, diced

1 medium bell pepper, any color, seeded and chopped

1 medium onion, chopped

1 clove garlic, minced

Pinch of fine sea salt

1 pound cooked boneless, skinless chicken breast, shredded

1 tablespoon Cajun Seasoning (page 58)

1 (10-ounce) can diced tomatoes with green chili peppers

1 cup chicken stock (see page 26)

⅓ cup heavy cream

Chopped fresh parsley, for garnish (optional)

• Melt the butter in a large pot over medium-high heat. Add the kielbasa and sauté until browned on all sides, about 5 minutes. Using a slotted spoon, transfer the kielbasa to a plate, leaving the drippings in the pot.

• To the drippings in the pot, add the celery, bell pepper, and onion and sauté, stirring occasionally, until the veggies are softened and just starting to brown, about 5 minutes. Add the garlic and salt and cook for 3 minutes more, until fragrant. Return the kielbasa to the pot and add the chicken and Cajun seasoning, then stir to combine. Pour in the tomatoes and chili peppers as well as the chicken stock and simmer for 10 minutes to blend the flavors.

• Stir in the cream. Taste and add more salt if needed. Garnish with chopped fresh parsley, if desired.

• Store leftovers in an airtight container in the fridge for up to 1 week.

PER SERVING
Calories **611** · Fat **41g** · Total Carbs **12g** · Net Carbs **9g** · Fiber **3g** · Protein **45g**

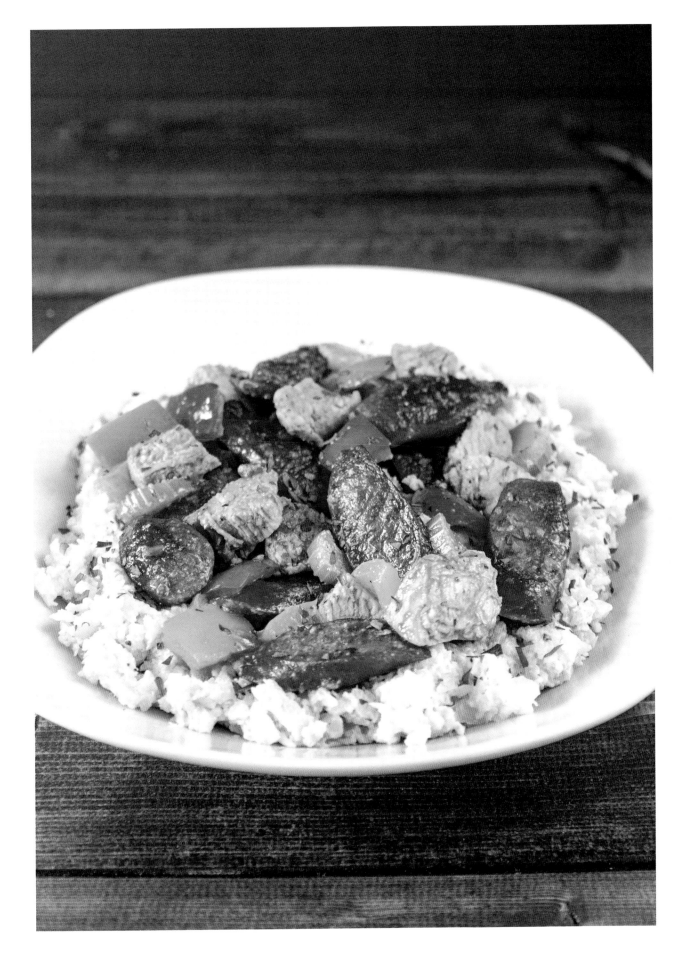

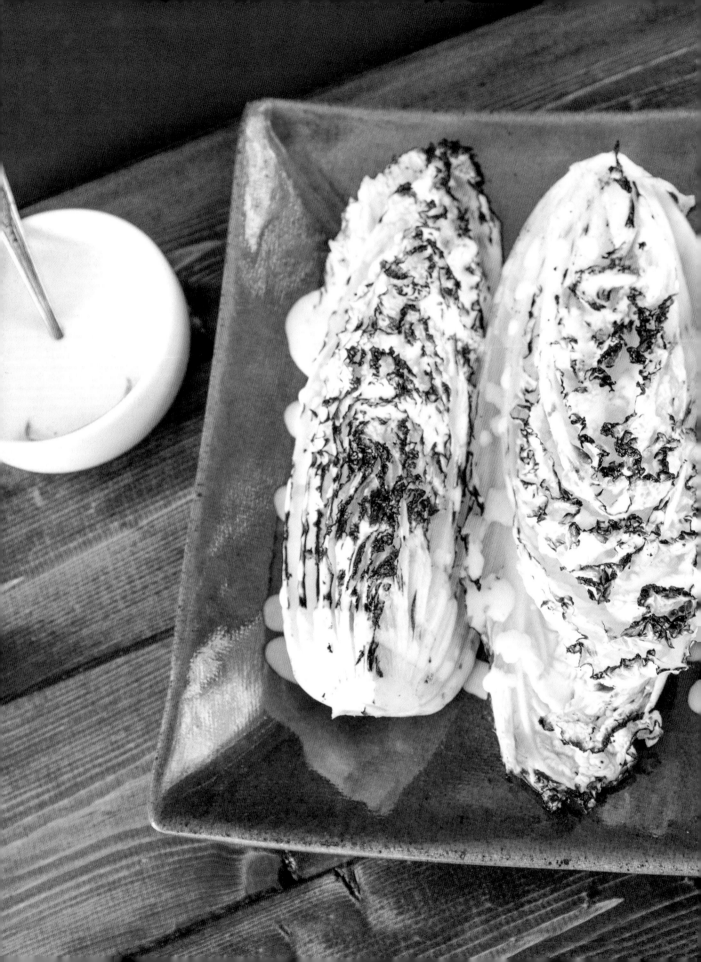

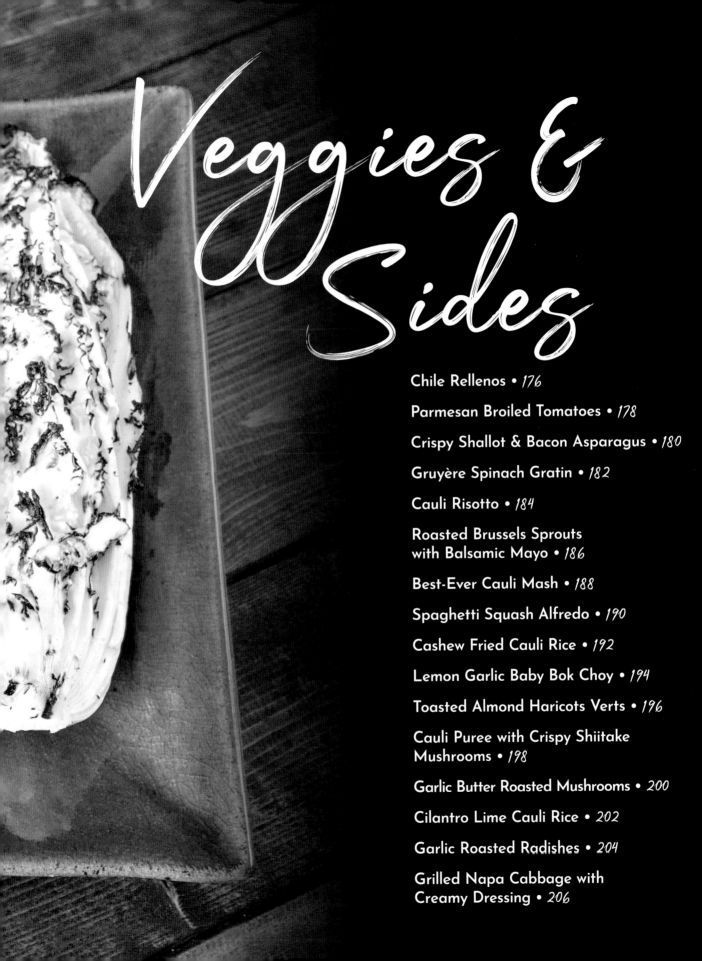

Veggies & Sides

CHILE RELLENOS

SERVES 4

Before I began eating keto, anytime I went to a Mexican restaurant, I always ordered a chile relleno. I just adore those cheese-stuffed smoky peppers wrapped in crispy goodness, and these keto-friendly versions couldn't be easier to make—they just require a little prep work. I serve these with my Authentic Enchilada Sauce (page 74), which makes them even more amazing. I'm partial to using light olive oil for all of my frying, but any high-heat-safe oil will work.

4 poblano peppers (about 1 pound)

2 cups shredded Monterey Jack cheese

4 large eggs, separated

¼ teaspoon fine sea salt

Light olive oil, for frying

1 cup Authentic Enchilada Sauce (page 74), warmed

· Position an oven rack directly under the broiler and turn the oven on to broil. Line a sheet pan with foil.

· Rinse the peppers and place them on a cutting board with the flattest side down. Cut a T into each pepper, being careful not to cut all the way through. Gently open each pepper and cut out the core, removing the seeds and membrane, then set them onto the prepared sheet pan.

· Broil the peppers until the skin blackens and blisters on all sides, about 10 minutes, flipping the peppers as needed. Remove the peppers from the oven (leave the foil on the pan) and place them in a medium-sized bowl, then cover the bowl tightly with plastic wrap to allow the peppers to steam and their skins to loosen. After 15 minutes, very gently remove and discard the skins, being careful not to tear the flesh.

· Carefully stuff each pepper with ½ cup cheese and close the flaps as much as possible. Set aside.

· Place a baking rack on the foil-lined sheet pan and set the oven to 250°F.

· In a small bowl, whisk the egg yolks and salt until pale yellow and frothy. In a separate small bowl, with a hand mixer on medium speed, beat the egg whites until stiff peaks form. Carefully fold the egg yolks into the egg whites until just combined.

· Heat a sauté pan over medium-high heat and pour in about an inch of oil. Test the temperature of the oil by dipping the handle of a wooden spoon in the oil. If the oil bubbles around the handle, it's ready. Once the oil is hot, add ½ cup of the egg mixture to the pan and use a spatula to spread it to about the same size as a pepper. Place one stuffed pepper cut side down on the batter and add another ½ cup of the egg mixture on top of the pepper, spreading it over the sides to completely encase the pepper. Don't worry about covering the very top of the pepper, with the stem.

PER SERVING

Calories **481** · Fat **40g** · Total Carbs **11g** · Net Carbs **5g** · Fiber **6g** · Protein **21g**

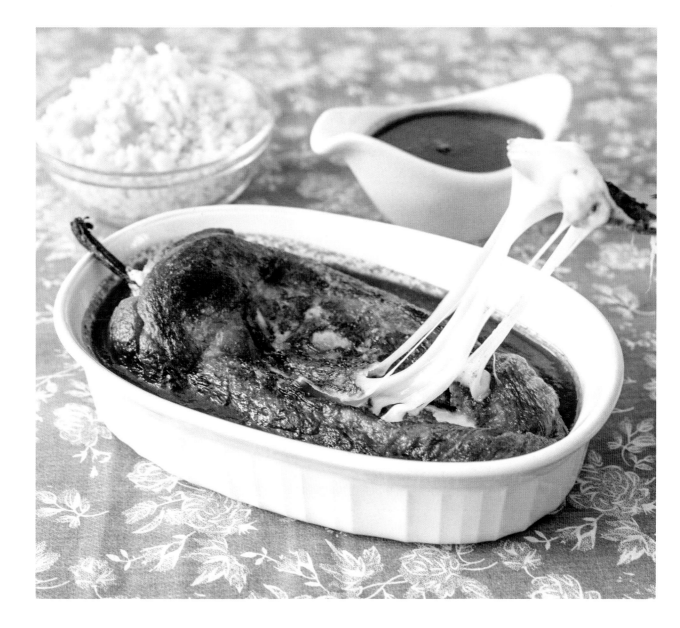

• Cook the pepper undisturbed until the bottom is golden brown, about 3 minutes. Using 2 spatulas, gently flip the pepper and cook on the other side until golden brown, an additional 3 minutes. If necessary, gently turn the uncooked sides of the pepper into the oil to brown. Place the cooked pepper on the rack over the sheet pan and sprinkle it with a pinch of salt. Place the sheet pan in the oven to keep the pepper warm. Repeat with the remaining peppers, placing them on the baking rack in the oven after they finish frying.

• Divide the enchilada sauce among 4 plates and place a pepper on each plate before serving.

• Store the peppers in an airtight container in the fridge for up to 1 week. These are best fresh, but they're still delicious when reheated in the microwave on high in 30-second increments.

PARMESAN BROILED TOMATOES

30 MINUTES or LESS

MAKES 4 TOMATOES
(1 per serving)

This tasty side has been a favorite with my family for quite some time. It's perfect for company and pairs beautifully with a simple entrée like grilled burgers. The delicious blend of basil and garlic with the salty Parmesan is always a crowd-pleaser.

4 firm Roma tomatoes

¼ cup grated Parmesan cheese

¼ cup mayonnaise (see page 43)

1 teaspoon dried basil

½ teaspoon garlic powder

⅛ teaspoon ground black pepper

- Position an oven rack about 5 inches under the broiler and turn the oven on to broil. Line a sheet pan with foil.

- Slice the tomatoes in half lengthwise and place them on the sheet pan cut side up.

- In a small bowl, stir together the remaining ingredients until well combined. Spread the mixture onto the tops of the tomato halves.

- Place the sheet pan under the broiler and bake until the tomatoes are softened and the topping is bubbly and browned, 3 to 5 minutes.

- Store in an airtight container in the fridge for 2 to 3 days.

PER SERVING
Calories **174** · Fat **15g** · Total Carbs **5g** · Net Carbs **3g** · Fiber **2g** · Protein **7g**

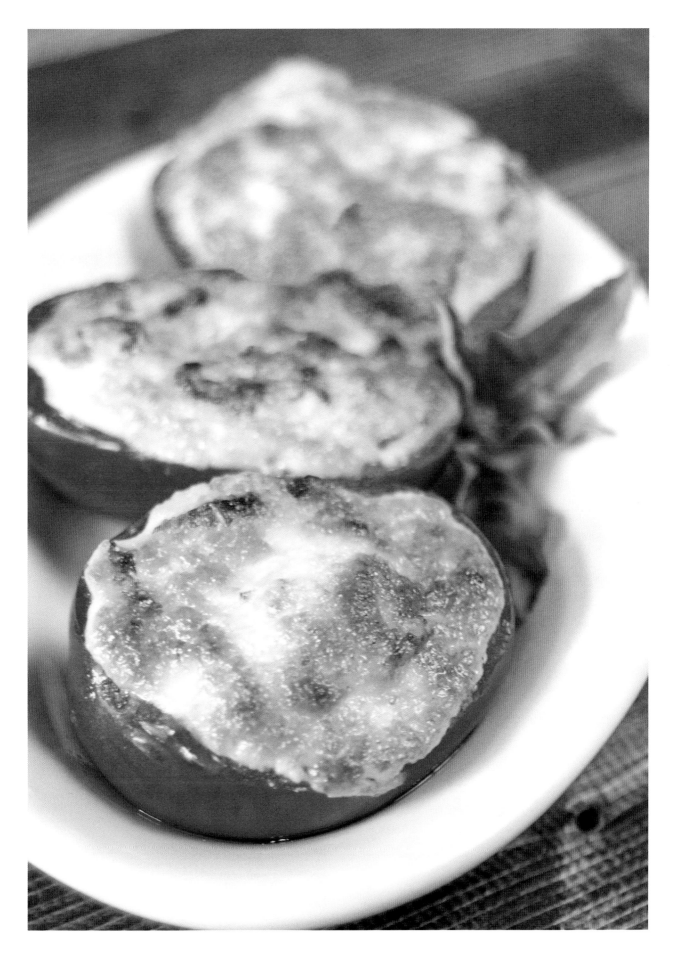

CRISPY SHALLOT & BACON ASPARAGUS

SERVES 4

The first time you have roasted asparagus, it's one of those aha moments when you can't believe you've gone your entire life without something. And when you add crispy shallots and bacon to these roasted gems, it elevates the dish into something truly special.

5 slices thick-cut bacon, cut into 1-inch pieces

1 small shallot, thinly sliced

1 pound asparagus, ends trimmed

1 tablespoon light olive oil

¼ teaspoon fine sea salt

• Preheat the oven to 400°F. Line a sheet pan with foil.

• Heat a skillet over medium-high heat. Place the bacon in the pan and cook, stirring occasionally, until crisp, about 15 minutes. Using a slotted spoon, transfer the bacon to a paper towel–lined plate and set aside. Pour most of the bacon drippings from the pan into a 1-pint glass jar to store for future use, but reserve 2 tablespoons of drippings in the skillet.

• Add the shallot to the skillet and sauté, stirring occasionally, until brown and crispy, about 10 minutes. Transfer the shallots to the plate with the bacon.

• Place the asparagus on the prepared sheet pan, drizzle with the oil, and sprinkle with the salt, then toss to coat. Place the asparagus in the oven and roast for 5 minutes, then flip the spears with tongs and roast until tender and browned, about 5 minutes more.

• Plate the asparagus and top it with the shallots and bacon.

• Store in an airtight container in the fridge for up to 1 week.

PER SERVING
Calories **72** · Fat **4g** · Total Carbs **7g** · Net Carbs **4g** · Fiber **3g** · Protein **3g**

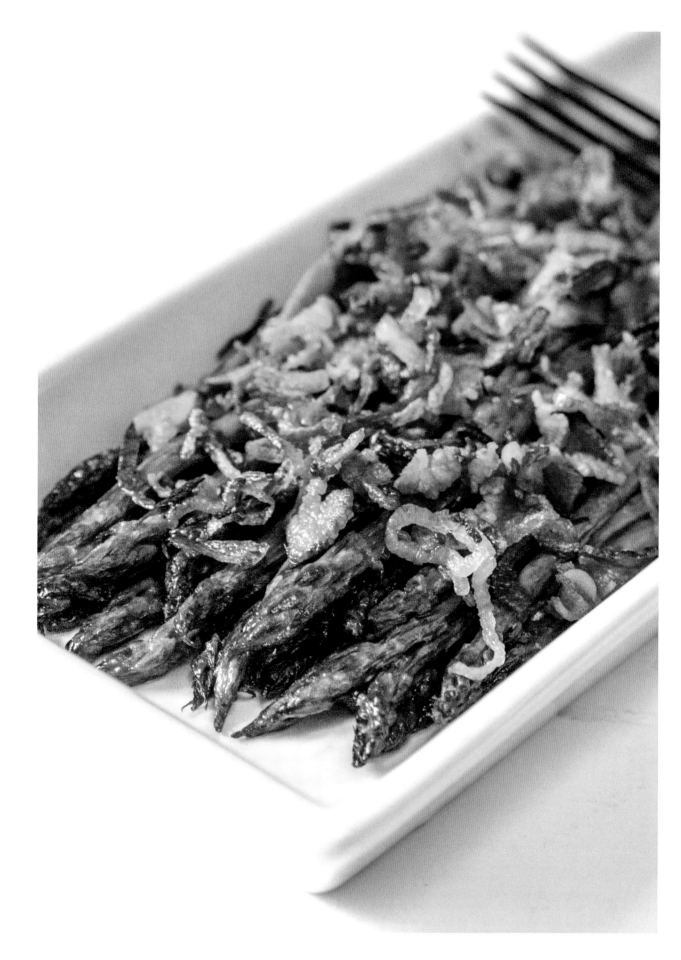

GRUYÈRE SPINACH GRATIN

30 MINUTES or LESS

SERVES **4**

Spinach is one of my favorite veggies, and what a great bonus that it's so packed with nutrients! I love a simple bowl of sautéed spinach with melted butter as a side, but sometimes a little more decadence is a nice change. This combination of spinach and a rich, creamy cheese sauce fits the bill.

2 tablespoons unsalted butter, softened

1 small shallot, minced

⅓ cup heavy cream

¼ cup shredded Parmesan cheese

1 ounce cream cheese (2 tablespoons), room temperature

⅛ teaspoon fine sea salt

⅛ teaspoon garlic powder

⅛ teaspoon ground white pepper

1 (12-ounce) bag frozen spinach, thawed, room temperature (see Note)

¼ cup shredded Gruyère cheese

- Preheat the oven to 400°F.

- Melt the butter in a saucepan over medium-high heat. Add the shallot and sauté until soft and just starting to brown, about 4 minutes. Turn the heat down to medium and stir in the cream, Parmesan cheese, cream cheese, salt, garlic powder, and pepper until combined.

- Squeeze the spinach in batches over a bowl to remove the excess water, then add it to the saucepan. Stir until all the spinach has been incorporated into the sauce. Transfer the spinach mixture to an au gratin baking dish that's about 1½ inches deep and top it with the Gruyère.

- Bake for 10 minutes, or until the top is brown and bubbly.

- Store in an airtight container in the fridge for up to 1 week.

Note : I recommend getting steam-in-the-bag frozen spinach. To thaw, just microwave it in the bag on high.

PER SERVING
Calories **173** · Fat **15g** · Total Carbs **2g** · Net Carbs **1g** · Fiber **1g** · Protein **6g**

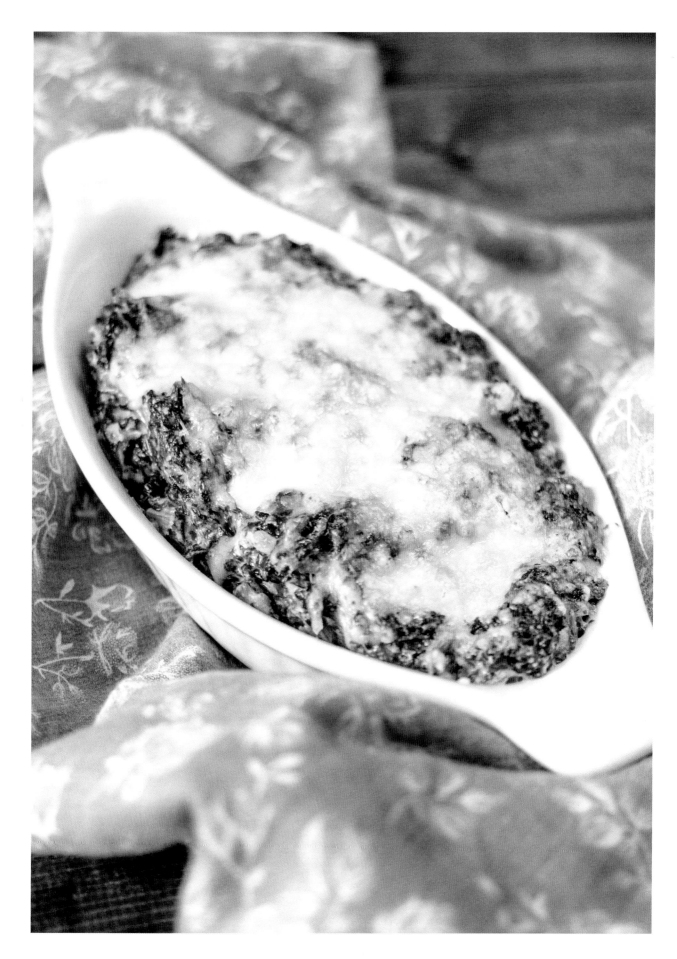

CAULI RISOTTO

SERVES 6

This cauli risotto is so creamy and decadent, it'll quickly become one of your favorites! The chardonnay gives it a wonderful flavor, but feel free to use chicken stock instead if you prefer. I have served this with many different entrées, and it is especially delicious with my Smoky Garlic Shrimp (page 288). The texture is so similar to ordinary risotto that you'd never know it's cauliflower!

1 medium head cauliflower (about 1½ pounds)

3 tablespoons unsalted butter

1 small onion, diced

2¼ teaspoons fine sea salt, divided

2 cloves garlic, minced

½ cup chardonnay or chicken stock (see page 26)

½ cup heavy cream

2 ounces cream cheese (¼ cup), room temperature

½ teaspoon ground black pepper

Chopped fresh parsley, for garnish (optional)

Note: All of my cauli rice recipes make a large batch for two reasons. The first is that they're so darn good that you're going to be happy you made a bunch. The second is that cauli rice freezes really well. You can absolutely cut this recipe in half if you prefer, but don't say I didn't warn ya!

• Rice the cauliflower: Chop the head into large chunks and, working in batches, pulse them in a food processor until the pieces are about the size of grains of rice. (Be sure to fill the food processor only halfway.) You can also rice them by hand with a hand grater.

• Melt the butter in a large sauté pan over medium heat. Add the onion and ¼ teaspoon of the salt and sauté until softened and lightly browned, about 3 minutes. Stir in the garlic and sauté until fragrant, about 2 minutes. Add the cauliflower and remaining 2 teaspoons of salt, stir, then add the wine. Cover and steam for 5 minutes, or until the cauliflower is slightly softened.

• Add the cream, cream cheese, and pepper, then stir to combine. Simmer, stirring occasionally, until the cauli rice is tender, about 5 minutes. Garnish with chopped fresh parsley, if desired.

• Store in an airtight container in the fridge for up to 1 week or in a sealed plastic bag in the freezer for up to 2 months. Defrost overnight in the fridge, then heat in the microwave on medium power until warmed through, about 3 to 5 minutes, stirring halfway through heating.

PER SERVING
Calories 202 · Fat 17g · Total Carbs 8g · Net Carbs 5g · Fiber 3g · Protein 3g

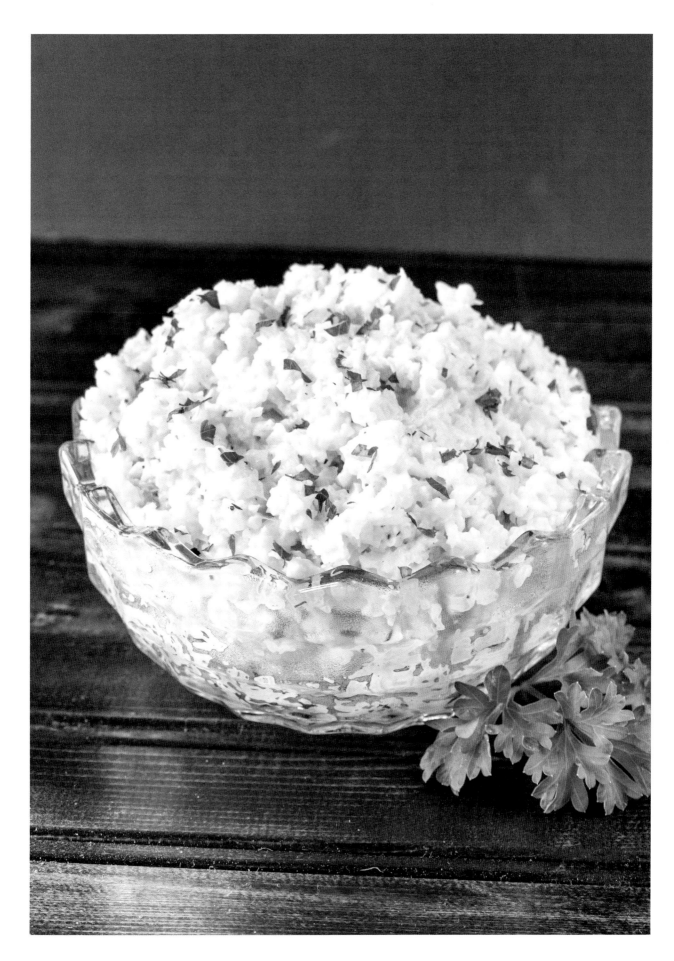

ROASTED BRUSSELS SPROUTS
with BALSAMIC MAYO

 30 MINUTES or LESS

SERVES 4

Man, if I had a nickel for everyone converted to loving Brussels sprouts after trying them roasted...! It's a life-changing experience, even more so when they're dipped in this luscious balsamic mayo.

1 pound fresh Brussels sprouts, trimmed and halved (see Note)

2 tablespoons extra-virgin olive oil

¼ teaspoon fine sea salt

FOR THE BALSAMIC MAYO:

¼ cup mayonnaise (see page 43)

½ tablespoon balsamic vinegar

¼ teaspoon powdered blended erythritol-stevia sweetener (see page 46)

Pinch of fine sea salt

Pinch of ground black pepper, plus more for garnish if desired

Note : It's important to use fresh Brussels sprouts in this recipe; frozen sprouts are too mushy and won't crisp properly.

• Preheat the oven to 450°F. Line a sheet pan with foil.

• Place the sprouts on the sheet pan, drizzle them with the olive oil and sprinkle them with the salt, then toss with your hands. Roast for 6 minutes, then shake the sheet pan to toss the sprouts and roast for another 6 minutes. The sprouts are ready when they are tender and deeply browned.

• While the sprouts are roasting, make the balsamic mayo: Whisk together all the balsamic mayo ingredients in a small bowl until combined. Sprinkle with fresh ground pepper, if desired.

• Serve the sprouts with the balsamic mayo on the side for dipping.

• Store in an airtight container in the fridge for 2 to 3 days.

PER SERVING
Calories **203** · Fat **18g** · Total Carbs **12g** · Net Carbs **6g** · Fiber **4g** · Protein **4g**

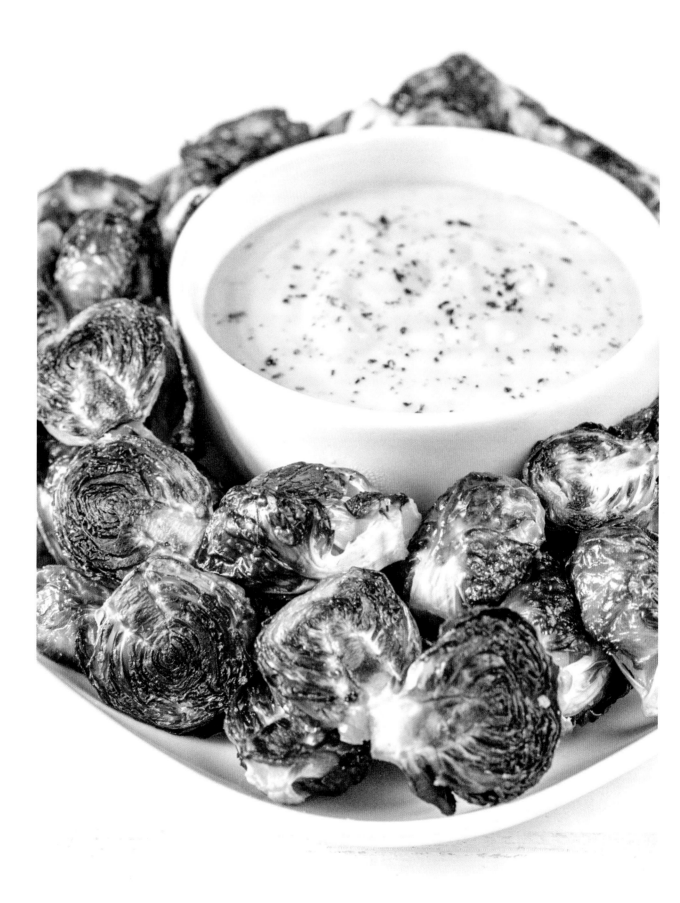

BEST-EVER CAULI MASH

30 MINUTES or LESS

SERVES 6

Mashed potatoes was always my favorite side dish, hands down. So when I started eating keto, I tried replacing it with mashed cauliflower, which is much lower in carbs. It took dozens of tries, but I finally came up with a recipe that results in an amazingly creamy and delicious dish. I don't even miss mashed potatoes!

1 medium head cauliflower (about 1½ pounds), cut into large chunks (see Note)

2 teaspoons water

4 ounces cream cheese (½ cup), room temperature

2 tablespoons heavy cream

2 tablespoons unsalted butter, softened, plus more for serving if desired

1¼ teaspoons fine sea salt

Chopped fresh parsley, for garnish (optional)

Note: You can use frozen cauliflower instead; look for the steam-in-the-bag variety. The bag will contain quite a bit of water after steaming, so be sure to use a slotted spoon to move the cauliflower to the blender or food processor and be careful not to transfer any water with it.

- Place the cauliflower in a large microwave-safe bowl and add the water. Cover the bowl tightly with plastic wrap and microwave on high for about 5 minutes, until the cauliflower is just fork-tender.

- Using a slotted spoon, transfer the cauliflower to a blender or food processor, being very careful not to transfer any water. Add the remaining ingredients and pulse until all the florets have been chopped into tiny pieces, then puree until smooth and thick, similar to mashed potatoes. The longer you puree it, the more velvety it will become.

- Spoon the mashed cauli into a serving bowl and top with additional butter if desired. Garnish with chopped fresh parsley, if desired.

- Store in an airtight container in the fridge for up to 1 week.

Variation: CHEESY GARLIC CAULI MASH

To the blender or food processor, add 1 teaspoon of garlic powder and 1 cup shredded sharp cheddar cheese.

PER SERVING
Calories **146** · Fat **12g** · Total Carbs **7g** · Net Carbs **4g** · Fiber **3g** · Protein **4g**

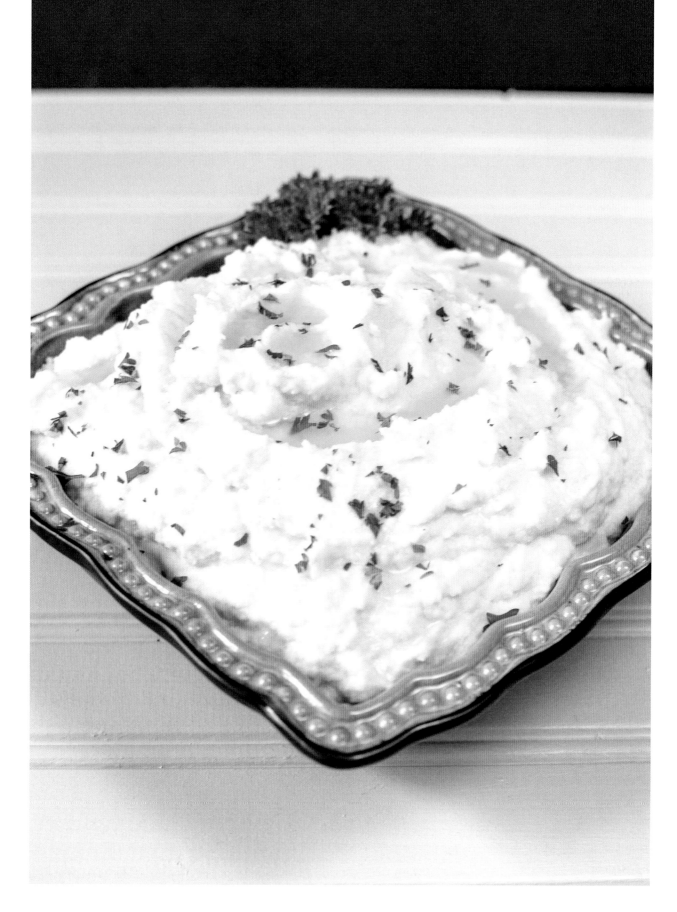

SPAGHETTI SQUASH ALFREDO

2 HOURS or LESS

SERVES 6

I have been eating spaghetti squash since I was a kid, and this is by far my favorite way to enjoy it. I like to roast spaghetti squash and separate it into noodles on the weekend so it's prepped for the week ahead. When the squash is already cooked, this delicious recipe comes together in no time—just heat the squash through in the skillet before making the alfredo sauce. Fresh Parmesan makes this dish even more decadent, but pregrated Parmesan will work as well.

1 medium spaghetti squash

⅓ cup heavy cream

⅓ cup grated Parmesan cheese

3 ounces cream cheese (¼ cup plus 2 tablespoons), room temperature

3 tablespoons unsalted butter

¾ teaspoon fine sea salt

¼ teaspoon ground black pepper

Chopped fresh parsley, for garnish (optional)

- Preheat the oven to 350°F. Prick the spaghetti squash all over with a small sharp knife. (These are vents for the steam, so the squash won't explode in the oven.) Place the squash on a sheet pan and roast it in the oven until it's tender when you press on it, 1 to 1½ hours. Remove it from the oven and let it cool. Once the squash is cool enough to handle, slice it in half crosswise and remove the seeds with a spoon. Gently pull the strands of squash from the rind with a fork.

- Heat the strands of spaghetti squash in a large sauté pan over medium heat just until warmed through, about 3 minutes. Push the squash to one side of the pan and add the rest of the ingredients, except the parsley, on the other side. Whisk the other ingredients until smooth and bubbly, about 3 minutes.

- Gently fold the spaghetti squash into the alfredo sauce until combined. Serve garnished with chopped parsley, if desired.

- Store in an airtight container in the fridge for up to 1 week.

PER SERVING
Calories **199** · Fat **17g** · Total Carbs **9g** · Net Carbs **7g** · Fiber **2g** · Protein **4g**

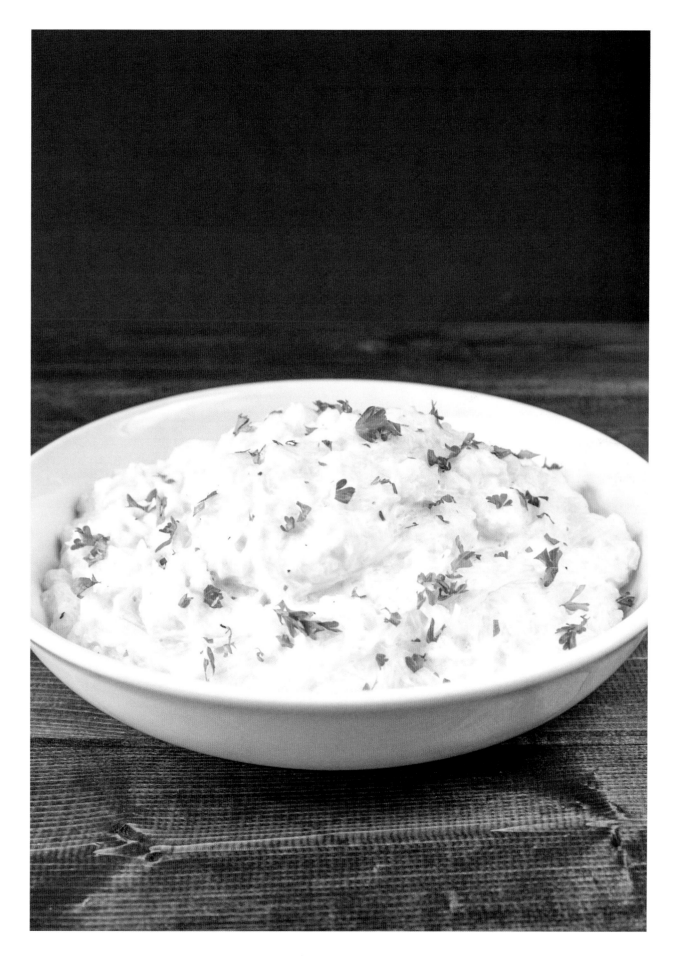

CASHEW FRIED CAULI RICE

30 MINUTES or LESS

SERVES 6

Bursting with sesame flavor and crunchy cashews, this is the perfect side dish for Asian dishes! It pairs beautifully with my Mongolian Beef (page 218), Spicy Garlic Pork (page 268), and Kung Pao Chicken (page 242).

1 medium head cauliflower (about 1½ pounds)

2 tablespoons peanut oil

1 small onion, diced

2 cloves garlic, minced

1 tablespoon coconut aminos

1 tablespoon soy sauce

1 teaspoon toasted sesame oil

½ teaspoon fine sea salt

2 large eggs

½ cup roasted unsalted cashews

1 scallion, sliced, for garnish

Note: All of my cauli rice recipes make a large batch for two reasons. The first is that they're so darn good that you're going to be happy you made a bunch. The second is that cauli rice freezes really well. You can absolutely cut this recipe in half if you prefer, but don't say I didn't warn ya!

• Rice the cauliflower: Chop the head into large chunks and, working in batches, pulse them in a food processor until the pieces are about the size of grains of rice. (Be sure to fill the food processor only halfway.) You can also rice them by hand with a hand grater. Set aside.

• Heat the peanut oil in a skillet over medium-high heat. Add the onion and a pinch of salt and sauté until softened and lightly browned, about 3 minutes. Stir in the garlic and cook until fragrant, about 2 minutes. Add the riced cauliflower, coconut aminos, soy sauce, sesame oil, and salt, then stir to combine. Cover and steam until the cauliflower is tender-crisp, 5 to 8 minutes.

• In a small bowl, whisk the eggs with a pinch of salt. Make a well in the center of the cauli rice and pour in the eggs. Scramble the eggs until completely cooked, about 2 minutes. Add the cashews and stir to combine.

• Garnish with sliced scallions before serving.

• Store in an airtight container in the fridge for up to 1 week or in a sealed plastic bag in the freezer for up to 2 months.

PER SERVING
Calories **162** · Fat **12g** · Total Carbs **10g** · Net Carbs **7g** · Fiber **3g** · Protein **7g**

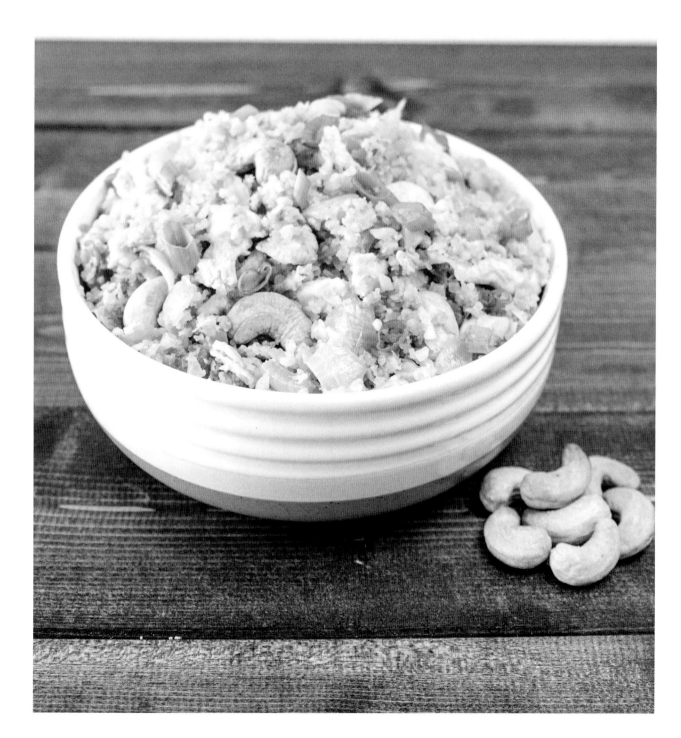

LEMON GARLIC BABY BOK CHOY

30 MINUTES or LESS

SERVES 4

I love the mild flavor of bok choy, and baby bok choy is honestly too cute to resist, so it's a win-win for me! Not only are these baby cabbages nutritional powerhouses, but I love how they sauté to a tender-crisp texture and take on flavors beautifully. Here, lemon and garlic make them even more mouthwatering.

1 tablespoon light olive oil

2 cloves garlic, thinly sliced

10 medium heads baby bok choy (about 20 ounces), halved lengthwise and thoroughly washed and dried

1 tablespoon unsalted butter

2 teaspoons lemon juice

¼ teaspoon fine sea salt

2 teaspoons grated lemon zest, for garnish

- Heat the oil in a large heavy-bottomed skillet over medium-high heat. Add the garlic and sauté, stirring constantly, until lightly browned and fragrant, about 2 minutes. Using a slotted spoon, transfer the garlic to a plate and set aside.

- Place the bok choy in the skillet cut side down and sear until golden brown, about 5 minutes. Flip the bok choy and add the butter, lemon juice, and salt and stir. Sauté the bok choy until crisp-tender, about 2 minutes.

- Transfer the bok choy to a serving dish, sprinkle with the garlic and lemon zest, and serve.

- Store in an airtight container in the fridge for up to 1 week.

PER SERVING
Calories **122** · Fat **6g** · Total Carbs **8g** · Net Carbs **2g** · Fiber **6g** · Protein **5g**

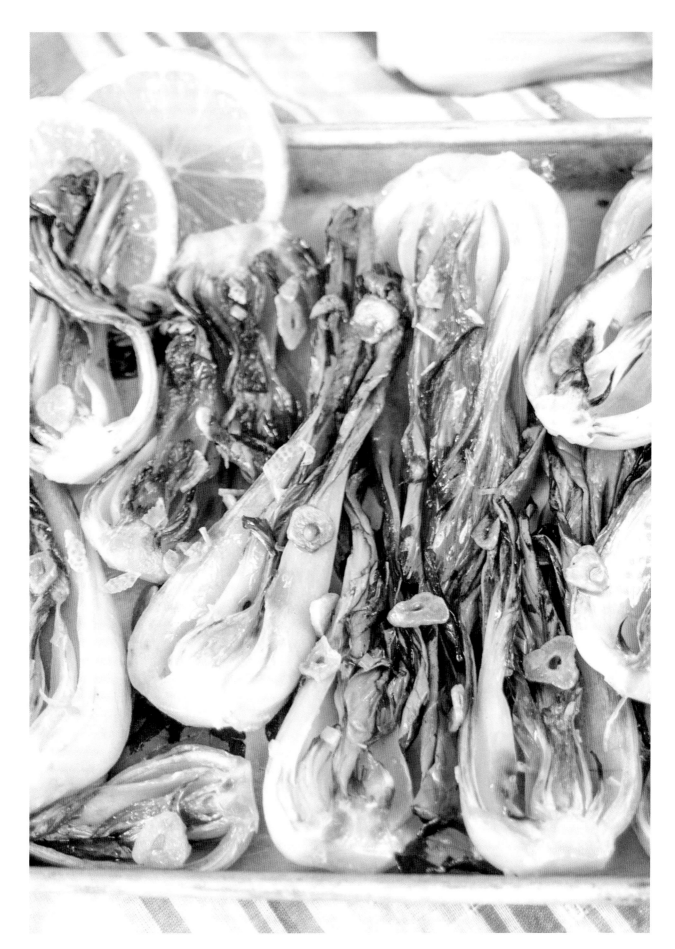

TOASTED ALMOND HARICOTS VERTS

MINUTES or LESS

SERVES 6

Haricots verts—also known as French green beans—are thinner and shorter than regular green beans. I'm not sure why they taste better, but they do! This dish infuses the beans with a smoky bacon flavor and tops them with crunchy toasted almonds. It cannot be missed.

1 cup water

1 pound haricots verts, trimmed

⅓ cup sliced almonds

2 tablespoons bacon grease

¼ teaspoon fine sea salt

• Bring the water to a boil in a sauté pan over high heat. Add the beans, cover, and cook until tender-crisp, about 5 minutes.

• While the beans cook, toast the almonds in a small dry skillet over medium heat, stirring frequently, until lightly browned, about 3 minutes.

• Drain the beans in a fine-mesh sieve over the sink. Return the pan to the stovetop and turn the heat down to medium. Put the bacon grease in the pan, add the beans, and stir to coat. Sauté the beans just until browned, 2 to 3 minutes, and sprinkle with the salt.

• Garnish with the toasted almonds before serving.

• Store in an airtight container in the fridge for up to 1 week.

PER SERVING
Calories **146** · Fat **12g** · Total Carbs **10g** · Net Carbs **5g** · Fiber **5g** · Protein **4g**

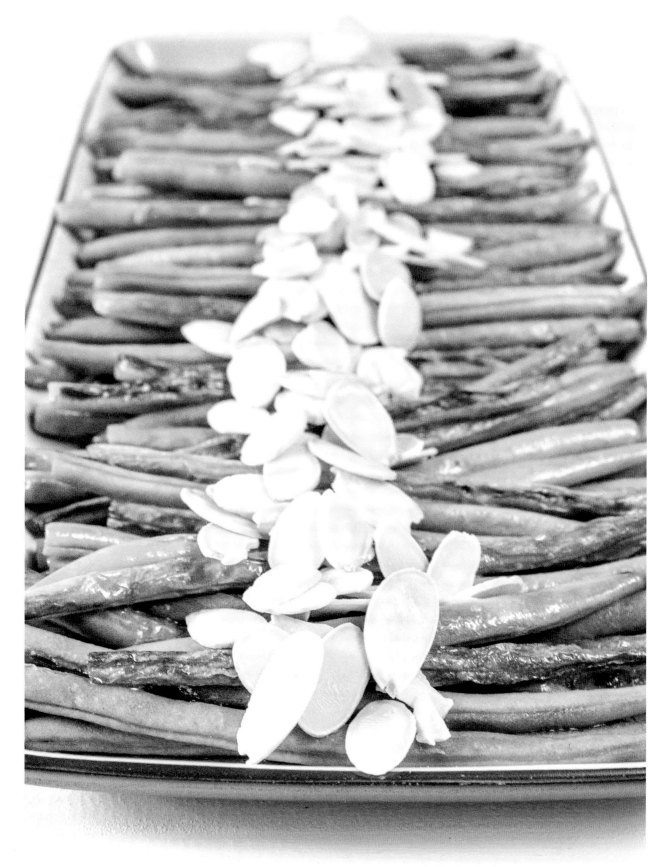

CAULI PUREE *with* CRISPY SHIITAKE MUSHROOMS

 30 MINUTES or LESS

SERVES **6**

In this dish, the rich and creamy cauliflower puree is nicely balanced by the crispy and meaty shiitake mushrooms. This pairs extremely well with my Garlic Roast Beef with Horseradish Cream (page 212).

1 tablespoon bacon grease

3½ ounces shiitake mushrooms, stemmed and cut into ½-inch pieces

1 medium head cauliflower (about 1½ pounds), cut into large chunks (see Note)

½ cup heavy cream

2 ounces cream cheese (¼ cup), room temperature

2 tablespoons unsalted butter, melted

2 teaspoons water

1¼ teaspoons fine sea salt

Chopped fresh parsley, for garnish (optional)

Note : You can use frozen cauliflower instead; look for the steam-in-the-bag variety. The bag will contain quite a bit of water after steaming, so be sure to use a slotted spoon to move the cauliflower to the blender or food processor and be careful not to transfer any water with it.

• Heat the bacon grease in a skillet over medium-high heat. Add the mushrooms and cook until crispy and golden, 6 to 8 minutes, stirring occasionally. Sprinkle with a pinch of salt, remove from the heat, and set aside.

• Place the cauliflower in a large microwave-safe bowl and add the water. Cover the bowl tightly with plastic wrap and microwave on high for about 5 minutes, until the cauliflower is just fork-tender.

• Using a slotted spoon, transfer the cauliflower to a blender or food processor, being very careful not to transfer any water. Add the remaining ingredients and pulse until all the florets have been chopped into tiny pieces, then puree until smooth and velvety.

• Spoon the cauliflower puree into a serving bowl and top with the mushrooms. Garnish with chopped fresh parsley, if desired.

• Store in an airtight container in the fridge for up to 1 week.

PER SERVING
Calories **182** · Fat **17g** · Total Carbs **7g** · Net Carbs **4g** · Fiber **3g** · Protein **3g**

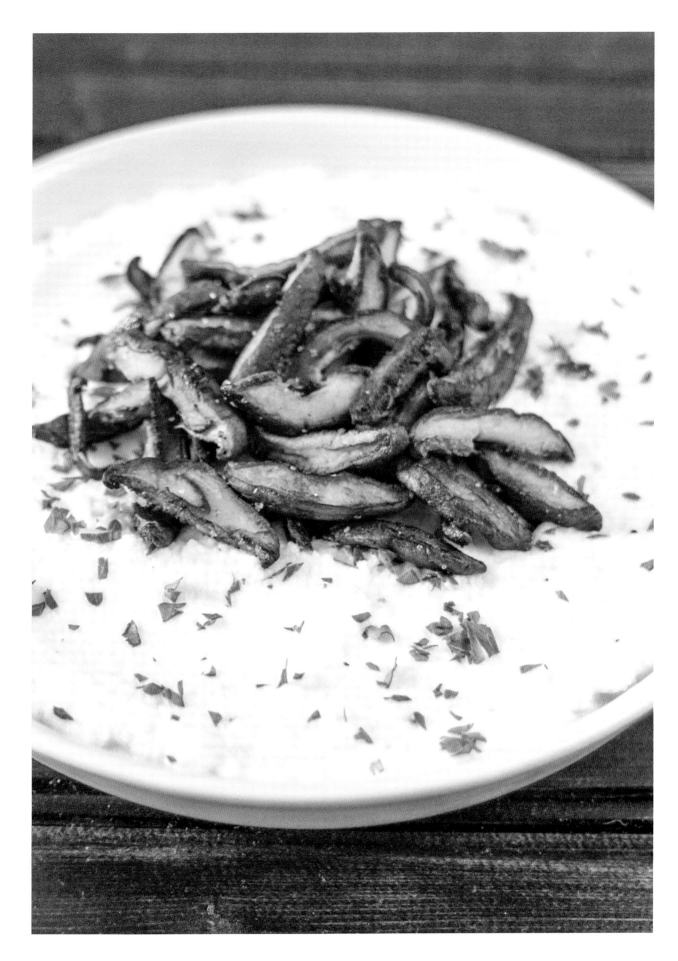

GARLIC BUTTER ROASTED MUSHROOMS

SERVES 6

Roasted mushrooms have an amazing rich and meaty flavor, along with the most exquisite texture. Pair them with warm garlic butter, and you've got the side dish to end all side dishes. I always serve these when I make my Garlic Roast Beef with Horseradish Cream (page 212).

1½ pounds button mushrooms, stems removed

2 tablespoons light olive oil

½ teaspoon fine sea salt

¼ teaspoon ground black pepper

2 tablespoons unsalted butter

2 cloves garlic, minced

1 tablespoon chopped fresh parsley, plus more for garnish if desired

• Preheat the oven to 450°F and line a sheet pan with foil.

• Place the mushroom caps on the sheet pan, drizzle them with the oil, and toss to coat. Roast for 15 minutes, then remove the pan from the oven and flip all the mushrooms over. Season them with the salt and pepper, then return them to the oven for another 10 minutes.

• Melt the butter in a small saucepan over medium heat and add the garlic. Sauté until the garlic is fragrant and just starting to brown, about 3 minutes.

• Transfer the mushrooms to a serving bowl. Stir the parsley and a pinch of salt into the garlic butter. Pour the garlic butter over the mushrooms and garnish with parsley if desired.

• Store in an airtight container in the fridge for up to 1 week.

PER SERVING
Calories **151** · Fat **13g** · Total Carbs **6g** · Net Carbs **4g** · Fiber **2g** · Protein **5g**

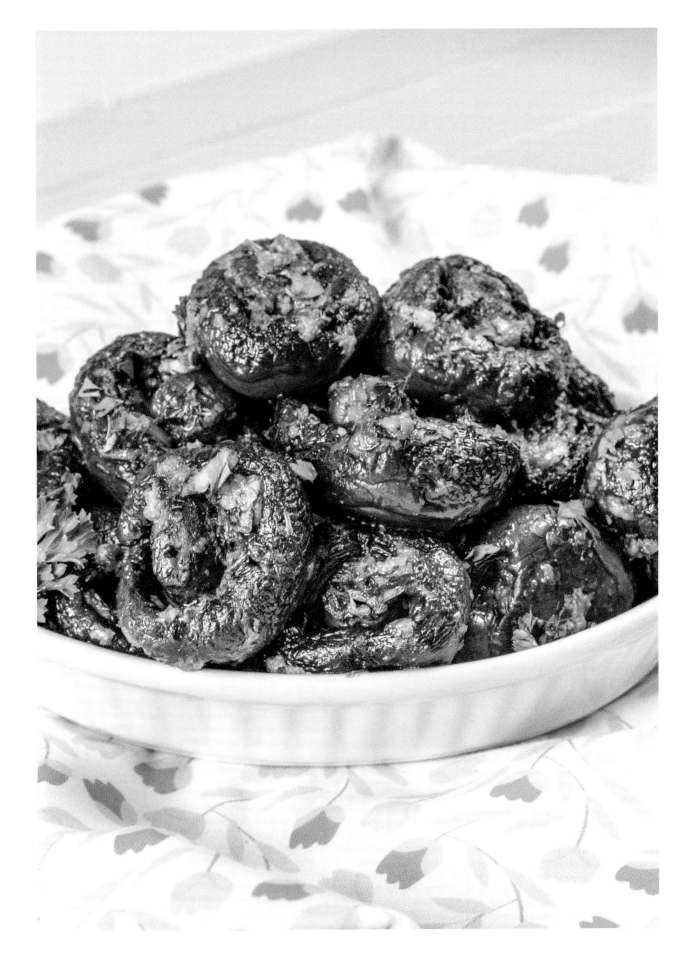

CILANTRO LIME CAULI RICE

30 MINUTES or LESS

SERVES 6

When I first started eating keto, I wasn't very impressed with cauli rice because, let's face it, it's not rice. However, I've discovered that it's really good when cooked and seasoned properly. There are so many different spices and seasonings you can add that the options are limitless! This is one of my favorite combinations, with tart lime and bright cilantro. It goes great with my Barbacoa (page 222), Carnitas (page 266), and Shrimp Fajitas (page 280).

1 medium head cauliflower (about 1½ pounds)

2 tablespoons bacon grease

¼ cup sliced scallions (about 3 stalks)

2 cloves garlic, minced

Grated zest from 1 lime

2 tablespoons lime juice

2 tablespoons chopped cilantro

1¼ teaspoons fine sea salt

¼ teaspoon ground black pepper

Note : All of my cauli rice recipes make a large batch for two reasons. The first is that they're so darn good that you're going to be happy you made a bunch. The second is that cauli rice freezes really well. You can absolutely cut this recipe in half if you prefer, but don't say I didn't warn ya!

· Rice the cauliflower: Chop the head into large chunks and, working in batches, pulse them in a food processor until the pieces are about the size of grains of rice. (Be sure to fill the food processor only halfway.) You can also rice them by hand with a hand grater.

· Heat the bacon grease in a sauté pan over medium-high heat. Add the scallions and garlic and sauté until softened and lightly toasted, about 3 minutes. Add the riced cauliflower and stir to combine. Cover and steam until the cauliflower is tender-crisp, 5 to 8 minutes.

· Transfer the cauli rice to a large bowl and add the lime zest, lime juice, cilantro, salt, and pepper. Stir until well combined. Serve immediately.

· Store in an airtight container in the fridge for up to 1 week or in a sealed plastic bag in the freezer for up to 2 months.

PER SERVING
Calories **69** · Fat **4g** · Total Carbs **7g** · Net Carbs **4g** · Fiber **3g** · Protein **2g**

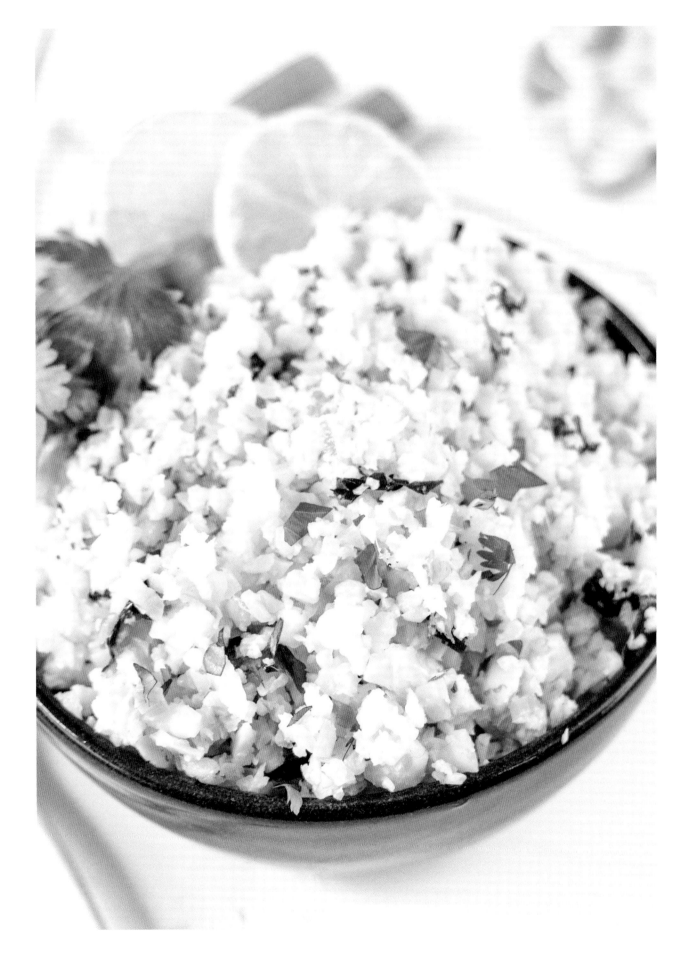

GARLIC ROASTED RADISHES

SERVES 4

Who knew that roasting radishes turned them into potatoes' pink cousins? They have a very potato-like texture, which makes them a great replacement for home fries, and they couldn't be easier to make.

1 bunch radishes (about 1 pound), trimmed

1 small onion, diced

2 cloves garlic, minced

2 tablespoons bacon grease

¼ teaspoon fine sea salt

⅛ teaspoon ground black pepper

• Preheat the oven to 400°F and line a sheet pan with foil.

• Cut larger radishes into quarters and smaller radishes in half. Place them in a medium-sized bowl, add the remaining ingredients, and toss well to combine. Spread the radish mixture in an even layer on the sheet pan and arrange the radishes cut side down.

• Roast for 15 minutes, or until the radishes are brown and crispy.

• Store in an airtight container in the fridge for up to 1 week.

PER SERVING
Calories **69** · Fat **6g** · Total Carbs **3g** · Net Carbs **2g** · Fiber **1g** · Protein **0g**

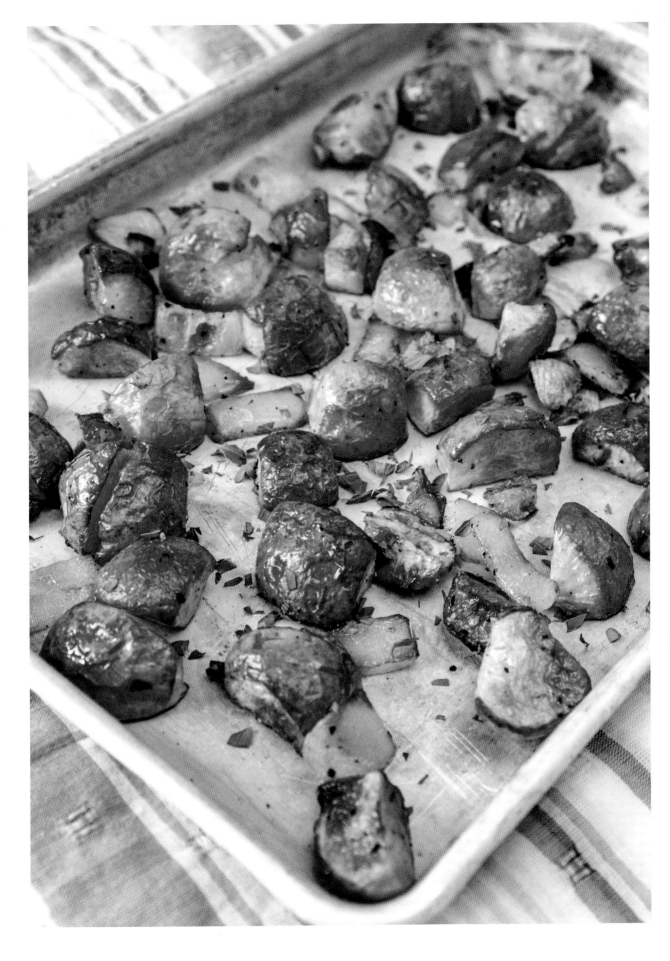

GRILLED NAPA CABBAGE
with CREAMY DRESSING

30 MINUTES or LESS

SERVES 4

I'm a big fan of napa cabbage, and I often shred it and use it in soups for a nice noodle-like addition. For this side dish, I've used a creamy sauce that has just the right amount of tang to complement the smokiness of the grilled cabbage.

FOR THE DRESSING:

3 tablespoons mayonnaise (see page 43)

1 tablespoon white wine vinegar

1 teaspoon Dijon mustard

⅛ teaspoon blended erythritol-stevia sweetener (see page 46)

⅛ teaspoon fine sea salt

⅛ teaspoon ground black pepper

1 large head napa cabbage (about 2 pounds), quartered

2 tablespoons light olive oil

Fine sea salt and ground black pepper

- Preheat a grill or cast-iron grill pan over medium-high heat.

- In a small bowl, whisk together all the dressing ingredients until well combined. Set aside.

- Generously brush the cut sides of the cabbage quarters with the oil, then sprinkle the cabbage with salt and pepper.

- Grill or sear the napa cabbage until lightly charred and softened, 3 to 5 minutes per side.

- Drizzle with the creamy dressing before serving.

- Store in an airtight container in the fridge for 2 to 3 days.

PER SERVING
Calories 141 · Fat 15g · Total Carbs 3g · Net Carbs 2g · Fiber 1g · Protein 1g

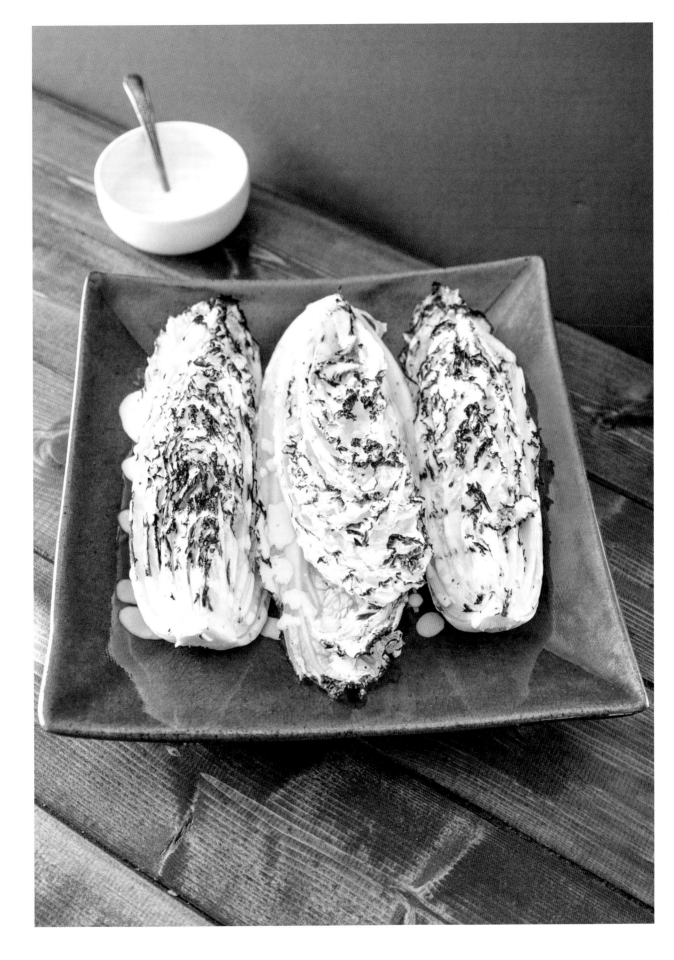

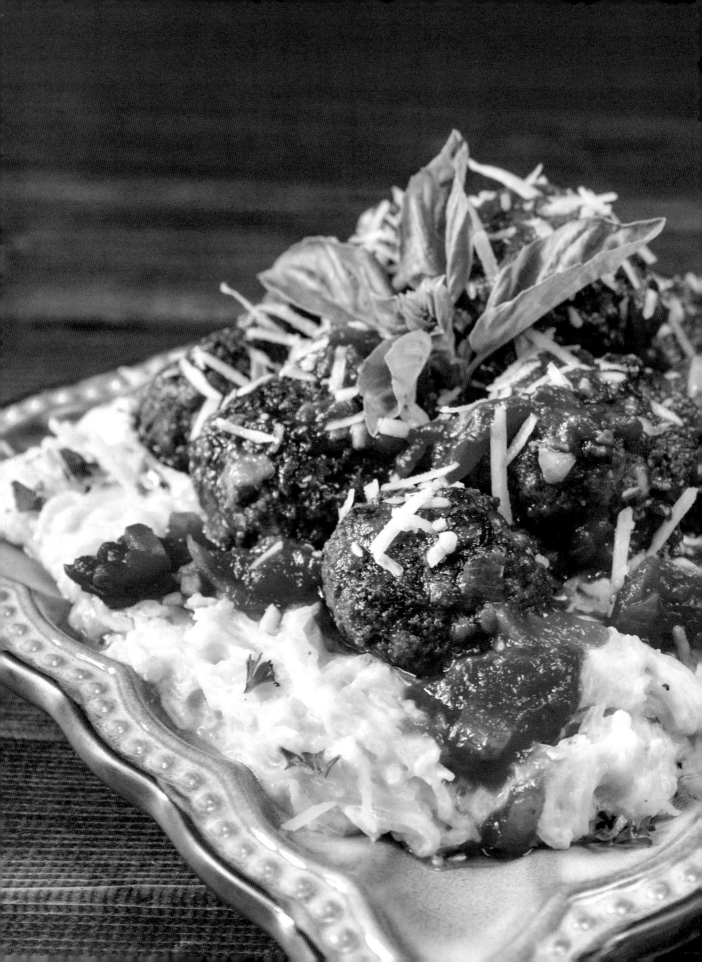

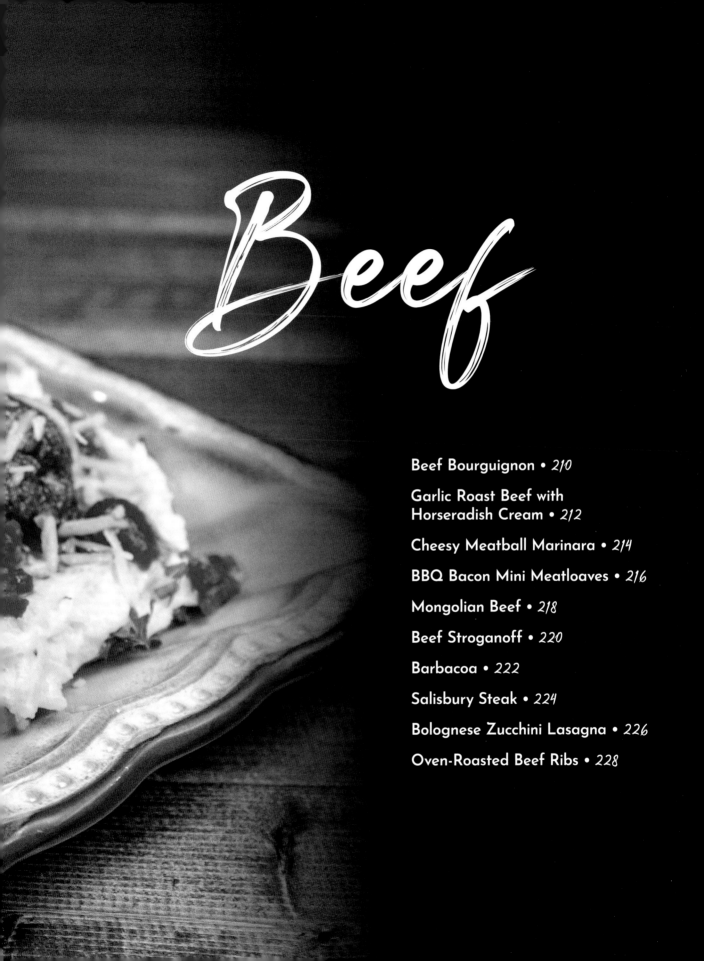

Beef

BEEF BOURGUIGNON

OVER 2 HOURS

SERVES 4

This recipe is a bit time-consuming, but it's not difficult at all, and it's so worth the time! It's like an upscale beef stew, full of the most amazing full-bodied flavors.

2 tablespoons unsalted butter

1 tablespoon light olive oil

2½ pounds boneless chuck roast, cut into bite-sized chunks

2½ teaspoons fine sea salt, divided

¼ teaspoon ground black pepper

2 stalks celery, cut lengthwise into quarters

1 medium carrot, peeled and cut lengthwise into quarters

1 medium shallot, diced

1 cup merlot (see Note)

2 cups beef stock

⅔ cup frozen pearl onions

⅓ cup heavy cream

Note : If you'd prefer not to use merlot, just use ½ cup of beef stock to deglaze the pan.

• Heat the butter and oil in a 6-quart Dutch oven over medium-high heat. Season the beef chunks with ½ teaspoon of the salt and the pepper. Working in batches to avoid overcrowding the pan, sear the beef until golden brown on all sides, about 3 minutes per side. Use a slotted spoon to transfer the beef to a plate, leaving the drippings in the pan. Set the beef aside.

• Cut the celery and carrot strips on the bias in 1-inch pieces. Add the celery, carrot, and shallot to the pan and stir to coat them in beef drippings. Sauté for 5 minutes, until the veggies are softened, stirring frequently. Add 1 teaspoon of the salt and stir. Using a slotted spoon, transfer the veggies to a bowl. Cover and set aside.

• Add the merlot to the pan and deglaze it, scraping the bottom of the pan to loosen all the brown bits. Turn the heat down to medium and simmer the merlot until it's reduced by half, about 5 minutes.

• Add the beef stock to the reduced merlot. Return the meat and any juices back to the pan and sprinkle with the remaining teaspoon of salt. Stir to combine. Bring to a boil, then turn the heat down to medium-low. Simmer the beef until tender, about 2 hours.

• Add the reserved sautéed veggies and frozen pearl onions to the pan and stir to combine. Cover and simmer for 30 minutes more, or until the onions are warmed through. Pour in the heavy cream and simmer until the sauce has thickened, about 5 minutes. Serve immediately.

• Store in an airtight container in the fridge for up to 1 week.

PER SERVING
Calories **833** · Fat **67g** · Total Carbs **6g** · Net Carbs **5g** · Fiber **1g** · Protein **50g**

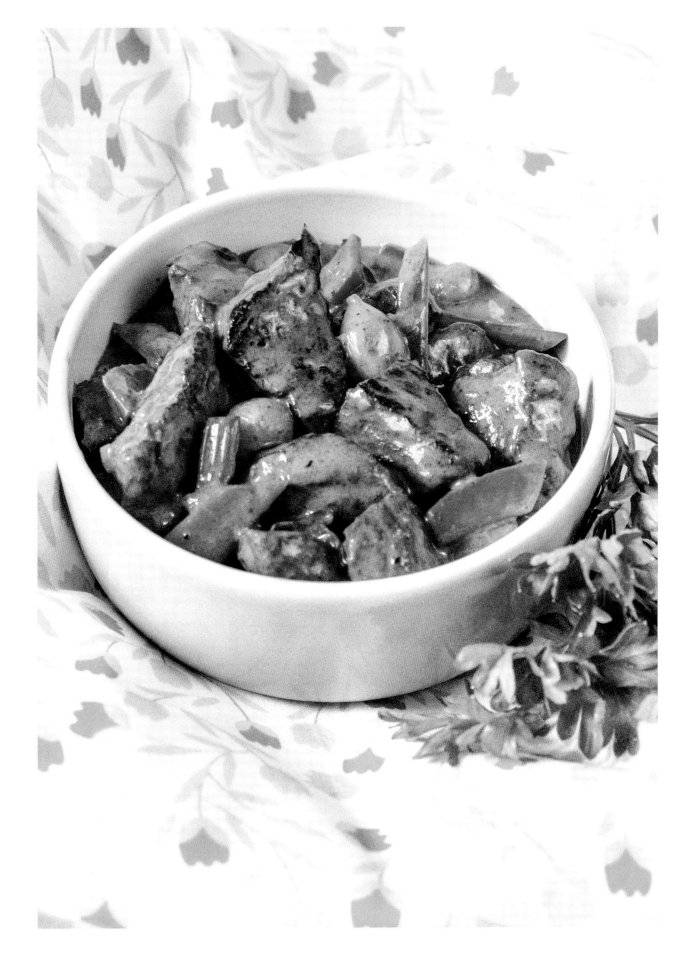

GARLIC ROAST BEEF *with* HORSERADISH CREAM

SERVES 4

My mom has been making this amazing garlicky roast beef all my life, and I've always loved it. The tangy, spicy horseradish cream is the perfect accompaniment to the roasted beef, and I really enjoy serving it with my Best-Ever Cauli Mash (page 188). Be sure to pull your roast out of the fridge an hour before you start cooking so it has time to come to room temperature—that will help it cook more evenly.

2½ pounds eye of round beef roast, room temperature

2 cloves garlic, peeled and cut into thin slivers

1 teaspoon fine sea salt

½ teaspoon ground black pepper

FOR THE HORSERADISH CREAM:

¼ cup mayonnaise (see page 43)

2 tablespoons prepared horseradish

2 tablespoons full-fat sour cream

1 teaspoon white wine vinegar

⅛ teaspoon blended stevia-erythritol sweetener (see page 46)

⅛ teaspoon fine sea salt

⅛ teaspoon ground black pepper

Chopped fresh parsley, for garnish (optional)

- Preheat the oven to 350°F.

- Using a sharp knife, pierce the roast all over with approximately twenty 1-inch-deep holes. Insert garlic slivers in each hole. Season the roast all over with the salt and pepper and place it in a roasting pan. Roast until the beef reaches an internal temp of 120°F for rare, 130°F for medium rare, 140°F for medium, or 150°F for well done, about 1 hour.

- While the beef is roasting, whisk all of the sauce ingredients together in a medium-sized bowl until smooth. Cover and chill in the fridge until you're ready to serve.

- Once the beef is done roasting, allow it to rest for 10 to 15 minutes before slicing. The internal temperature of the beef will increase by 5 degrees while resting.

- Cut the beef into thin slices and place it on a serving platter. Serve immediately with the chilled horseradish cream. Garnish with chopped fresh parsley, if desired.

- Store leftovers in an airtight container in the fridge for up to 1 week.

Note : My favorite thing to do with leftover roast beef is to cube it, sauté it with chopped onions and bell peppers for about 5 minutes over medium-high heat, and then serve it with over-easy eggs and hollandaise sauce. It makes for a very quick but impressive meal.

PER SERVING
Calories **589** · Fat **37g** · Total Carbs **2g** · Net Carbs **2g** · Fiber **0g** · Protein **58g**

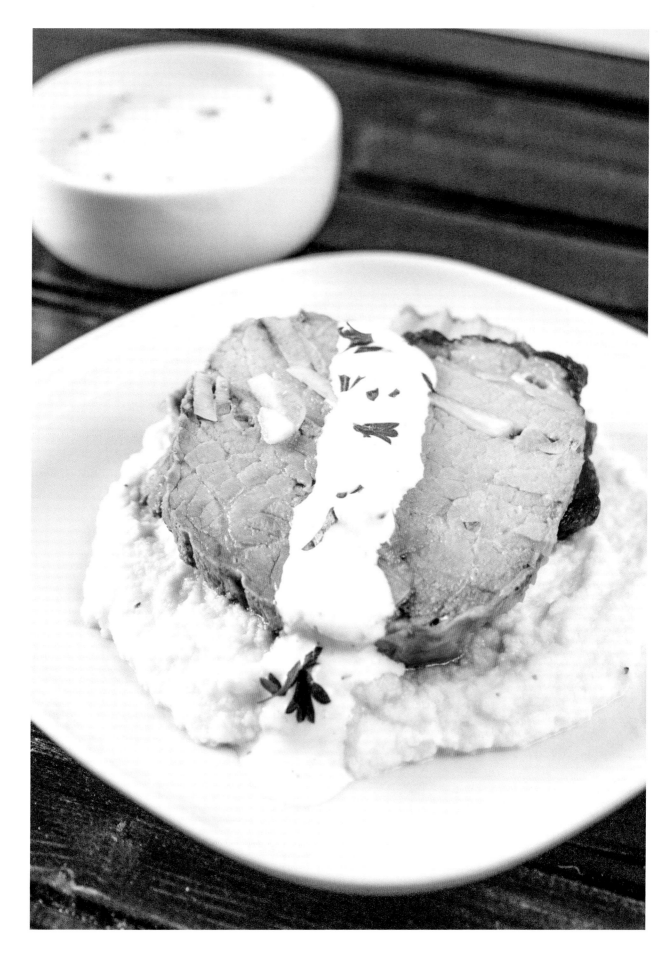

CHEESY MEATBALL MARINARA

1 HOUR or LESS

SERVES 4

I don't think I've ever met a person who doesn't love meatballs. These cheesy meatballs in particular are a huge hit with my kids, and they're absolutely dynamite on top of my Spaghetti Squash Alfredo (page 190).

FOR THE SAUCE:

2 tablespoons light olive oil

½ medium onion, diced

2 cloves garlic, minced

½ teaspoon fine sea salt

⅛ teaspoon crushed red pepper

1 (28-ounce) can whole San Marzano tomatoes (including liquid)

FOR THE MEATBALLS:

1 tablespoon unsalted butter

⅓ cup crushed pork rinds

1 pound ground beef, 90% lean

1 large egg

⅓ cup shredded mozzarella

1 tablespoon minced fresh parsley

1 teaspoon fine sea salt

¼ teaspoon garlic powder

¼ teaspoon ground black pepper

¼ cup light olive oil, for frying

¼ cup freshly grated Parmesan, for garnish

Sprig of fresh basil, for garnish (optional)

Note : Be sure to use 90% lean ground beef. The frying oil is mixed into the sauce, and using beef with a higher percentage of fat would make it greasy.

- Make the sauce: Heat the 2 tablespoons of oil in a large nonreactive saucepan over medium-high heat. Add the onion and sauté until translucent, about 3 minutes. Add the garlic and sauté until fragrant, about 3 minutes more. Add the salt and crushed red pepper and stir.

- Hold the tomatoes over the pot and carefully crush them by hand so the juice doesn't spray everywhere. Drop the tomatoes into the pot and pour in the liquid from the can. Bring to a boil, then turn the heat down to medium-low and simmer while you make the meatballs.

- Make the meatballs: Melt the butter in a skillet over medium-high heat and add the pork rind crumbs. Toast, stirring frequently, until golden brown, about 4 minutes. Transfer the toasted crumbs to a large bowl and set aside to cool for a few minutes.

- Once the crumbs are cool enough to handle, add the rest of the meatball ingredients and mix thoroughly with your hands. Using a 2-tablespoon cookie scoop, scoop up a portion of the meatball mixture and roll it into a ball, then repeat with the rest of the mixture. You should end up with approximately 16 meatballs.

- Heat the ¼ cup of oil over medium-high heat in a medium-sized sauté pan. Working in batches to avoiding overcrowding the pan, fry the meatballs until golden brown all over, about 5 minutes per batch. As the meatballs finish frying, add them to the simmering sauce.

- Once all the meatballs have been fried and added to the sauce, pour the frying oil into the sauce and stir well. Simmer, still over medium-low heat, until all the oil has been absorbed into the sauce, about 30 minutes. Plate and garnish with freshly grated Parmesan and a sprig of fresh basil, if desired.

- Store leftovers in an airtight container in the fridge for up to 1 week.

PER SERVING
Calories **552** · Fat **42g** · Total Carbs **10g** · Net Carbs **8g** · Fiber **2g** · Protein **46g**

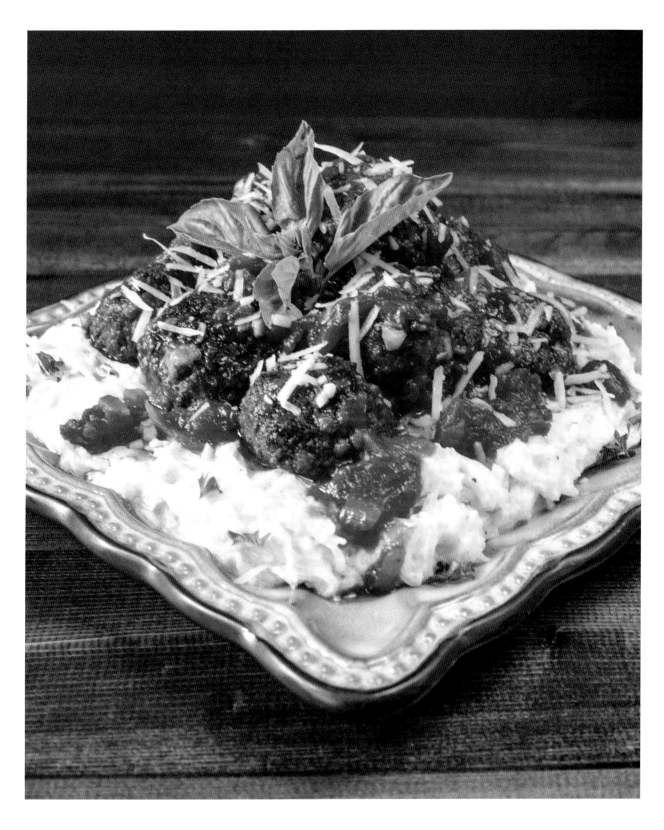

Switch It Up:

Substitute fresh grated Pecorino Romano or Parmigiano-Reggiano for the mozzarella in the meatballs for a sharp and robust flavor.

BBQ BACON MINI MEATLOAVES

HOUR or LESS

SERVES 4

Meatloaf is great, but mini meatloaves are oh-so-cute! These savory meatloaves are perfectly paired with sweet-and-spicy BBQ sauce and smoky bacon. You'll want to make extras for leftovers, trust me!

FOR THE MEATLOAF MIXTURE:

1½ teaspoons unsalted butter

½ cup crushed pork rinds

1 pound ground beef, 80% lean

½ cup diced onions

1 large egg

1 tablespoon dried parsley

1 teaspoon fine sea salt

½ teaspoon ground black pepper

½ teaspoon garlic powder

½ teaspoon paprika

4 strips bacon, cut in half crosswise

½ cup sugar-free barbecue sauce, homemade (page 66) or store-bought

• Preheat the oven to 350°F. Line a sheet pan with foil.

• Melt the butter in a skillet over medium-high heat and add the crushed pork rinds. Toast, stirring frequently, until golden brown, about 4 minutes. Transfer the toasted crumbs to a large bowl and set aside to cool for a few minutes.

• Once the crumbs are cool enough to handle, add the rest of the meatloaf ingredients and mix thoroughly with your hands. Form the mixture into 4 individual loaves and place them on the prepared sheet pan.

• Top each loaf with 2 half-strips of bacon and bake for 25 minutes, or until the internal temperature reaches 160°F. Position an oven rack directly under the broiler, turn on the broiler, and move the meatloaves to under the broiler. Broil for 3 to 5 minutes to crisp the bacon.

• Remove the meatloaves from the oven (leave the broiler on). Remove the crisped bacon from the loaves and set aside. Spread one-quarter of the barbecue sauce on top of each loaf, then return the loaves to the oven and broil for 2 to 3 minutes more, until the sauce is warmed and bubbly.

• Remove the loaves from the oven and place the bacon back on top before serving.

• Store leftovers in an airtight container in the fridge for up to 1 week.

PER SERVING
Calories **421** · Fat **32g** · Total Carbs **4g** · Net Carbs **4g** · Fiber **0g** · Protein **28g**

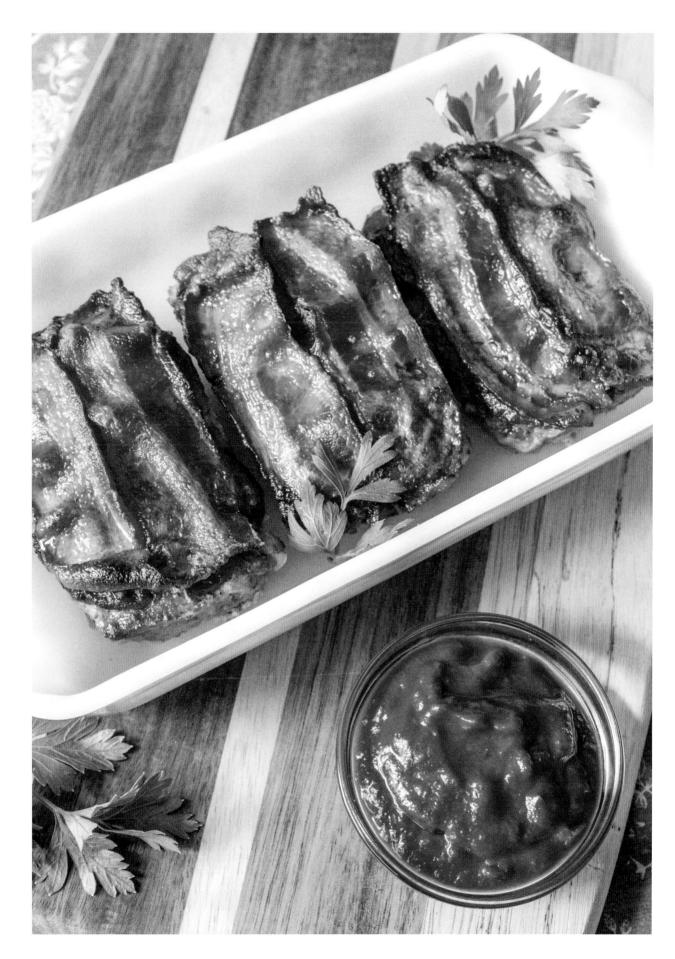

MONGOLIAN BEEF

MINUTES or LESS

SERVES 4

Asian dishes are my favorite, especially Mongolian beef. I love the rich and slightly sweet yet savory sauce and the tender pieces of beef—delicious! I highly recommend serving this atop my Cashew Fried Cauli Rice (page 192).

6 tablespoons light olive oil, divided

1½ pounds flank steak, thinly sliced against the grain, on the bias

Fine sea salt and ground black pepper

2 cloves garlic, minced

2 teaspoons grated ginger

FOR THE SAUCE:

2 tablespoons coconut aminos (see Note)

1 tablespoon soy sauce

1 tablespoon unseasoned rice vinegar

1 tablespoon water

½ teaspoon blended erythritol-stevia sweetener (see page 46)

4 scallions, cut on the bias into 3-inch-long pieces

Sliced scallions, for garnish (optional)

Note: I really recommend using coconut aminos in this recipe, but if you are unable to find them, add another tablespoon of soy sauce (2 tablespoons total) and ¼ teaspoon blended erythritol-stevia sweetener (¾ teaspoon total) in their place.

• Heat ¼ cup of the oil in a large heavy-bottomed saucepan or wok over medium-high heat. Season the beef with a pinch each of salt and pepper. Working in batches to avoid overcrowding the pan, sear the beef until golden brown on both sides, about 5 minutes per side. Using a slotted spoon, transfer the beef to a plate and set aside.

• While the beef is cooking, whisk together the sauce ingredients in a small bowl.

• Once all the beef is seared and out of the pot, turn the heat down to medium and pour in the remaining 2 tablespoons of oil. Add the garlic and ginger and cook, stirring constantly, until fragrant, about 2 minutes. Add the sauce and stir to combine. Simmer until the sauce has thickened, about 5 minutes, then return the meat and any juices back to the pan. Add the scallions and stir to combine. Cook until the scallions have wilted, about 3 minutes. Garnish with sliced scallions, if desired, and serve immediately.

• Store leftovers in an airtight container in the fridge for up to 1 week.

Variation: **SPICY MONGOLIAN BEEF**

Add a few whole dried red chili peppers or sliced fresh chili peppers with the garlic and ginger to make this spicy!

PER SERVING
Calories **463** · Fat **35g** · Total Carbs **3g** · Net Carbs **3g** · Fiber **0g** · Protein **36g**

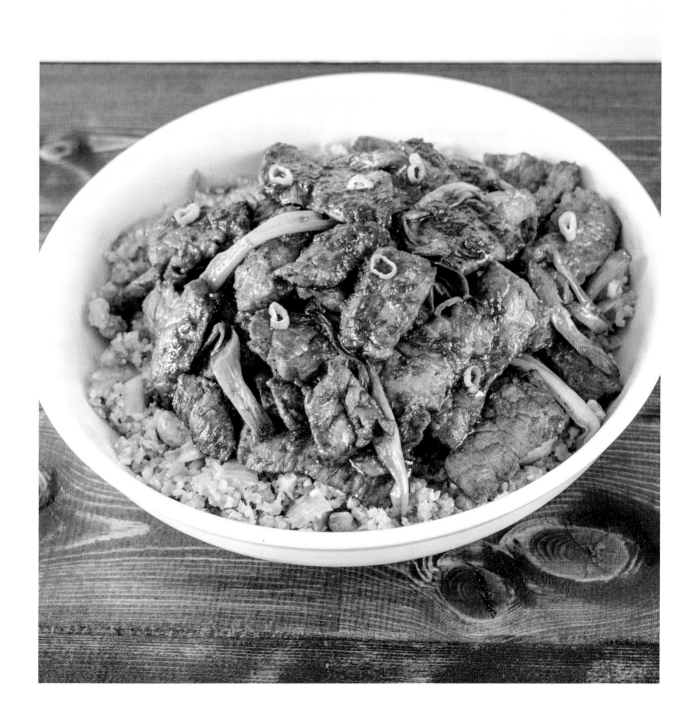

BEEF STROGANOFF

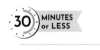

30 MINUTES or LESS

SERVES 4

As much as I love the tender chunks of beef in this rich and creamy sauce, I really think the buttered cabbage noodles steal the show. They add a touch of sweetness with a perfect al dente bite that pairs so well with the stroganoff.

FOR THE STROGANOFF:

1 tablespoon light olive oil

1 tablespoon unsalted butter

1 pound sirloin, cut into bite-sized pieces

¾ teaspoon fine sea salt, divided

¼ teaspoon ground black pepper

8 ounces white mushrooms, cleaned, stemmed, and quartered

1 medium shallot, thinly sliced

2 tablespoons cooking sherry

2 teaspoons Worcestershire sauce

½ cup beef stock

¼ cup heavy cream

FOR THE NOODLES:

2 tablespoons unsalted butter

1 small head cabbage, cut into long, thin strips

Chopped fresh parsley, for garnish (optional)

· Heat the oil and butter in a large heavy-bottomed sauté pan over medium-high heat. Season the sirloin with ½ teaspoon of the salt and the pepper. Add the sirloin to the pan and sear until golden brown on all sides, about 5 minutes. Transfer the seared meat to a plate and set aside.

· Add the mushrooms to the pan and sauté until brown, about 10 minutes. Add the shallot and the remaining ¼ teaspoon of the salt and stir to combine. Sauté for about 3 minutes, until the shallot is softened.

· Add the sherry and Worcestershire sauce and deglaze the pan, scraping up any browned pieces on the bottom. Pour in the beef stock and heavy cream and stir to combine. Return the meat to the pan, along with any juices. Turn the heat down to medium-low and simmer until the sauce thickens, about 10 minutes.

· While the stroganoff is simmering, make the noodles: Melt the butter in a large skillet and sauté the cabbage strips until tender-crisp, about 10 minutes.

· Divide the cabbage noodles evenly among 4 plates and spoon the stroganoff over the top. Garnish with chopped fresh parsley, if desired, and serve immediately.

· Store leftovers in an airtight container in the fridge for up to 1 week.

PER SERVING
Calories **409** · Fat **26g** · Total Carbs **15g** · Net Carbs **10g** · Fiber **5g** · Protein **27g**

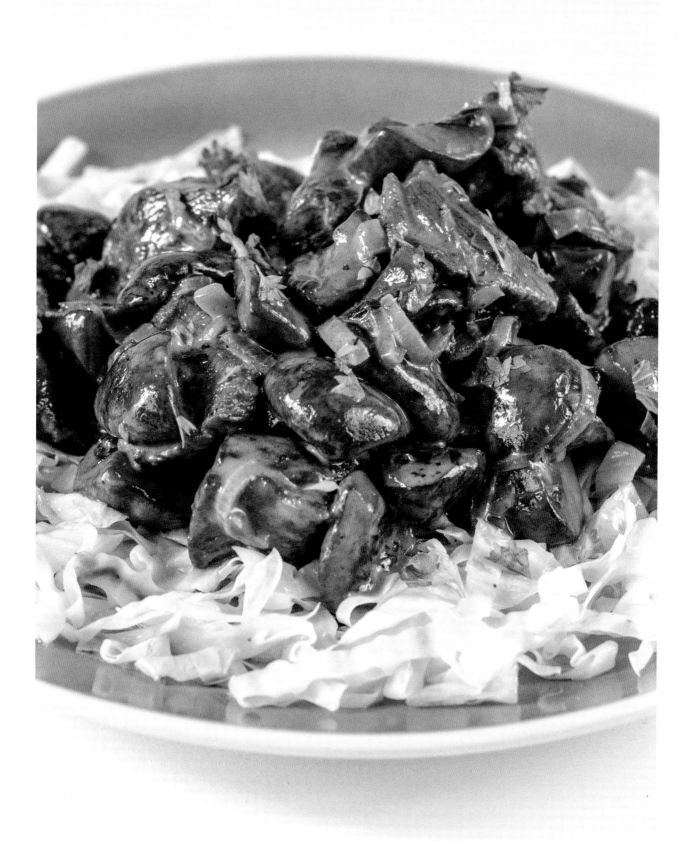

BARBACOA

SERVES 6

Oh, how I love barbacoa! This method of slow-cooking meat traditionally involves an underground oven, but it's equally delicious made in an ordinary oven. It's incredible served with taco-style toppings (you can even wrap it in a lettuce leaf for the full taco experience), but if you're like me, you'll eat it straight from the pot. I really love to serve this alongside or on top of my Cilantro Lime Cauli Rice (page 202).

2 tablespoons light olive oil or bacon grease

3 pounds boneless chuck roast

2 teaspoons fine sea salt

1 teaspoon ground black pepper

1 cup beef stock

Juice of 1 lime

1 tablespoon ancho chili powder

1 tablespoon ground cumin

2 teaspoons garlic powder

TOPPINGS (OPTIONAL):

Cilantro Chimichurri (page 70)

Fresh chopped cilantro

Sliced jalapeño

Sliced red onion

· Preheat the oven to 300°F.

· Heat the oil in a heavy-bottomed Dutch oven over medium-high heat. Season both sides of the chuck roast with the salt and pepper. Sear the chuck roast in the Dutch oven until it's browned on both sides, about 5 minutes per side.

· While the meat is cooking, in a medium-sized bowl, combine the beef stock, lime juice, and spices and whisk until well blended. Once the meat is browned, pour the mixture over the meat. Cover and transfer the Dutch oven to the oven.

· Roast until the meat is tender, about 3 hours. Once the meat shreds easily with a fork, remove it from the oven and shred it completely.

· You can serve the barbacoa just like this, but if you prefer it crispy, as I do, increase the oven temperature to 400°F, line a sheet pan with foil, and spread the shredded beef on the sheet pan. Place it in the oven and roast until the meat is crispy around the edges, about 10 minutes.

· To serve, top with cilantro, jalapeño slices, red onion slices, and sour cream, if desired.

· Store leftovers in an airtight container in the fridge for up to 1 week.

Note: This barbacoa is spectacular served in crispy cheese taco shells and piled high with your favorite toppings, especially my Cilantro Chimichurri (page 70).

To make crispy cheese taco shells, preheat the oven to 350°F and line a sheet pan with parchment paper. Place mounds of ¼ cup shredded cheese (any mild variety will do: cheddar, Jack, Colby, etc.) a few inches apart so they have room to spread. Bake until the edges are brown, about 5 minutes. Suspend a wooden spoon between 2 tall cups, hang the still-pliant cheese over the spoon, and allow the cheese to cool and harden for about 5 minutes to create a taco shell. The hot cheese can also be draped over other objects to form different shapes: for instance, place it over the bottom of a bowl to form a bowl or a small cup to form a cup.

PER SERVING
Calories **635** · Fat **48g** · Total Carbs **4g** · Net Carbs **4g** · Fiber **0g** · Protein **44g**

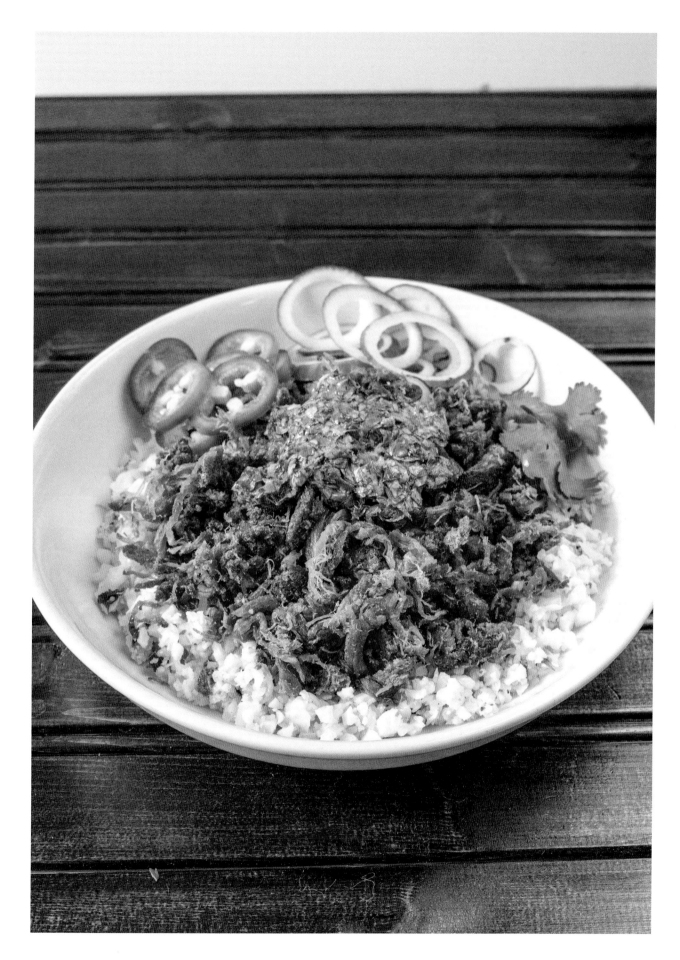

SALISBURY STEAK

SERVES 4

Salisbury steak is classic comfort food, and this recipe will fill you with nostalgic memories. Be sure to serve this over my Best-Ever Cauli Mash (page 188) for the full experience.

FOR THE STEAK:

1 tablespoon unsalted butter

½ cup crushed pork rinds

1 pound ground beef, 80% lean (see Note)

1 large egg

½ medium onion, diced

1 tablespoon Worcestershire sauce

1 teaspoon fine sea salt

¼ teaspoon ground black pepper

¼ teaspoon garlic powder

FOR THE GRAVY:

2 tablespoons unsalted butter

8 ounces sliced white mushrooms

2 tablespoons cooking sherry

1 teaspoon Worcestershire sauce

½ cup heavy cream

¼ teaspoon fine sea salt

Note : You can substitute ground turkey, chicken, pork, or even lamb for the ground beef if you like.

• Melt the butter in a medium-sized skillet over medium-high heat and add the crushed pork rinds. Toast, stirring frequently, until golden brown, about 4 minutes. Transfer the toasted crumbs to a large bowl to cool for about 5 minutes.

• Once the crumbs are cool enough to handle, add the rest of the steak ingredients to the bowl and mix thoroughly with your hands. Form the mixture into 4 equal-sized patties.

• Place the patties in a large heavy-bottomed skillet over medium-high heat. Sear the patties on both sides until golden brown, about 5 minutes per side. Transfer the seared patties to a plate, leaving the drippings in the pan.

• Make the gravy: Add the 2 tablespoons of butter to the drippings in the pan and melt over medium-high heat. Add the mushrooms and sauté, stirring occasionally, until soft and golden brown, about 10 minutes. Add the sherry and deglaze the pan, scraping up any browned bits from the bottom of the pan. Add the Worcestershire sauce, cream, and salt, stirring well to combine.

• Return the steak patties to the pan, along with any juices. Spoon the gravy over the patties and turn the heat down to medium. Simmer the patties in the gravy until their internal temperature reaches 160°F or no pink remains in the center, about 10 minutes. Transfer the patties to serving plates and spoon the gravy over the top. Serve immediately.

• Store leftovers in an airtight container in the fridge for up to 3 days.

PER SERVING
Calories **466** · Fat **36g** · Total Carbs **5g** · Net Carbs **4g** · Fiber **1g** · Protein **32g**

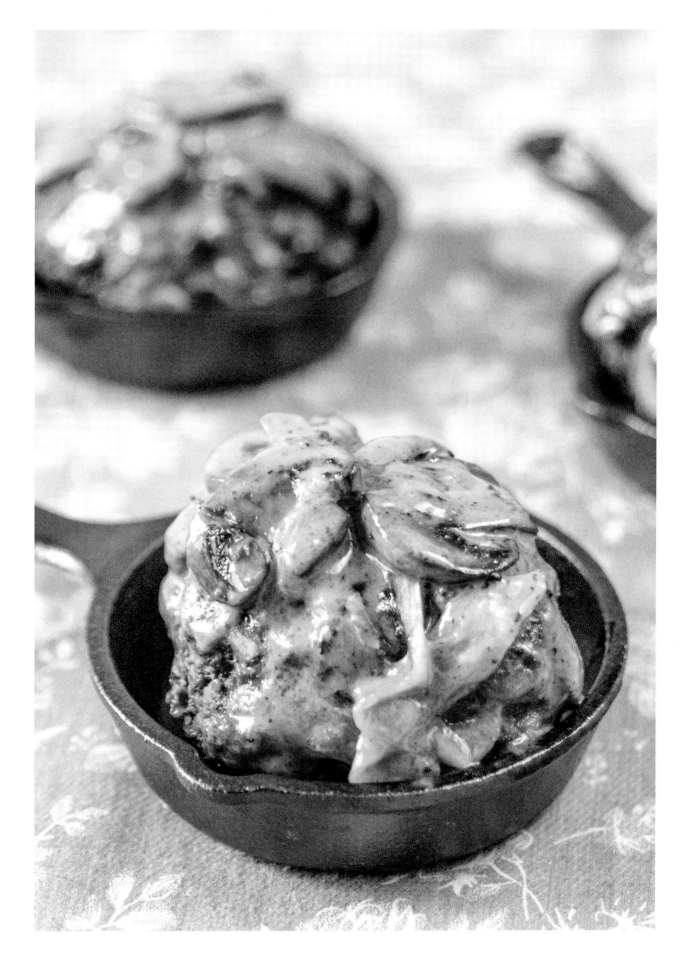

BOLOGNESE ZUCCHINI LASAGNA

SERVES 4

Mmm, lasagna! This recipe is so rich and cheesy, and the zucchini adds a nice light flavor and great texture to the dish, along with more nutrients. I always serve this with my Cheesy Garlic Butter Breadsticks (page 120).

3 large zucchini (see Notes)

1 tablespoon light olive oil

Fine sea salt and ground black pepper

FOR THE BOLOGNESE:

1 tablespoon light olive oil

1 small shallot, minced

1 clove garlic, minced

1 pound ground beef, 80% lean

1 teaspoon fine sea salt

½ teaspoon ground black pepper

2 cups sugar-free marinara (see Notes)

FOR THE RICOTTA LAYER:

1 cup whole-milk ricotta

2 tablespoons shredded Parmesan cheese

4 fresh basil leaves, chiffonaded

Pinch of fine sea salt

Pinch of ground black pepper

2 cups shredded mozzarella cheese

Notes : *Feel free to substitute summer squash for the zucchini; it works just as well.*

I always use Rao's brand marinara sauce for this recipe. It's full of flavor and has no added sugar!

- Preheat the oven to 350°F. Lightly grease an oven-safe 11 by 7-inch casserole dish.

- First, cook the zucchini: Trim the ends of the zucchini and cut them in half crosswise. Slice each half into 4 to 5 slices, each about ¼ inch thick. In a medium-sized bowl, toss the zucchini with the oil and season lightly with salt and pepper. Place the zucchini in a medium-sized sauté pan and cook over medium-high heat until lightly browned and slightly softened, about 3 minutes per side. Remove from the heat and set aside.

- Make the sauce: Heat the oil in a medium-sized saucepan over medium-high heat, add the shallot, and sauté until softened, about 3 minutes. Add the garlic and sauté, stirring occasionally, until fragrant, about 2 minutes. Add the ground beef, salt, and pepper and stir to combine. Cook until the ground beef is browned, about 7 minutes. Once the beef is browned, remove any excess grease with a large spoon. Add the marinara, turn the heat down to low, and simmer for 15 minutes, stirring occasionally.

- While the sauce simmers, combine all of the ingredients for the ricotta layer in a medium-sized bowl.

- Assemble the lasagna: Spoon about one-quarter of the sauce into the bottom of the casserole dish, then place half of the zucchini slices in a layer on top of the sauce. Spoon half of the ricotta mixture over the zucchini, then spoon another quarter of the sauce over the ricotta mixture. Sprinkle half of the mozzarella over the sauce. Repeat these layers once more—sauce, zucchini, ricotta, sauce, cheese. Bake until brown and bubbly, about 25 minutes.

- Store leftovers in an airtight container in the fridge for up to 1 week.

Variation : **ITALIAN SAUSAGE ZUCCHINI LASAGNA**

Replace the ground beef with 1 pound of bulk sweet or hot Italian sausage (see page 254) for a different flavor profile.

PER SERVING
Calories **620** · Fat **48g** · Total Carbs **13g** · Net Carbs **11g** · Fiber **2g** · Protein **44g**

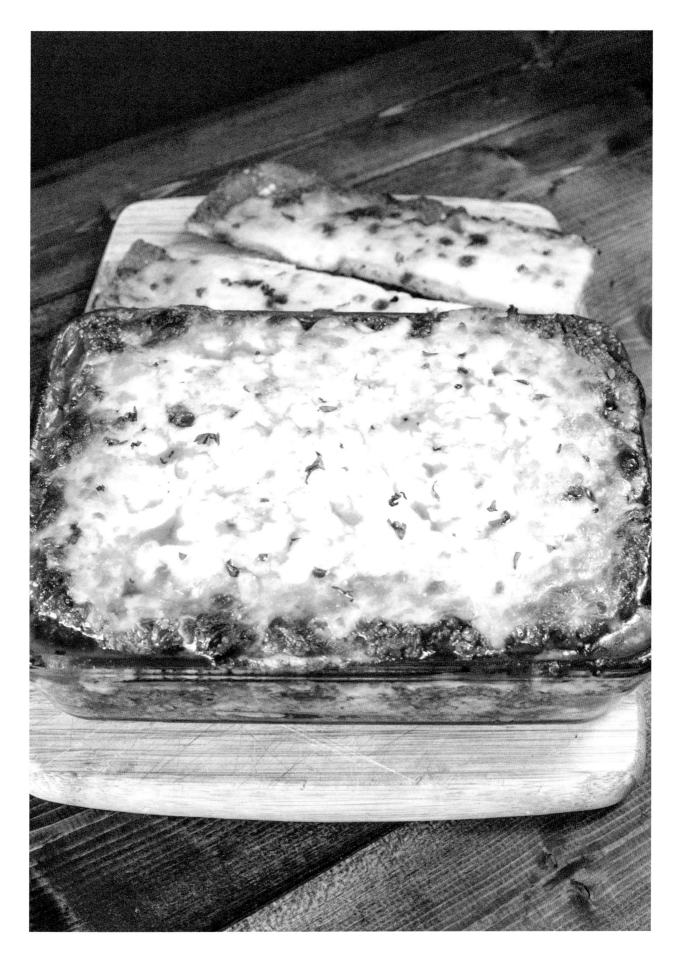

OVEN-ROASTED BEEF RIBS

OVER 2 HOURS

2+

SERVES 4

Pork ribs are great, but beef ribs are my favorite. I love the rich, meaty flavor they get after a long, slow roast in the oven. I always serve these with my Sweet Dijon Coleslaw (page 146), which perfectly balances the richness of the ribs.

2 racks beef short ribs (about 6 pounds)

¼ cup Smoky BBQ Rub (page 60)

1 cup Chipotle BBQ Sauce (page 66)

• Preheat the oven to 250°F.

• Line a large sheet pan with foil and place both racks of ribs on it. Massage each side of the ribs with 1 tablespoon of the spice rub. Cover the ribs tightly with foil and bake until the meat pulls away from the bone and is very tender, about 3½ hours.

• Remove the foil and brush the top of each rack with ½ cup of the BBQ sauce. Position an oven rack directly under the broiler and turn the oven to broil. Broil the ribs, uncovered, until the sauce bubbles and caramelizes, about 3 minutes. Serve immediately.

• Store leftovers in an airtight container in the fridge for up to 1 week.

Variation : **OVEN-ROASTED PORK RIBS**

Substitute pork ribs for the beef ribs for a milder and almost sweet flavor profile.

PER SERVING
Calories **562** · Fat **40g** · Total Carbs **7g** · Net Carbs **7g** · Fiber **0g** · Protein **45g**

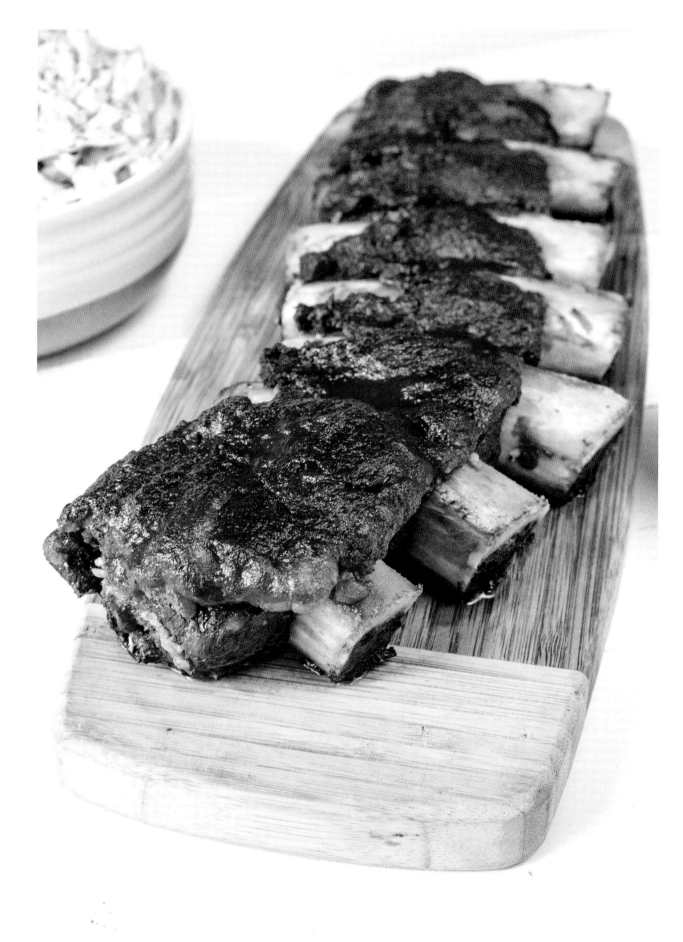

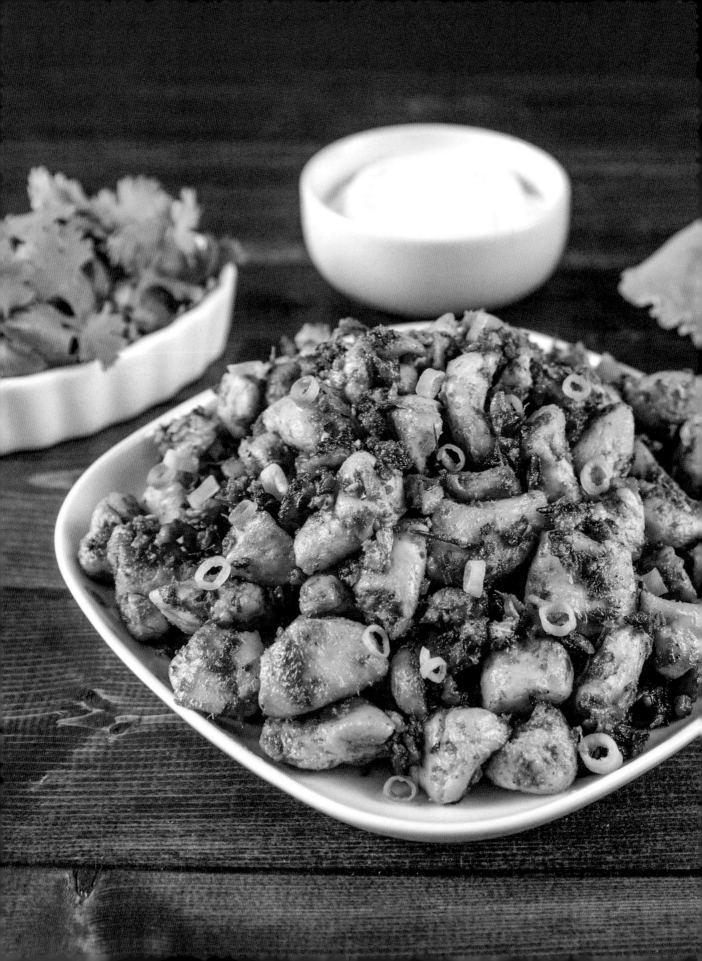

Poultry

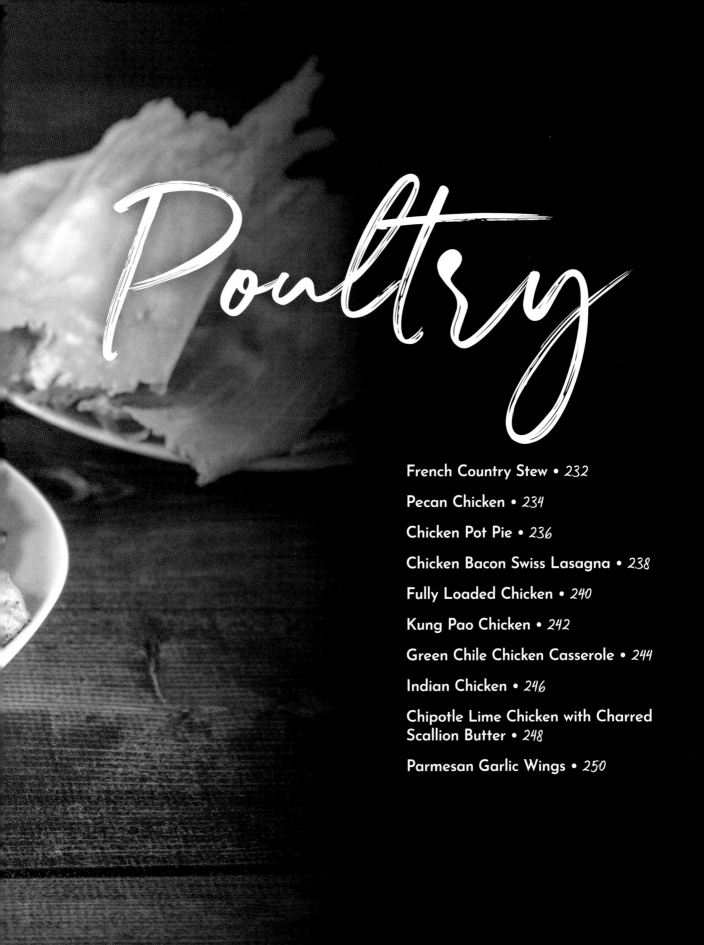

FRENCH COUNTRY STEW

1 HOUR or LESS

SERVES 4

This French-inspired dish is as impressive as it is delicious. It's my take on classic coq au vin, with different veggies and white wine instead of red. The chicken thighs are fall-off-the-bone tender from stewing in the luscious sauce. This is phenomenal served with my Cauli Risotto (page 184).

2 tablespoons bacon grease

8 bone-in chicken thighs

2 tablespoons unsalted butter

1 leek, cleaned (see page 41) and thinly sliced

2 stalks celery, halved lengthwise and sliced in ¼-inch pieces

1 medium carrot, halved lengthwise and sliced in ¼-inch pieces

1 teaspoon fine sea salt

1 cup dry white wine (see Notes)

1 cup chicken stock (see page 26)

Juice of ½ lemon

Chopped fresh parsley, for garnish (optional)

Notes : This tastes even better the next day!

If you'd prefer not to use wine, add ½ cup of chicken stock (for a total of 1½ cups).

• Heat the bacon grease in a heavy-bottomed Dutch oven over medium-high heat. Lightly season the chicken thighs with salt and pepper and add them to the pot, skin side down. Sear the chicken until golden brown, about 4 minutes, then flip them to sear the other side, about 4 minutes more. Use a slotted spoon to transfer the chicken thighs to a plate and set aside. Do not wash the pan.

• Add the butter to the chicken drippings in the pan and allow it to melt, then add the leek and stir to coat it in the butter. Sauté, stirring occasionally, for 3 minutes, then add the celery and carrot. Sauté for 3 minutes more, or until softened. Add the salt, then add the wine and deglaze the pan, scraping up the browned bits from the bottom. Simmer until the wine is reduced by half, about 10 minutes.

• Pour in the chicken stock, stir, and return the chicken thighs and their juices back to the pot, skin side up. Turn the heat down to medium-low and cover. Simmer for 30 minutes, then add the lemon juice. Simmer, uncovered, until the sauce has thickened, about 10 minutes. Divide among 4 bowls, garnish with chopped fresh parsley, if desired, and serve immediately.

• Store leftovers in an airtight container in the fridge for up to 1 week.

Variation : KETO COQ AU VIN

Use red wine instead of white for a richer and more robust flavor profile—one that's closer to classic coq au vin.

PER SERVING
Calories **687** · Fat **52g** · Total Carbs **5g** · Net Carbs **4g** · Fiber **1g** · Protein **35g**

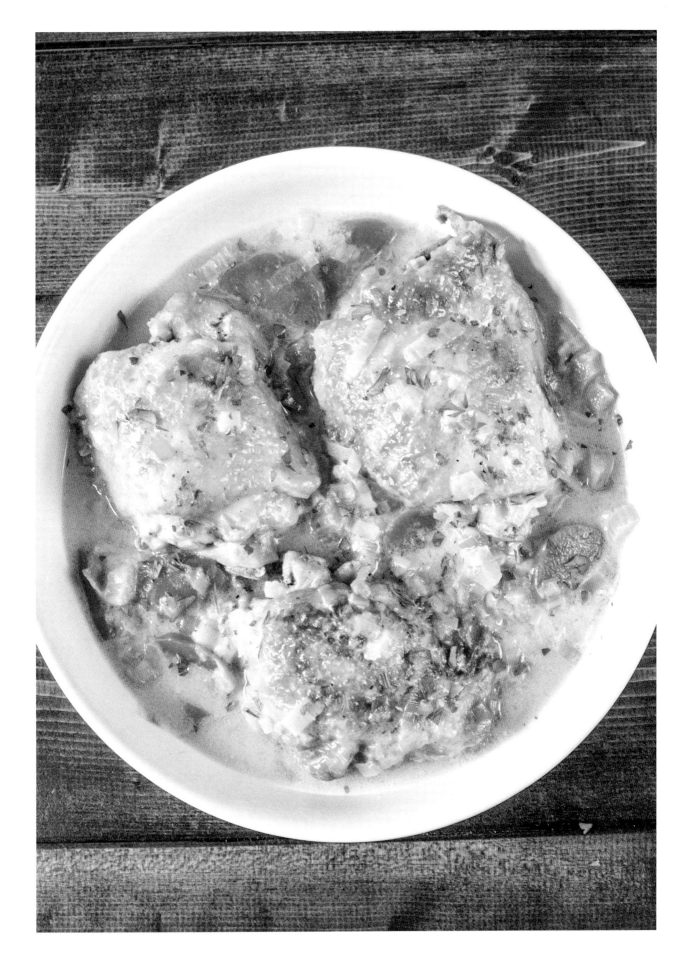

PECAN CHICKEN

30 MINUTES or LESS

SERVES 4

This is a dish that my mom made for me when I got home from the hospital from having my son, and I instantly fell in love! I actually begged her to make it three times in a single week, and when I transitioned to keto, it was one of the first things that I made keto-friendly because I can't live without it. Once you try this moist chicken in a crispy coating with an incredible toasted nutty flavor, you'll see why! This dish is wonderful served with my Best-Ever Cauli Mash (page 188) and Crispy Shallot & Bacon Asparagus (page 180).

2 large boneless, skinless chicken breasts (about 1 pound total), trimmed of fat (see Notes)

FOR THE BREADING:

¾ cup chopped raw pecans

¾ cup crushed pork rinds

½ cup grated Parmesan cheese

1 tablespoon dried dill weed

1 teaspoon garlic powder

1 teaspoon ground black pepper

FOR THE EGG WASH:

1 large egg

Splash of heavy cream

Pinch of fine sea salt

Pinch of ground black pepper

½ cup light olive oil, for frying

Chopped fresh parsley, for garnish (optional)

Notes: If the chicken is less than 1 pound, use 3 breasts to get as close to that weight as possible.

To avoid batter buildup on your fingers, use one hand to dip the chicken cutlets in the egg and the other hand to bread them.

• Slice both chicken breasts lengthwise in thirds to make 6 thin cutlets. This will allow the chicken to cook perfectly so the breading doesn't burn.

• In a medium-sized bowl, mix together all of the breading ingredients until well combined, then pour the mixture onto a large plate. In a shallow bowl, whisk together the egg wash ingredients.

• Heat the oil in a large sauté pan over medium-high heat.

• While the oil heats, bread the chicken: Dip a chicken cutlet into the egg wash and then into the breading. Using clean hands, scoop the breading over the cutlet and press down, then flip the cutlet over and repeat on the other side to ensure that the chicken is well covered. Set the breaded chicken aside on a large plate. Repeat with the remaining cutlets.

• To test the oil temperature, sprinkle in a few pork rind crumbs; if they sizzle, it's ready. Working in batches to avoid overcrowding the pan, shallow-fry the breaded chicken cutlets until golden brown on both sides and the internal temperature reaches 165°F, about 5 minutes per side. Transfer the chicken to a paper towel–lined plate and sprinkle with salt.

• If you have breading left over, fry it in the oil until crispy, about 5 minutes, and transfer it to a plate to cool. Once it's cool, sprinkle the crispy breading over the chicken; it's delicious!

• Garnish with chopped fresh parsley before serving, if desired.

• Store leftovers in an airtight container in the fridge for up to 1 week.

PER SERVING
Calories **655** · Fat **57g** · Total Carbs **4g** · Net Carbs **2g** · Fiber **2g** · Protein **36g**

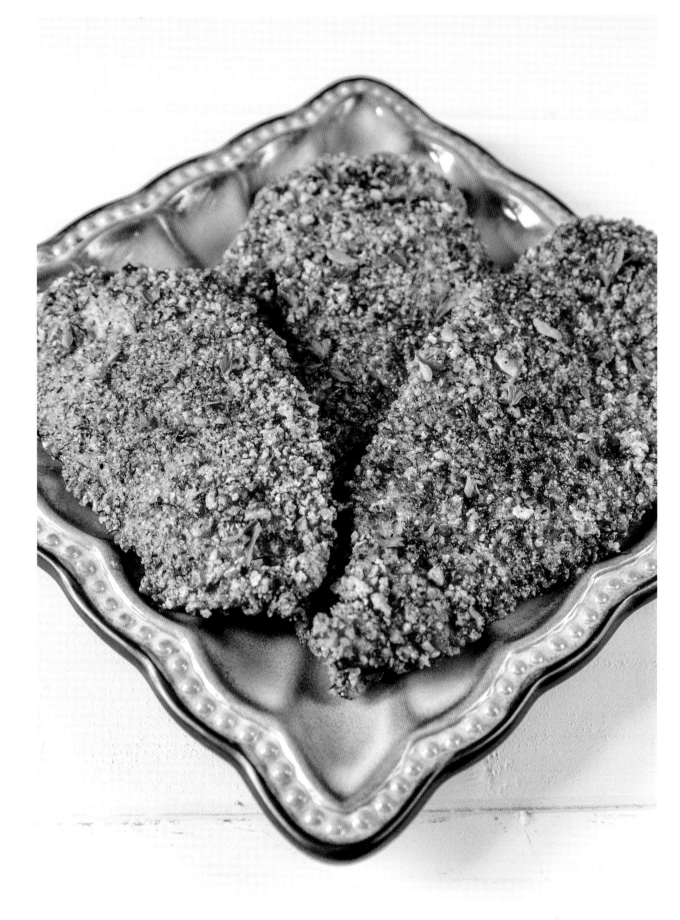

CHICKEN POT PIE

 30 MINUTES or LESS

SERVES 4

In this rich and creamy chicken dish, I've used my Best-Ever Cauli Mash (page 188) as a topping in place of the traditional high-carb pie crust. You'll never miss it!

¼ cup (½ stick) unsalted butter

2 stalks celery, cut into ¼-inch pieces

1 medium zucchini, chopped

1 large carrot, shredded

1 cup frozen pearl onions

1 teaspoon fine sea salt

1 pound cooked boneless, skinless chicken breasts, shredded

FOR THE SAUCE:

1 cup chicken stock (see page 26)

4 ounces cream cheese (½ cup), room temperature

½ cup heavy cream

1 teaspoon fine sea salt

½ teaspoon ground black pepper

2 cups Best-Ever Cauli Mash (page 188), for topping

- Preheat the oven to 350°F.

- Melt the butter in a sauté pan over medium heat and add the celery. Sauté for 2 minutes, until slightly softened, then add the zucchini, carrot, pearl onions, and salt and stir well to combine. Sauté for 3 minutes, until the veggies are softened and the onions are thawed, then stir in the chicken. Remove from the heat.

- Make the sauce: Place all the sauce ingredients in a small saucepan over medium heat and whisk together until smooth. Simmer the sauce until it has thickened and reduced slightly, about 10 minutes.

- Once the sauce has thickened, pour the sauce into the pan with the chicken and veggies and mix to combine, then spoon the mixture into a 9 by 9-inch baking dish or 4 ramekins and top with the cauli mash.

- Bake until the casserole is heated through and the top is golden brown, about 15 minutes. Serve immediately.

- Store leftovers in an airtight container in the fridge for up to 1 week.

PER SERVING
Calories **554** · Fat **44g** · Total Carbs **12g** · Net Carbs **9g** · Fiber **3g** · Protein **29g**

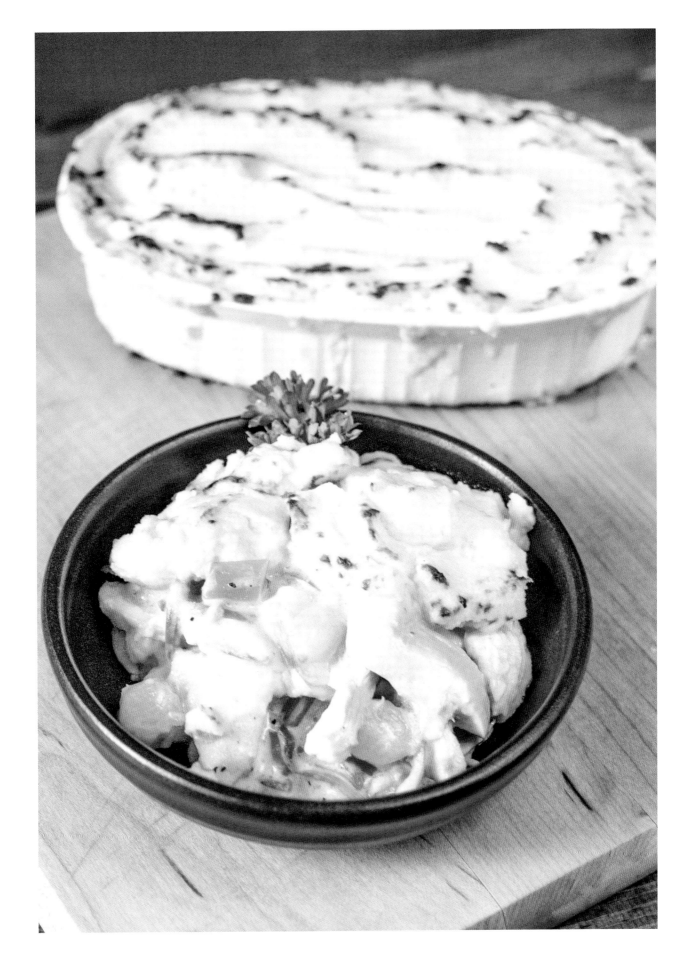

CHICKEN BACON SWISS LASAGNA

SERVES 4

This is one of those recipes where you'll be amazed at just how delicious it is. Everyone who has tried it has absolutely adored it. Seared zucchini layered with chicken and bacon, then covered in a rich and creamy Swiss cheese sauce—does it get any better than that?

5 slices bacon, cut into 1-inch pieces

2 large cooked boneless, skinless chicken breasts, shredded

½ teaspoon fine sea salt

¼ teaspoon garlic powder

¼ teaspoon ground black pepper

2 large zucchini (see Note)

1 tablespoon light olive oil

FOR THE SAUCE:

1 cup heavy cream

4 ounces cream cheese (½ cup), room temperature

3 cups shredded Swiss cheese (reserve ½ cup for the top)

½ teaspoon fine sea salt

¼ teaspoon ground black pepper

Note : Feel free to substitute 2 large summer squash for the zucchini; it works just as well. You want about 1½ pounds total.

- Preheat the oven to 350°F and grease a 9 by 5-inch loaf pan.

- Heat a medium-sized skillet over medium-high heat and drop in the bacon pieces. Cook the bacon until it's brown and crispy, about 10 minutes. Using a slotted spoon, transfer the crisped bacon to a paper towel–lined plate and set aside.

- To the bacon drippings in the pan, add the chicken, salt, garlic powder, and pepper, stirring well to combine. Sauté until the chicken is warmed through, about 5 minutes. Remove the pan from the heat and set aside.

- Trim the zucchini and slice them in half crosswise. Slice each half into 4 or 5 slices, each about ¼ inch thick. Toss the zucchini slices with the oil in a medium-sized bowl and season with a sprinkle of salt and pepper. In a medium-sized sauté pan over medium-high heat, sear the zucchini on both sides until lightly browned and slightly softened, about 3 minutes per side. Remove from the heat and set aside.

- Make the sauce: Pour the heavy cream into a saucepan over medium heat, then add the cream cheese. Whisk until smooth, then whisk in 2½ cups of the Swiss cheese, the salt, and the pepper. Cook, whisking continuously, until the sauce is bubbly and starts to thicken, about 5 minutes, then remove the saucepan from the heat.

- Place a layer of zucchini on the bottom of the prepared loaf pan, then add a layer of chicken, a layer of bacon, and a layer of sauce. Repeat these layers with the remaining components, reserving a little bacon for garnish, and top with the reserved Swiss cheese. Bake until the top is bubbly and browned, about 25 minutes. Remove from the oven and sprinkle with the reserved bacon. Slice and serve immediately.

- Store leftovers in an airtight container in the fridge for up to 1 week.

Variation : CHICKEN BACON CHEDDAR LASAGNA

Try using different cheese, like sharp cheddar or pepper Jack, for a sharper or spicy flavor profile.

PER SERVING
Calories **840** · Fat **66g** · Total Carbs **11g** · Net Carbs **9g** · Fiber **2g** · Protein **56g**

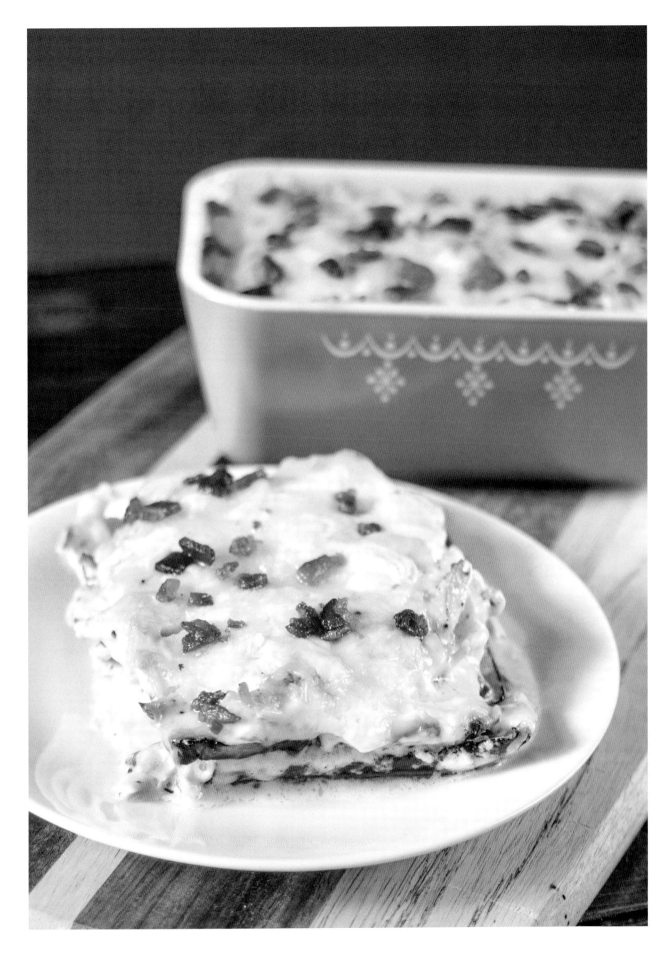

FULLY LOADED CHICKEN

1 HOUR or LESS

SERVES 4

If something is good, it's even better fully loaded, right? This chicken brings together bacon, butter, cheese, and mushrooms for a rich, filling dish. I love it because it's quick and easy as well as delicious. Be sure to have my Bloom Sauce (page 68) to dip the loaded chicken in; it takes it to a whole other level!

2 large boneless, skinless chicken breasts

1 tablespoon plus 1 teaspoon Smoky BBQ Rub (page 60)

4 slices thick-cut bacon

1 small onion, sliced

2 tablespoons unsalted butter, divided

8 ounces button mushrooms, sliced

Pinch of fine sea salt

1 cup shredded Colby Jack cheese

¼ cup plus 2 tablespoons Bloom Sauce (page 68), for serving

• Preheat the oven to 425°F and line a sheet pan with aluminum foil.

• Slice the chicken breasts in half lengthwise to form 4 cutlets. Season each cutlet with 1 teaspoon of the spice rub and set aside.

• Cook the bacon in a medium-sized skillet over medium-high heat until crispy, about 10 minutes. Using a slotted spoon, transfer the bacon to a paper towel–lined plate and set aside.

• Add the onion to the bacon drippings in the skillet and sauté until softened and lightly browned, about 5 minutes. Transfer the onion to a plate and set aside.

• In the same skillet, still over medium-high heat, melt 1 tablespoon of the butter. Add the mushrooms and sauté until golden brown, about 10 minutes. Season with the salt, stir, and transfer the mushrooms to the plate with the onion.

• Melt the remaining tablespoon of butter in the skillet. Add the chicken cutlets and sear until golden brown on both sides, 3 to 4 minutes per side. Place the seared chicken on the prepared sheet pan and top each cutlet with 1 slice of bacon broken in half. Spoon the mushrooms and onion slices evenly over the chicken cutlets, on top of the bacon. Top each cutlet with ¼ cup of cheese.

• Bake for 10 minutes, or until the cheese is melted and the chicken's internal temperature reaches 165°F. Serve immediately with the sauce on the side for dipping.

• Store leftovers in an airtight container in the fridge for up to 1 week.

Variation: PIZZA SUPREME CHICKEN

Substitute 24 slices of pepperoni for the bacon, 1 small bell pepper for the onion, 8 ounces of canned sliced black olives for the mushrooms, and 1 cup shredded mozzarella for the Colby Jack cheese. Use no-sugar-added marinara for the dipping sauce.

PER SERVING
Calories **430** · Fat **32g** · Total Carbs **7g** · Net Carbs **6g** · Fiber **1g** · Protein **26g**

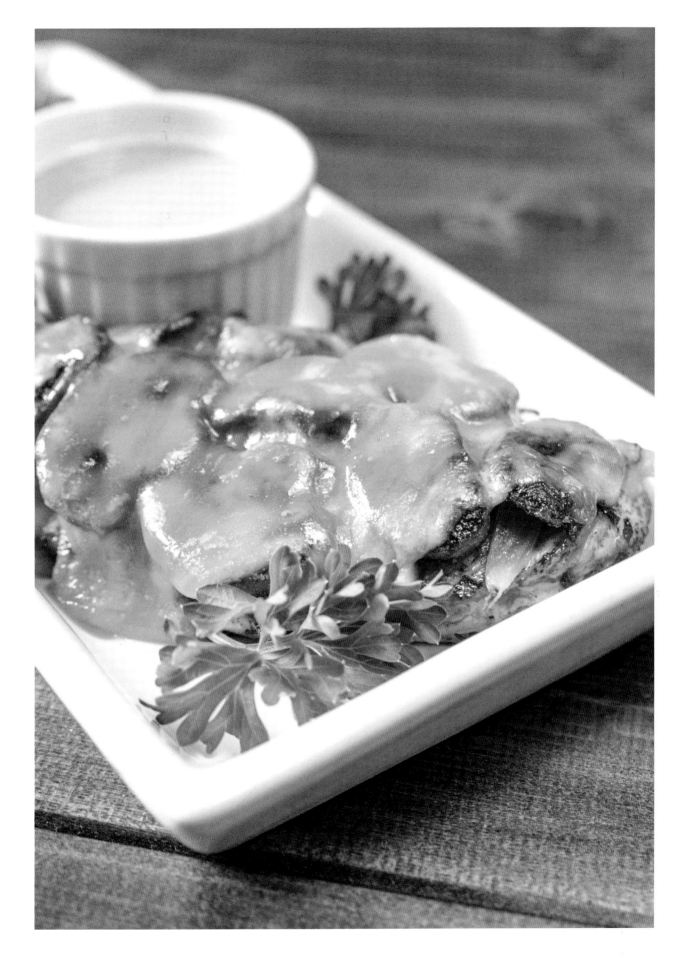

KUNG PAO CHICKEN

30 MINUTES or LESS

SERVES 4

Tender chunks of chicken in a light sweet-and-savory sauce along with crunchy peanuts and a touch of spice—you can't beat kung pao chicken! My Cashew Fried Cauli Rice (page 192) goes really well with this recipe.

FOR THE MARINADE:

1 tablespoon soy sauce

2 teaspoons cooking sherry

¼ teaspoon fine sea salt

⅛ teaspoon ground white pepper

1½ pounds boneless, skinless chicken breasts, cut into bite-sized pieces

FOR THE SAUCE:

1 tablespoon balsamic vinegar

1 teaspoon coconut aminos

1 teaspoon soy sauce or tamari

½ teaspoon blended erythritol-stevia sweetener (see page 46)

½ teaspoon ground Szechuan pepper (see Note, page 260)

¼ cup plus 2 tablespoons light olive oil, divided

4 dried red chili peppers (see Note)

2 cloves garlic, minced

2 teaspoons grated ginger

2 scallions, sliced, green and white parts separated

⅓ cup unsalted roasted peanuts

Note: For less heat, replace the chili peppers with a red bell pepper cut into large chunks.

- In a large bowl, combine all of the ingredients for the marinade and stir well to combine. Add the chicken and stir to coat, then set aside to marinate for a few minutes while you make the sauce.

- In a medium-sized bowl, whisk together the sauce ingredients. Set aside.

- Heat ¼ cup of the oil in a large skillet or wok over medium-high heat. Add the chicken and sauté, stirring constantly, until the chicken is about halfway cooked, about 5 minutes. Transfer the chicken to a plate and set aside.

- Add the remaining 2 tablespoons of oil to the pan. Add the chili peppers, garlic, and ginger and sauté until fragrant, about 2 minutes. Add the white parts of the scallions and the sauce, turn the heat down to medium, and simmer until the mixture starts to thicken, about 3 minutes.

- Return the chicken and any juices on the plate to the pan and stir well to coat the chicken in the sauce. Cook until the chicken is cooked through, about 5 minutes. Remove the pan from the heat and stir in the peanuts. Garnish with the reserved green parts of the scallions before serving.

- Store leftovers in an airtight container in the fridge for up to 1 week.

PER SERVING
Calories **384** · Fat **28g** · Total Carbs **3g** · Net Carbs **2g** · Fiber **1g** · Protein **34g**

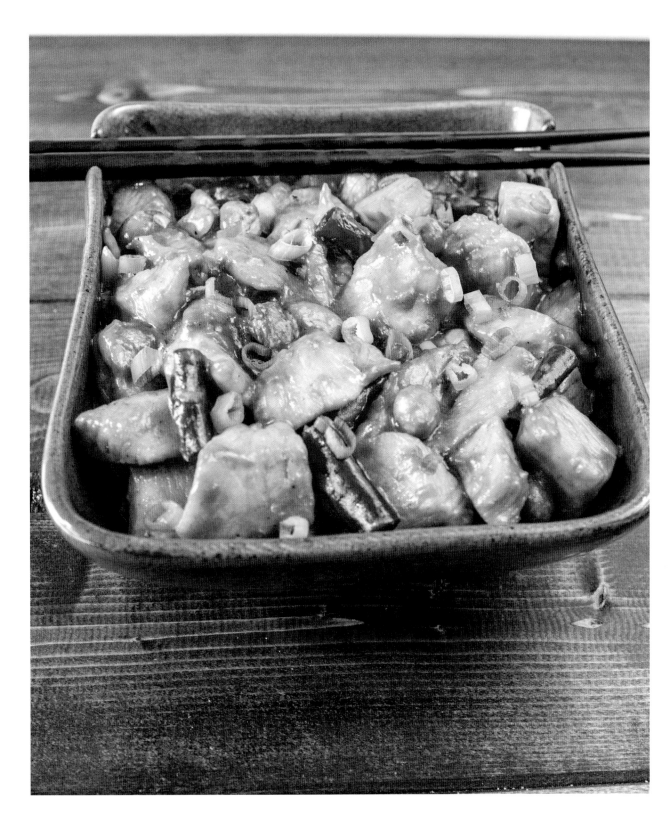

GREEN CHILE CHICKEN CASSEROLE

SERVES 4

This rich casserole is a crowd-pleaser! Everyone who has tried it has asked for the recipe, and my kids beg for it weekly. It has a gentle heat and is full of smoky flavor.

6 medium Anaheim peppers

FOR THE CHICKEN:

2 tablespoons unsalted butter

½ cup diced white onions

1½ pounds cooked boneless, skinless chicken breast, shredded

½ teaspoon fine sea salt

¼ teaspoon garlic powder

¼ teaspoon smoked paprika

FOR THE SAUCE:

2 tablespoons unsalted butter

4 jalapeño peppers, seeded and minced

4 ounces cream cheese (½ cup)

½ cup heavy cream

½ teaspoon fine sea salt

½ teaspoon smoked paprika

¼ teaspoon garlic powder

¼ teaspoon ground white pepper

2 cups shredded Monterey Jack cheese

Note: You can easily make one large casserole by greasing a 9 by 9-inch casserole dish and layering the ingredients as instructed. The bake time stays the same.

- Place an oven rack directly under the broiler, turn the oven to the broil setting, and line a sheet pan with aluminum foil.

- Place the Anaheim peppers on the lined sheet pan and set it directly under the broiler. Broil the peppers until the skin blackens and blisters on all sides, about 10 minutes, flipping the peppers as needed. Remove the peppers from the oven and place them in a medium-sized bowl, then cover the bowl tightly with plastic wrap. The peppers will steam in the bowl, causing the skin to loosen. After 15 minutes, remove and discard the outer skin, seeds, and stems. Slice the Anaheim peppers into long strips and set aside.

- Preheat the oven to 350°F. Grease four 8-ounce ramekins.

- Make the chicken: Melt the butter in a medium-sized saucepan over medium-high heat. Add the onions and sauté, stirring occasionally, until softened and translucent, about 5 minutes. Add the chicken, salt, garlic powder, and paprika and stir to combine. Sauté for a few minutes to heat through, then transfer the chicken and onions to a plate.

- Make the sauce: Melt the butter in the pot, still over medium-high heat. Add the jalapeños and sauté until they just start to brown, about 5 minutes. Whisk in the rest of the sauce ingredients. Turn the heat down to medium-low and simmer for 5 minutes, then remove from the heat.

- Assemble the casserole: Divide one-third of the chicken mixture among the prepared ramekins. Layer on one-third of the Anaheim peppers, again divided equally among the ramekins, then spoon one-third of the sauce on top. Divide ⅔ cup of the cheese among the ramekins. Repeat all layers in this order— chicken, peppers, sauce, cheese—twice more

- Bake for 25 minutes, or until the top is bubbly.

- Store leftovers in an airtight container in the fridge for up to 1 week.

PER SERVING

Calories **714** · Fat **53g** · Total Carbs **12g** · Net Carbs **11g** · Fiber **1g** · Protein **51g**

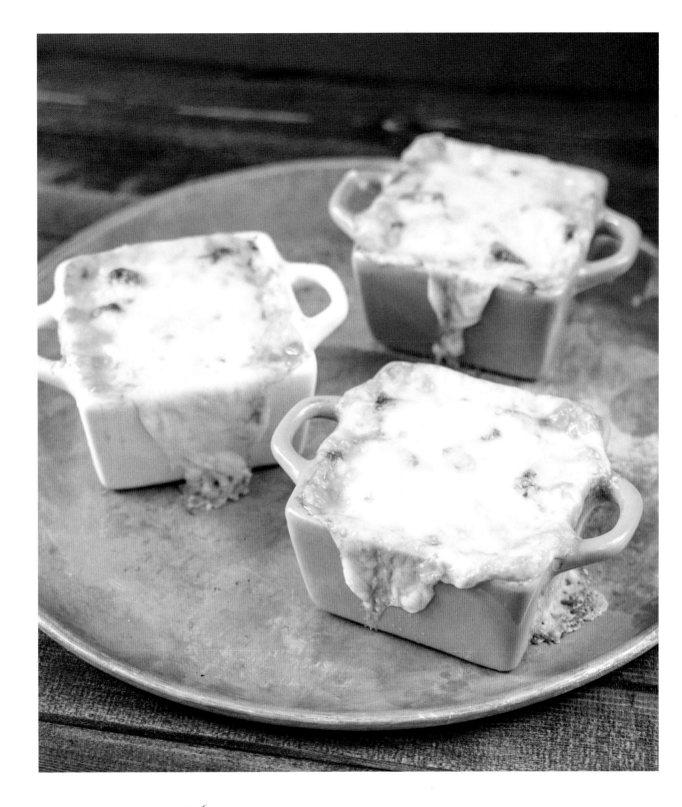

Variation: GREEN CHILE CHICKEN STUFFED PEPPERS

Prepare all the components as instructed, but instead of layering the ingredients in a casserole dish, mix everything together in a large bowl. Core and seed 4 bell peppers and stuff them with the casserole mixture. Bake in a preheated 350°F oven for 25 minutes, or until the tops are lightly browned and bubbly.

INDIAN CHICKEN

SERVES 4

A dear friend showed me how to make this dish years ago, and she didn't measure anything. Over the years I have figured out amounts that work consistently, and let me tell you, it is glorious! It's got the most incredible depth of flavor, and the heat can be tailored to your taste—my friend's would light your mouth on fire, but this version has a very gentle heat. Simply double or even triple the cayenne pepper for a spicier dish.

FOR THE GINGER GARLIC PASTE:

4 cloves garlic, peeled

1 (2-inch) piece of fresh ginger, peeled and roughly chopped

2 teaspoons light olive oil

FOR THE MARINADE:

½ teaspoon fine sea salt

½ teaspoon turmeric powder

¼ teaspoon cayenne pepper

Half of the ginger garlic paste (from above)

1½ pounds boneless, skinless chicken breasts, cut into bite-sized pieces

6 tablespoons light olive oil, divided

6 whole cloves

½ teaspoon ground cinnamon

1 small onion, diced

1 large Roma tomato, diced

1 teaspoon ground coriander

½ teaspoon fine sea salt

½ teaspoon turmeric powder

¼ teaspoon cayenne pepper

Sliced scallions, for garnish

FOR SERVING:

1 head iceberg lettuce, leaves separated

Chopped fresh cilantro

Full-fat sour cream

· Place all the ginger garlic paste ingredients in a small food processor and pulse until they form a smooth paste. Set aside.

· In a large bowl, combine all of the marinade ingredients. Add the chicken and stir well to coat it in the marinade. Cover and set aside to marinate on the counter for 30 minutes.

· While the chicken is marinating, heat ¼ cup of the oil in a large skillet over medium-high heat. Add the cloves and cinnamon and toast, stirring frequently, for about 2 minutes. Remove the cloves and discard. Add the onion to the fragrant oil and sauté until softened, about 5 minutes. Add the remaining half of the ginger garlic paste, stirring to combine. Sauté until fragrant, about 2 minutes, then add the tomato, ground coriander, salt, turmeric, and cayenne, stirring well. Turn the heat down to medium and continue to cook for an additional 5 minutes, stirring occasionally.

· While the veggie mixture is cooking, heat the remaining 2 tablespoons of oil in another skillet over medium-high heat. Add the marinated chicken and sauté until golden brown and cooked through, about 10 minutes. Transfer the cooked chicken to the veggie mixture and stir well to coat.

· Continue cooking, stirring occasionally, until the veggie mixture turns from pale yellow to reddish brown, 15 to 20 minutes. Garnish with sliced scallions and serve with lettuce leaves for wrapping and cilantro and sour cream for topping.

· Store leftovers in an airtight container in the fridge for up to 1 week.

Note: For the ginger garlic paste, if you don't have a food processor, you can mince the garlic and grate the ginger, omitting the oil. But making the paste with a food processor gives you even more flavor because each ingredient is broken down more.

PER SERVING
Calories **454** · Fat **33g** · Total Carbs **7g** · Net Carbs **5g** · Fiber **2g** · Protein **35g**

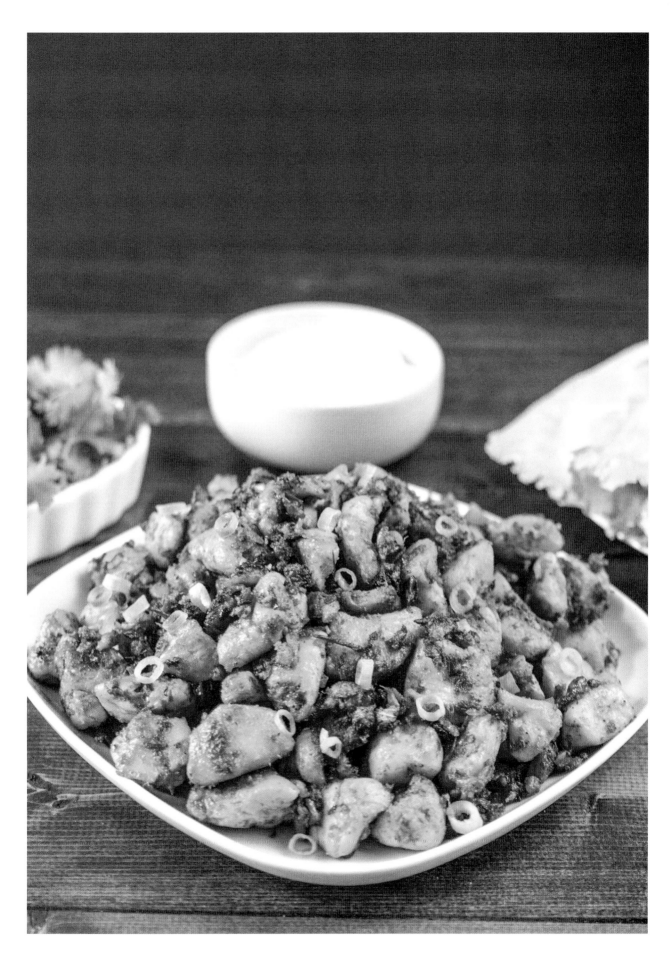

CHIPOTLE LIME CHICKEN *with* CHARRED SCALLION BUTTER

1 HOUR or LESS

+ TIME TO REST

SERVES 4

I have met quite a few people who have never had split chicken breasts, which come with the breastbone intact and skin still on. I love getting chicken breasts this way because you get the yummy skin, and cooking the breasts on the bone keeps them so tender and juicy—plus, you can use the bones for stock (see page 26). A huge bonus is that these are really cheap on sale! Win-win-win!

FOR THE CHICKEN:

2½ teaspoons lime juice

2 teaspoons grated lime zest

1 teaspoon fine sea salt

½ teaspoon chili powder

½ teaspoon chipotle powder

½ teaspoon garlic powder

¼ teaspoon ground black pepper

½ teaspoon smoked paprika

4 bone-in, skin-on split chicken breasts

FOR THE CHARRED SCALLION BUTTER:

4 scallions

½ cup (1 stick) unsalted butter, softened

2 teaspoons lime juice

1 teaspoon grated lime zest

¼ teaspoon chipotle powder

¼ teaspoon fine sea salt

¼ teaspoon ground black pepper

Note: This recipe will also work great with bone-in chicken thighs instead of breasts; just reduce the cook time to about 35 minutes.

• Preheat the oven to 400°F and line a sheet pan with aluminum foil.

• In a small bowl, mix all of the chicken seasonings into a paste. Slide your fingers carefully under the skin of the chicken breasts just to loosen it from the meat; do not remove the skin. Rub the seasoning paste under the skin of each breast, directly onto the meat. Try not to get any of the paste onto the outer skin, as it will burn during cooking.

• Place the chicken on the lined sheet pan, skin side up, and set it aside for 20 minutes to allow the seasonings to soak into the meat. After 20 minutes, put the chicken in the oven and roast until the skin is crispy and the internal temperature reaches 160°F, about 45 minutes.

• While the chicken is roasting, make the scallion butter: Heat a skillet over medium-high heat. Place the scallions in the pan and cook until they are starting to char all over, about 5 minutes, turning frequently for even charring. Remove the scallions from the skillet and set aside to cool.

• In a medium-sized bowl, whisk together the butter, lime juice and zest, chipotle powder, salt, and pepper until thoroughly combined. Mince the scallions and stir them into the butter mixture. Cover and leave on the counter until time to serve.

• Serve each split chicken breast with a scoop of the scallion butter.

• Store leftovers in an airtight container in the fridge for up to 1 week.

PER SERVING
Calories **473** · Fat **29g** · Total Carbs **2g** · Net Carbs **1g** · Fiber **1g** · Protein **49g**

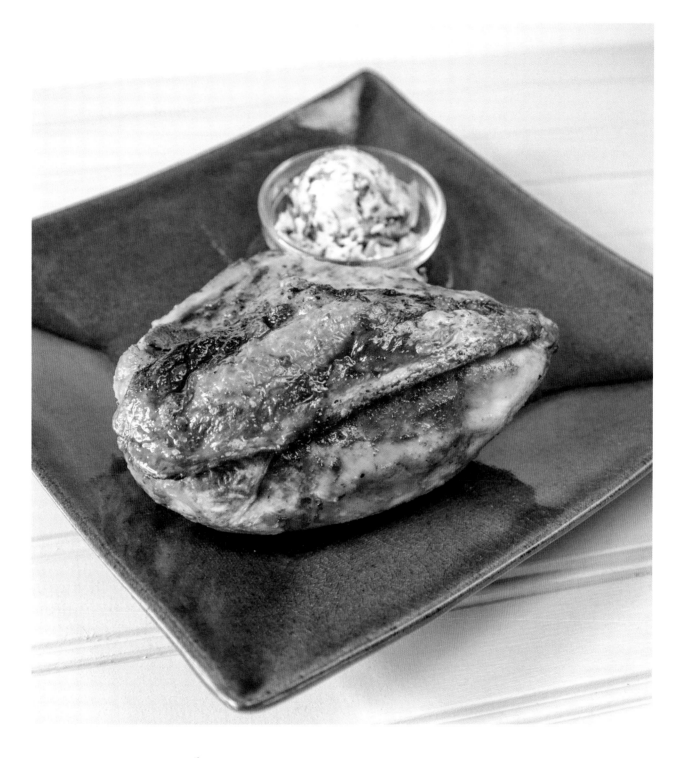

Variation: LEMON GARLIC CHICKEN WITH LEMON BASIL BUTTER

Substitute grated lemon zest for the lime zest and omit the smoked paprika from the chicken seasoning. Instead of charring scallions, just chiffonade 2 tablespoons of fresh basil leaves and add them to the rest of the butter ingredients. Omit the chipotle powder from both the chicken seasoning and the scallion butter; instead, in the seasoning, use 1 teaspoon garlic powder (total), and in the scallion butter, use ¼ teaspoon garlic powder.

PARMESAN GARLIC WINGS

HOUR or LESS

MAKES 32 WINGS
(8 per serving)

I love wings, and while I generally go for hot Buffalo-style wings, these Parmesan garlic ones have a very special place in my heart. With a sinfully rich and delicious flavor, these wings will quickly become a favorite of yours.

32 chicken wingettes and drummettes

¼ cup (½ stick) unsalted butter

2 cloves garlic, minced

¼ cup grated Parmesan cheese (see Note), divided

1 tablespoon chopped fresh parsley

¼ teaspoon fine sea salt

Note : I've found that pregrated, shelf-stable Parmesan—especially Kraft brand, the kind that comes in a shaker with a green top—results in the perfect texture and flavor. Grating your own will work, but it won't be quite as good.

• Preheat the oven to 400°F.

• Line a sheet pan with parchment paper, then place the wings on the pan in a single layer.

• Bake the wings until the exterior is crispy and the juices run clear, 35 to 45 minutes, flipping halfway through.

• Once the wings are cooked, melt the butter in a small saucepan over medium heat. Add the garlic and cook for 1 to 2 minutes, just until the garlic is lightly golden. Remove from the heat and stir in 2 tablespoons of the Parmesan cheese, the parsley, and the salt.

• Transfer the wings to a large bowl, then pour the garlic butter over them and toss to coat.

• Plate the wings and top with the remaining 2 tablespoons of Parmesan cheese.

PER SERVING
Calories **634** · Fat **54g** · Total Carbs **5g** · Net Carbs **4g** · Fiber **1g** · Protein **39g**

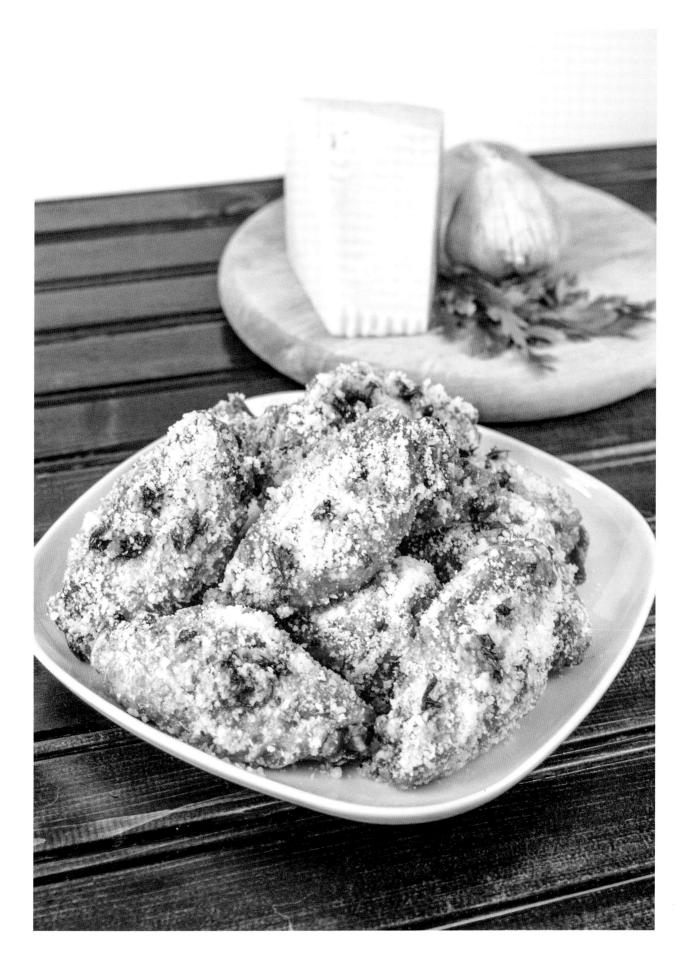

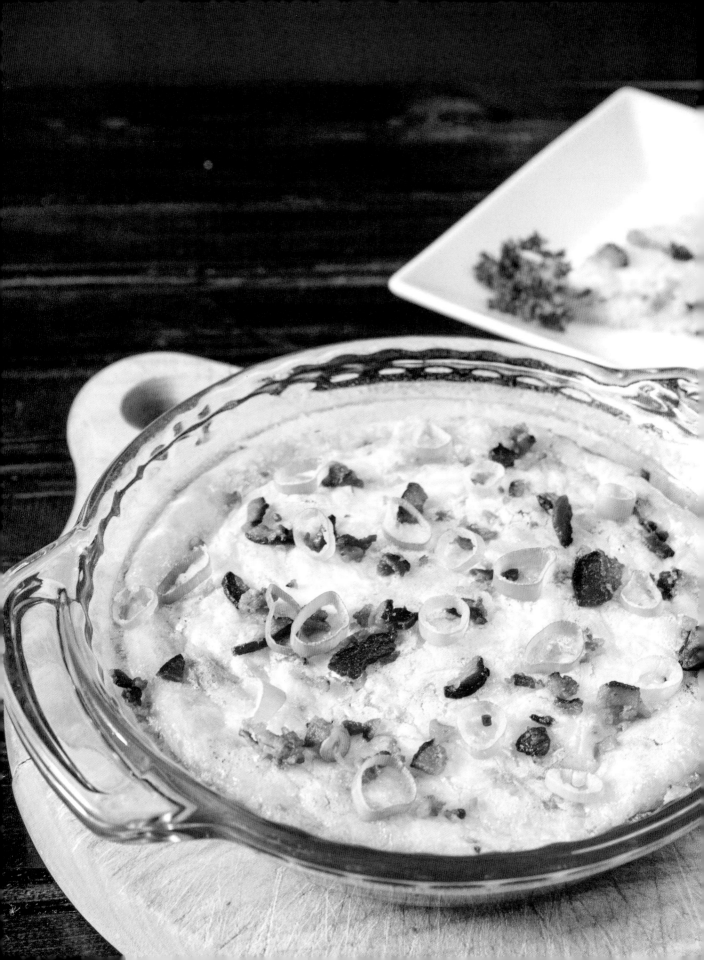

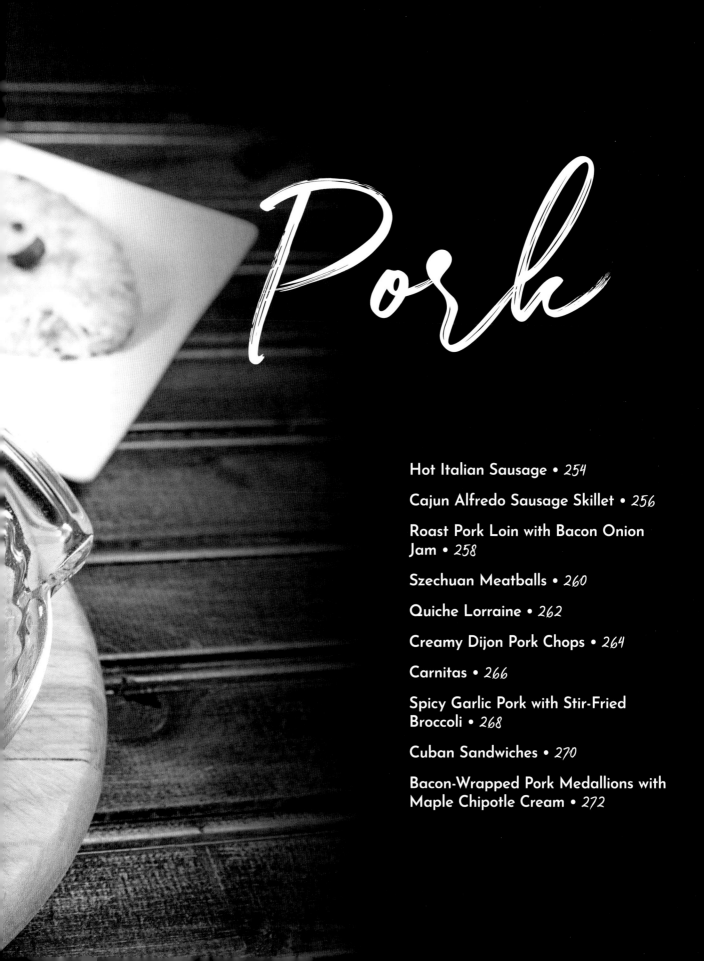

Pork

HOT ITALIAN SAUSAGE

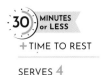

30 MINUTES or LESS

+ TIME TO REST

SERVES 4

One day I just got tired of going without sausage because it contained corn syrup and sometimes even MSG, so I decided to figure out how to make it myself. It's really easy to do, and homemade sausage has great flavor with no additives. Plan ahead for this recipe: it really needs to sit in the fridge overnight before cooking to become properly seasoned. This is wonderful shaped into patties for breakfast sausages or stirred into marinara for a meat sauce, and it's a must for my Cajun Alfredo Sausage Skillet (page 256).

2½ teaspoons sweet paprika

1 teaspoon crushed red pepper

1 teaspoon dried parsley

1 teaspoon fine sea salt

1 teaspoon garlic powder

1 teaspoon onion flakes

½ teaspoon crushed fennel seeds

¼ teaspoon ground dried oregano

¼ teaspoon ground black pepper

¼ teaspoon ground white pepper

⅛ teaspoon dried thyme leaves

Pinch of cayenne pepper

1 pound ground pork, room temperature

- In a medium-sized bowl, combine all of the seasonings and mix well. Add the pork and use your hands or a fork to mix it with the seasonings. Cover the bowl tightly with plastic wrap and refrigerate overnight so flavors have time to develop.

- This mix can be cooked as crumbled sausage or formed into patties. To cook as crumbled sausage, place in a skillet over medium-high heat and cook, breaking the meat apart with a wooden spoon, until no pink remains, about 5 minutes. To cook as patties, form into 2-inch patties and place in a skillet over medium-high heat. Cook until both sides are golden brown, about 3 minutes per side.

- Store in an airtight container in the fridge for up to 1 week.

Variation : MILD ITALIAN SAUSAGE

For a version with less heat, omit the crushed red pepper and cayenne.

PER SERVING
Calories **271** · Fat **20g** · Total Carbs **2g** · Net Carbs **2g** · Fiber **0g** · Protein **20g**

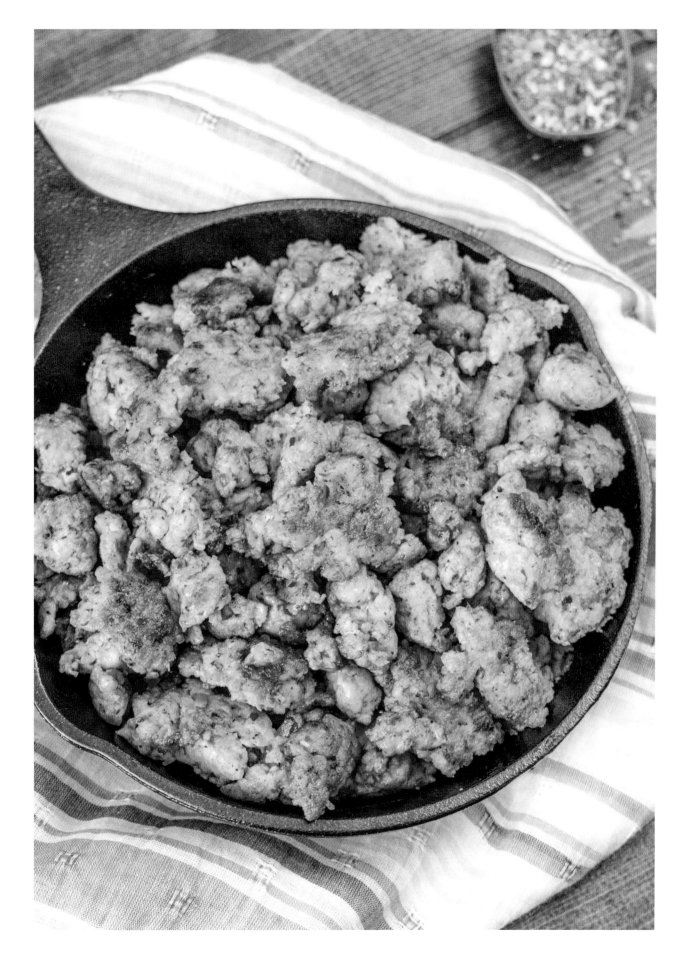

CAJUN ALFREDO SAUSAGE SKILLET

MINUTES or LESS

SERVES 4

This is a recipe I have been making for years, and before I started eating keto, I used jarred alfredo sauce and served the entire dish over pasta. Turns out it was never the pasta that made this dish so amazing! It's delicious served over a bed of spaghetti squash noodles or riced cauliflower, but it's also magnificent eaten all by itself.

2 tablespoons unsalted butter, divided

8 ounces sliced mushrooms

Fine sea salt

1 large bell pepper, cut in ¼-inch-wide slices

1 medium onion, cut into ½-inch-wide slices

1 batch Hot Italian Sausage (page 254)

1 cup heavy cream

4 ounces cream cheese (½ cup)

2 teaspoons Cajun Seasoning (page 58)

Chopped fresh parsley, for garnish (optional)

• Melt 1 tablespoon of the butter in a skillet over medium-high heat. Add the mushrooms, stirring to coat them in the butter, and sauté until softened and lightly brown, about 10 minutes. Sprinkle the mushrooms with salt, remove them from the pan, and set aside.

• Melt the remaining tablespoon of butter in the skillet. Add the bell pepper and sauté, stirring occasionally, until it starts to soften, about 5 minutes. Add the onion and continue to sauté until both onion and pepper are starting to brown around the edges, about 5 minutes more. Sprinkle the veggies with salt, remove them from the pan, and set aside.

• Add the sausage to the skillet and cook until warmed through while stirring to break it up. (If you're using raw sausage mixture, cook until no pink remains, about 10 minutes.) Push the sausage to one side of the skillet. On the other side, place the cream, cream cheese, and Cajun seasoning and whisk together until smooth. Once the sauce starts to bubble and thicken, about 3 minutes, stir it into the sausage until well combined. Add the reserved mushrooms, pepper, and onion to the skillet and stir to combine. Simmer for just a few minutes to heat through. Plate, garnish with chopped fresh parsley, if desired, and serve immediately.

• Store leftovers in an airtight container in the fridge for up to 1 week.

Variation : GARLIC ALFREDO SAUSAGE SKILLET

For a garlicky version, substitute 1 teaspoon garlic powder and ⅛ teaspoon fine sea salt for the Cajun seasoning.

PER SERVING
Calories **660** · Fat **57g** · Total Carbs **13g** · Net Carbs **11g** · Fiber **2g** · Protein **26g**

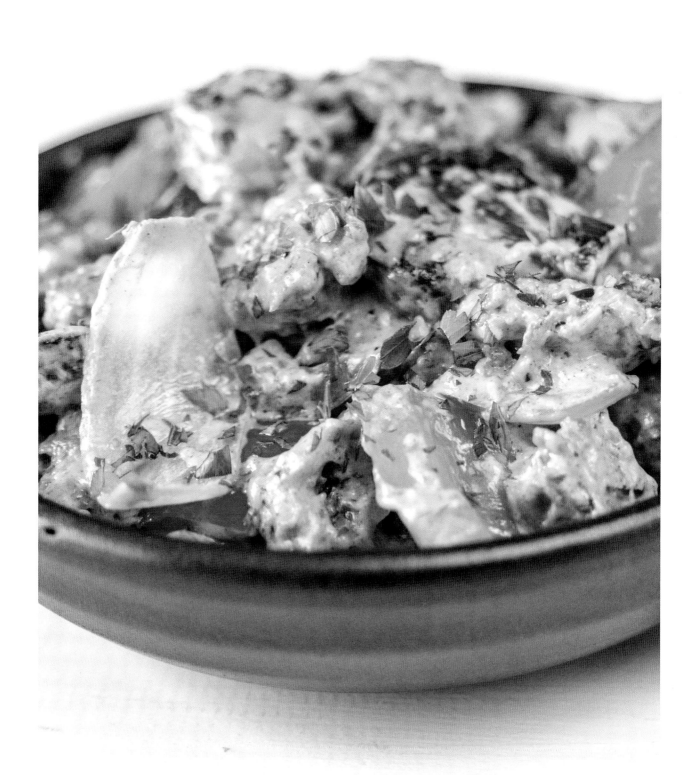

ROAST PORK LOIN
with BACON ONION JAM

2 HOURS or LESS

SERVES 6

I love roasting meat—it becomes so succulent. This pork loin is no exception. It's delicious just by itself, but the bacon onion jam really amplifies the pork and turns it into a truly stunning meal. I enjoy serving this with my Gruyère Spinach Gratin (page 182).

2 tablespoons bacon grease or light olive oil

2 pounds boneless pork loin with a nice fat cap

1 teaspoon fine sea salt

½ teaspoon ground black pepper

1 batch Bacon Onion Jam (page 80), for serving

Note : Leftover pork loin is perfect for cutting into thin slices and making Cuban Sandwiches (page 270).

- Preheat the oven to 350°F.

- Heat the bacon grease in a heavy-bottomed skillet over medium-high heat. Season the pork loin with the salt and pepper, add it to the skillet, and sear it on all sides until golden brown all over, about 3 minutes per side.

- Transfer the pork to a roasting pan, place it in the oven, and roast until the internal temperature reaches 145°F, about 1 hour. Let the pork loin rest for 10 minutes before slicing. Serve with the bacon onion jam.

- Store leftovers in an airtight container in the fridge for up to 1 week.

PER SERVING
Calories **483** · Fat **32g** · Total Carbs **4g** · Net Carbs **3g** · Fiber **1g** · Protein **45g**

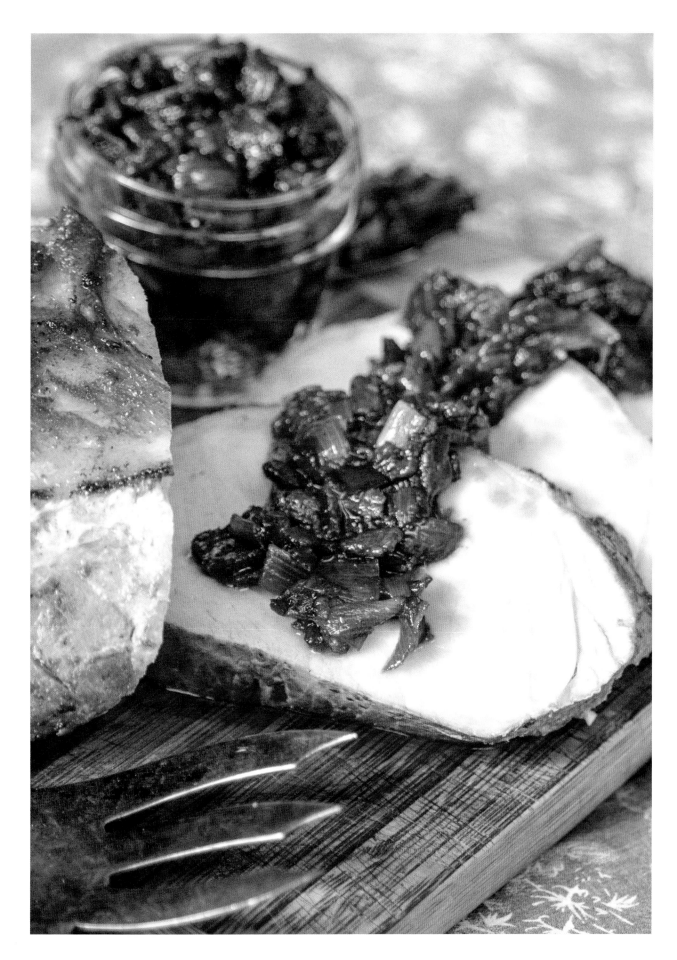

SZECHUAN MEATBALLS

MAKES ABOUT 16 MEATBALLS
(4 per serving)

Words cannot describe how much my kids and I love these meatballs. The Szechuan pepper and the Chinese five-spice powder really make them special, with flavors of spicy citrus, star anise, and cloves. These are even more wonderful when served with my Cashew Fried Cauli Rice (page 192).

FOR THE MEATBALLS:

1 tablespoon unsalted butter

½ cup crushed pork rinds

1 pound ground pork

1 large egg

1 scallion, both white and green parts, minced

1 teaspoon fine sea salt

¼ teaspoon Chinese five-spice powder

¼ teaspoon ground Szechuan pepper (see Notes)

¼ teaspoon toasted sesame oil

2 tablespoons light olive oil

FOR THE SAUCE:

1 scallion, both white and green parts, minced

1 clove garlic, minced

2 tablespoons water

1 tablespoon coconut aminos

1 tablespoon rice wine vinegar

1 tablespoon sambal oelek (see Notes)

1 tablespoon soy sauce

½ teaspoon blended erythritol-stevia sweetener (see page 46)

¼ teaspoon Chinese five-spice powder

¼ teaspoon ground Szechuan pepper (see Notes)

Minced cilantro, for garnish

- Melt the butter in a skillet over medium heat and stir in the crushed pork rinds. Toast the crushed pork rinds, stirring occasionally, until they're crispy and golden, about 3 minutes. Transfer the toasted crumbs to a large bowl and set aside to cool.

- Once the toasted crumbs are cool, add the rest of the meatball ingredients except the olive oil and mix well. With your hands, form about 2 tablespoons of the mixture into a meatball and set aside. Repeat with the rest of the mixture; you should end up with about 16 meatballs.

- Heat the olive oil in the same skillet over medium-high heat. Working in batches if necessary to avoid overcrowding the pan, add the meatballs and shallow-fry, shaking the skillet often to spin them, until they are golden brown on all sides, about 10 minutes. Use a slotted spoon to transfer the meatballs to a plate and set aside. Do not wash the pan.

- Make the sauce: To the meatball drippings and remaining oil in the pan, add the scallion and garlic. Cook, stirring constantly, until fragrant, about 3 minutes. Add the rest of the sauce ingredients and stir to combine. Deglaze the pan, scraping all the good browned bits off the bottom. Turn the heat down to medium-low and simmer until the sauce thickens, about 5 minutes.

- Return the meatballs to the skillet and roll them around in the sauce to coat. Cook for a few minutes to heat the meatballs through. Serve garnished with minced cilantro.

- Store in an airtight container in the fridge for up to 1 week.

Notes: Sambal oelek is a Southeast Asian chili pepper sauce. There's really no substitute for it in this recipe, but you should be able to find it in the international-foods aisle of your grocery store.

If you can't find ground Szechuan pepper, you can also use ground sansho pepper (also known as Japanese pepper), which is available at most grocery stores.

PER SERVING
Calories **454** · Fat **36g** · Total Carbs **1g** · Net Carbs **1g** · Fiber **0g** · Protein **30g**

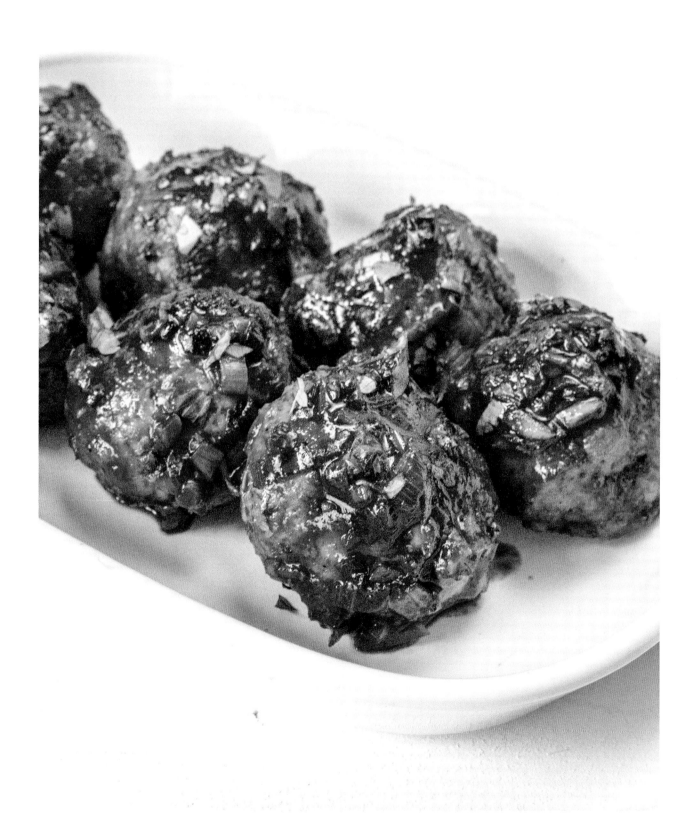

QUICHE LORRAINE

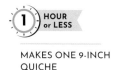

1 HOUR or LESS

MAKES ONE 9-INCH QUICHE
(4 servings)

Quiche Lorraine is traditionally made with just bacon, but now that it's relatively easy to find no-sugar-added ham, I've added that for an even more filling and delicious quiche.

10 slices bacon, cut into 1-inch pieces

8 ounces no-sugar-added ham, chopped

4 scallions, both white and green parts, sliced, plus more for garnish

1 cup shredded Swiss cheese

6 large eggs

1 cup heavy cream

½ teaspoon fine sea salt

¼ teaspoon ground black pepper

Note : This reheats so well that I often double the recipe and bake it in a 9 by 13-inch casserole dish. After it cools, cut it into individual servings, wrap, and refrigerate.

- Preheat the oven to 350°F. Line a plate with paper towels.

- Heat a skillet over medium-high heat and drop in the bacon pieces. Cook until the bacon is brown and crispy, about 10 minutes. Using a slotted spoon, transfer the bacon to the paper towel–lined plate and set aside.

- Add the ham and scallions to the bacon drippings in the pan and sauté until the scallions wilt, about 3 minutes. Transfer the ham and scallions to a 9-inch pie pan and top with reserved bacon pieces and the Swiss cheese.

- In a medium-sized bowl, beat together the eggs, cream, salt, and pepper until light and frothy. Pour the egg mixture slowly over the ham, bacon, and cheese.

- Bake for 25 minutes, or until lightly browned on top and set in the middle. Garnish with sliced scallion and serve immediately.

- Store leftovers in an airtight container in the fridge for up to 1 week.

Variation : **HAM, ASPARAGUS & CHEDDAR QUICHE**

There are so many options when it comes to quiche, but another one of my favorite variations is using asparagus and cheddar in the recipe above. Make it as instructed above, but omit the bacon, add 1 cup cooked chopped asparagus, and replace the Swiss cheese with cheddar.

PER SERVING
Calories **687** · Fat **54g** · Total Carbs **5g** · Net Carbs **5g** · Fiber **0g** · Protein **45g**

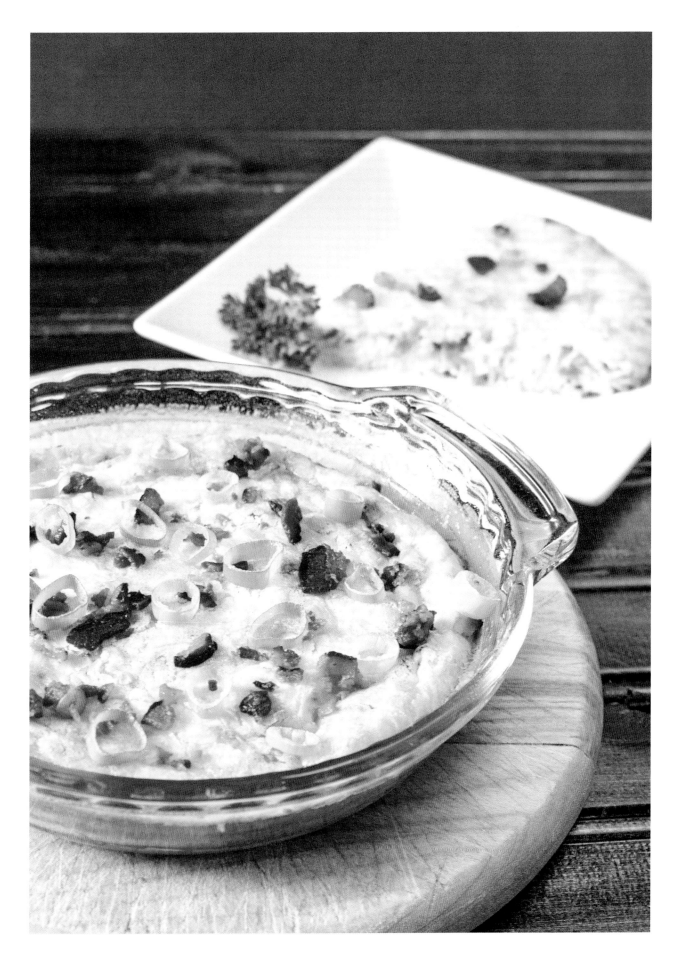

CREAMY DIJON PORK CHOPS

30 MINUTES or LESS

SERVES **6**

I usually buy a huge pork loin from a warehouse store and cut it down into roasts and chops of whatever size I want. But you can easily use boneless pork loin chops that you'll find precut at your grocery store, too.

1 tablespoon light olive oil

6 boneless pork loin chops, each ½ inch thick

1 teaspoon fine sea salt

½ teaspoon ground black pepper

2 tablespoons unsalted butter

1 medium shallot, minced

½ cup dry white wine

½ cup chicken stock (see page 26)

½ cup heavy cream

2 teaspoons Dijon mustard

Chopped fresh parsley, for garnish (optional)

• Heat the oil in a heavy-bottomed skillet over medium-high heat. Season both sides of the pork chops with the salt and pepper, add the pork to the pan, and sear until golden brown on all sides, about 3 minutes per side. Transfer the chops to a plate and set aside. Do not wash the pan.

• Melt the butter in the skillet, then add the shallot and sauté until softened, about 5 minutes. Add the wine and deglaze the skillet, scraping up the browned bits at the bottom of the pan. Turn the heat down to medium and simmer until the wine reduces by half, about 5 minutes.

• Add the chicken stock and return the pork chops to the pan, along with their juices. Simmer for 15 minutes. Using a slotted spoon or tongs, transfer the chops to a serving plate and cover with foil to keep warm.

• Whisk the heavy cream and Dijon mustard into the sauce in the pan and simmer until the sauce starts to thicken, about 3 minutes.

• Serve the pork chops with the Dijon sauce poured over the top or on the side. Garnish with chopped fresh parsley, if desired.

• Store leftovers in an airtight container in the fridge for up to 1 week.

PER SERVING
Calories **355** · Fat **26g** · Total Carbs **2g** · Net Carbs **2g** · Fiber **0g** · Protein **4g**

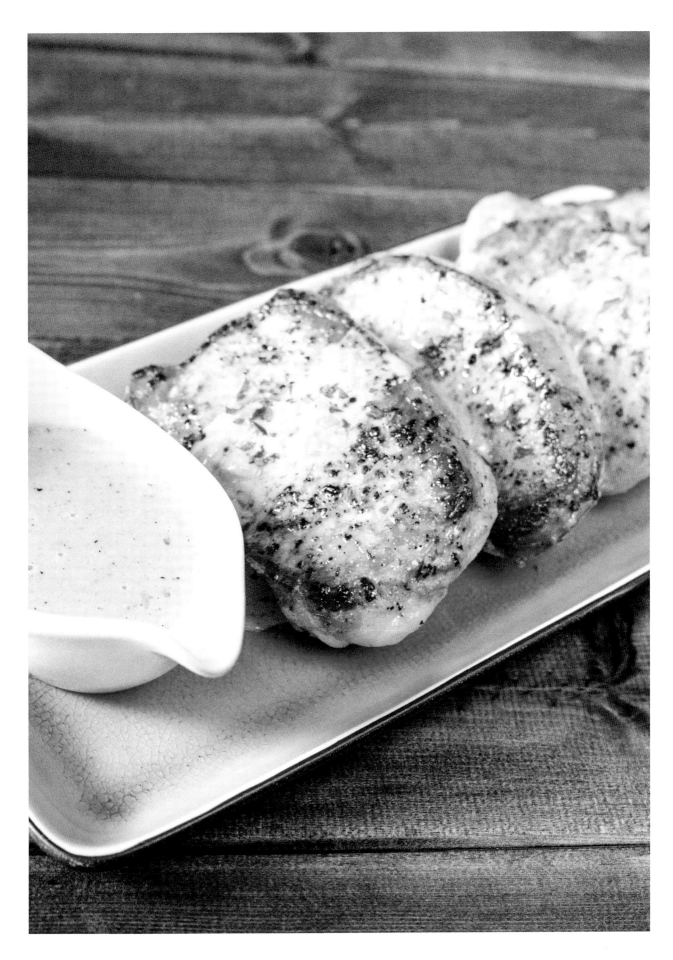

CARNITAS

SERVES 6

Everyone loves carnitas! Slow-roasted and seasoned pulled pork fried to a delicious crunch and served with all of your favorite toppings—what could be better? I always serve this with my Cilantro Lime Cauli Rice (page 202), and it's also wonderful with my Cilantro Chimichurri (page 70).

2 tablespoons light olive oil or bacon grease

3 pounds boneless pork butt, cut into 3-inch chunks

2 teaspoons fine sea salt

1 teaspoon ground black pepper

1 cup chicken stock (see page 26)

Juice of 1 lime

1 tablespoon chili powder

1 teaspoon garlic powder

½ teaspoon dried Mexican oregano leaves

½ teaspoon ground cumin

FOR SERVING (OPTIONAL):

Chopped fresh cilantro

Cilantro Chimichurri (page 70)

Lime wedges

Sliced jalapeño

Sliced red onion

- Preheat the oven to 300°F.

- Heat the oil in a heavy-bottomed Dutch oven over medium-high heat.

- While the oil heats, place the pork chunks in a large bowl, sprinkle with the salt and pepper, and toss to coat. In a medium-sized bowl, mix together the chicken stock, lime juice, and seasonings and whisk to blend.

- Once the oil is hot, sear the seasoned pork chunks in the Dutch oven until browned on all sides, about 5 minutes per side. Pour the sauce over the pork, cover, and transfer to the oven.

- Roast until the meat is tender, about 3 hours. Once the pork shreds easily with a fork, remove it from the oven and shred the pork.

- You can serve the carnitas just like this, but if you prefer them crispy, as I do, raise the oven temperature to 400°F, line a sheet pan with foil, and spread the shredded pork on the sheet pan in an even layer. Place it in the oven and cook until the pork is crispy around the edges, about 10 minutes.

- Garnish with fresh cilantro and serve with sour cream, lime wedges, sliced jalapeño, and sliced red onion.

- Store leftovers in an airtight container in the fridge for up to 1 week.

Note : For an amazing brunch, serve these carnitas on top of cheese-filled omelets sprinkled with chopped jalapeños. Kick it up a notch by drizzling the omelets with a spicy mayo made with 3 tablespoons mayo, 3 teaspoons Sriracha, ⅛ teaspoon blended erythritol-stevia sweetener, and 2 drops of toasted sesame oil.

PER SERVING
Calories **537** · Fat **38g** · Total Carbs **3g** · Net Carbs **2g** · Fiber **1g** · Protein **30g**

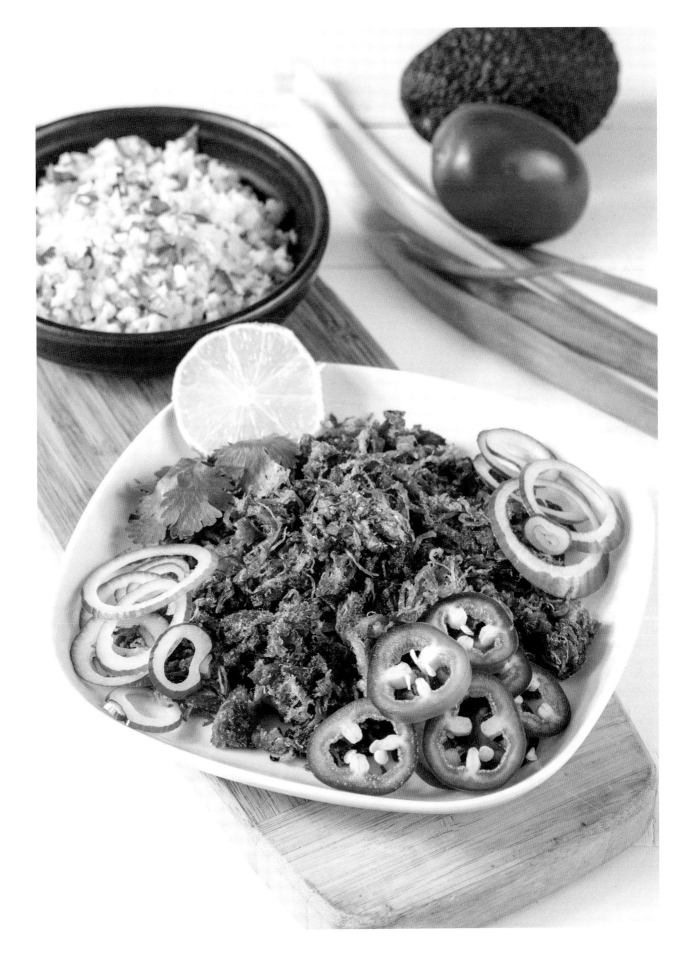

SPICY GARLIC PORK
with STIR-FRIED BROCCOLI

SERVES 4

This dish is oh-so-delicious, but it's quite spicy. If you'd prefer a milder version, reduce the sambal oelek by half or eliminate it altogether. This dish is fantastic served over my Cashew Fried Cauli Rice on page 192.

4 tablespoons light olive oil, divided

1 broccoli crown (about 7 ounces), cut into florets

2 tablespoons water

1½ pounds pork, julienned

½ teaspoon fine sea salt

¼ teaspoon ground white pepper

FOR THE SAUCE:

2 tablespoons light olive oil

2 cloves garlic, minced

2 teaspoons grated fresh ginger (about one ¼-inch piece)

¼ cup sambal oelek (see Notes, page 260)

1 tablespoon unseasoned rice wine vinegar

1 teaspoon blended erythritol-stevia sweetener (see page 46)

Sliced scallions, for garnish (optional)

- Heat 2 tablespoons of the oil in a skillet or wok over medium-high heat and add the broccoli, stirring to coat it in the oil. Sauté until the broccoli is browned around the edges, about 3 minutes. Add the water and continue to cook, stirring occasionally, until the broccoli is crisp-tender, about 5 minutes.

- While the broccoli is cooking, season the pork all over with the salt and pepper.

- Once the broccoli is cooked, transfer it to a plate and loosely cover it with foil to keep it warm.

- Pour the remaining 2 tablespoons of oil into the skillet, still over medium-high heat, and add the pork. Cook, stirring constantly, until cooked through, about 5 minutes. Using a slotted spoon, transfer the pork to a plate and set aside. Do not wash the pan.

- Make the sauce: Pour the oil into the pan, still over medium-high heat, then add the garlic and ginger. Cook, stirring constantly, until fragrant, about 3 minutes. Add the sambal oelek, vinegar, and sweetener and turn the heat down to medium. Simmer until the sauce starts to thicken, about 5 minutes, then return the pork to the skillet and toss it with the sauce. Simmer until the pork is heated through, about 2 minutes.

- To serve, arrange the broccoli in a circle on a plate and place the pork in the middle. Garnish with sliced scallions if desired.

- Store leftovers in an airtight container in the fridge for up to 1 week.

PER SERVING
Calories **361** · Fat **30g** · Total Carbs **4g** · Net Carbs **3g** · Fiber **1g** · Protein **24g**

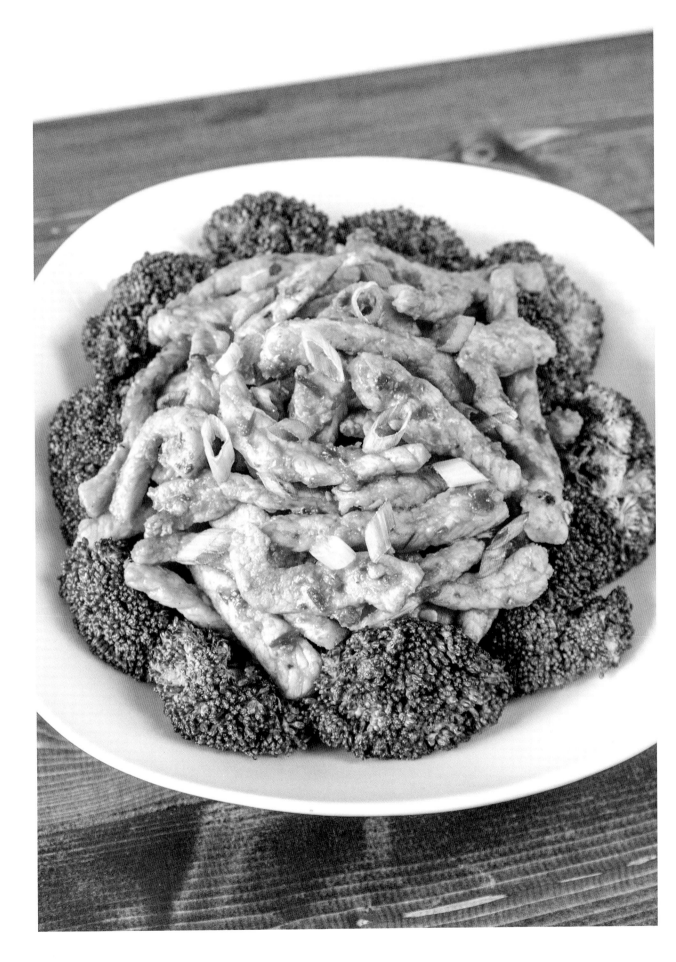

CUBAN SANDWICHES

 MINUTES or LESS

MAKES 4
SANDWICHES
(1 per serving)

I love Cuban sandwiches, those flavorful variations on ham-and-cheese, and these low-carb ones really hit the spot! So easy to make, and they work wonderfully with my Best-Ever Flax Buns (page 112). I pretty much always make these after I make my Roast Pork Loin with Bacon Onion Jam (page 258) because it is a perfect and delicious use of the leftover pork!

1 batch Best-Ever Flax Buns (page 112), made into 4 buns

2 tablespoons plus 2 teaspoons prepared yellow mustard

8 slices Swiss cheese

16 slices roast pork loin, each about ⅛ inch thick

12 thin slices no-sugar-added ham

24 dill pickle chips

2 tablespoons unsalted butter

· Slice each bun in half lengthwise. Spread 1 teaspoon of mustard onto each side and add a slice of Swiss cheese on each side. To each of the bottom buns, add 4 slices of roast pork, 3 slices of ham, and 6 pickle chips. Put the cheese-topped top buns onto the piled-high bottom buns.

· Melt the butter in a large skillet over medium heat and add all 4 sandwiches, bottom side down. Once the cheese starts to melt, carefully flip the sandwiches to the other side. Cook until the buns are golden brown and the cheese is melted, about 10 minutes. You may need to flip the sandwiches a few times to cook evenly. Transfer the sandwiches to a cutting board and cut in half before serving.

· Store in an airtight container in the fridge for up to 3 days.

PER SERVING
Calories **511** · Fat **43g** · Total Carbs **10g** · Net Carbs **5g** · Fiber **5g** · Protein **36g**

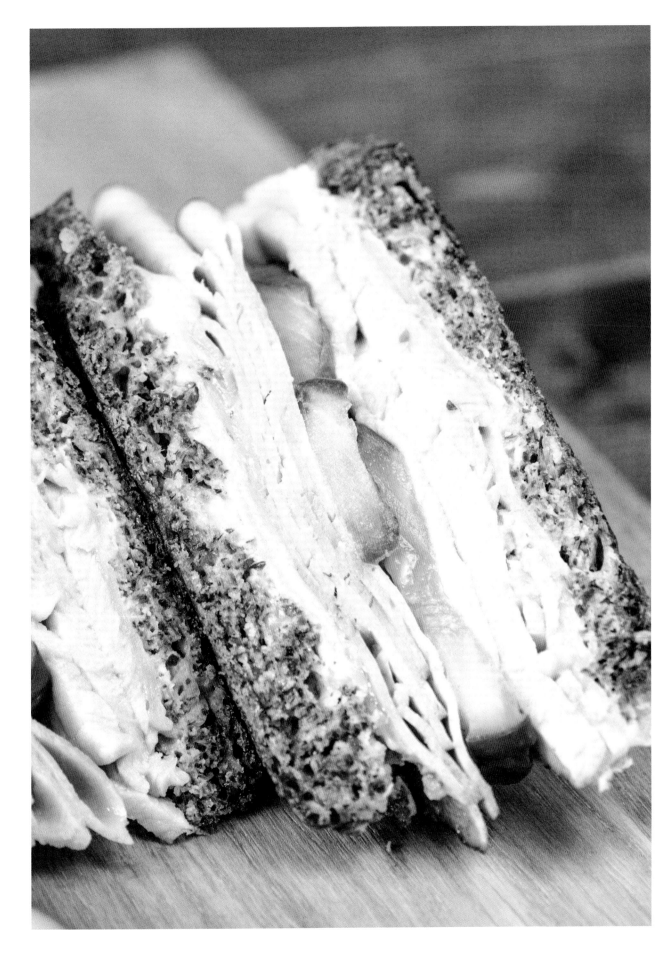

BACON-WRAPPED PORK MEDALLIONS
with MAPLE CHIPOTLE CREAM

MAKES 6 MEDALLIONS
(1½ per serving)

This recipe is so easy, and it's one of my favorites. The pork is extremely tender and juicy, and it's so well complemented by the smoky bacon and spicy Maple Chipotle Cream.

6 slices thick-cut bacon

2 pounds pork tenderloin, cut into 6 equal pieces

1 teaspoon fine sea salt

½ teaspoon ground black pepper

FOR THE MAPLE CHIPOTLE CREAM:

¼ cup full-fat sour cream

¼ cup mayonnaise (see page 43)

¼ cup no-sugar-added chipotle sauce

¼ teaspoon blended erythritol-stevia sweetener (see page 46)

⅛ teaspoon fine sea salt

⅛ teaspoon garlic powder

⅛ teaspoon maple extract

• Preheat the oven to 350°F and line a sheet pan with foil.

• Lay the bacon on the sheet pan and par-cook for 15 minutes. The bacon should be no longer raw but not yet starting to brown. Move the bacon to a plate and pour the bacon drippings from the sheet pan into a glass bowl and set aside. Raise the oven temperature to 400°F.

• Season the pork medallions with the salt and pepper. Wrap a slice of bacon around the circumference of each medallion and secure it with a toothpick. Heat an oven-safe skillet or cast-iron skillet over high heat and pour in the reserved bacon drippings. Place the pork medallions in the very hot skillet and sear for 2 minutes, then flip them over and immediately put the skillet into the oven.

• Roast the medallions until the internal temperature reaches 145°F and the bacon starts to crisp, about 20 minutes. Remove from the oven and allow to rest for 5 minutes.

• While the pork is roasting, whisk together all of the chipotle cream ingredients in a medium-sized bowl.

• Serve the pork medallions with a side of Maple Chipotle Cream for dipping.

• Store leftovers in an airtight container in the fridge for up to 1 week.

PER SERVING
Calories **458** · Fat **28g** · Total Carbs **2g** · Net Carbs **1g** · Fiber **1g** · Protein **50g**

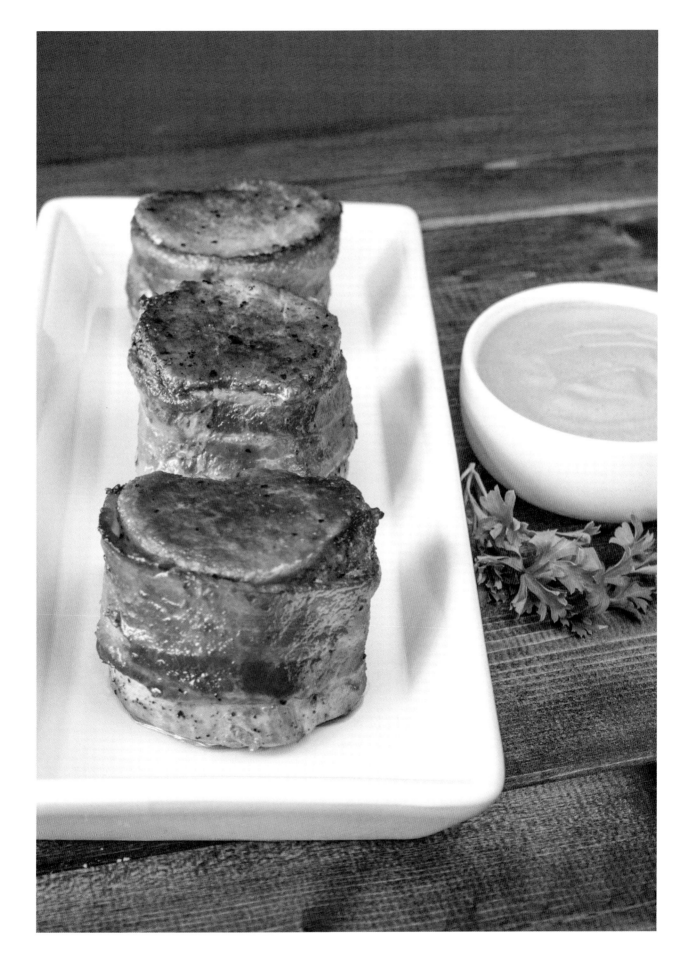

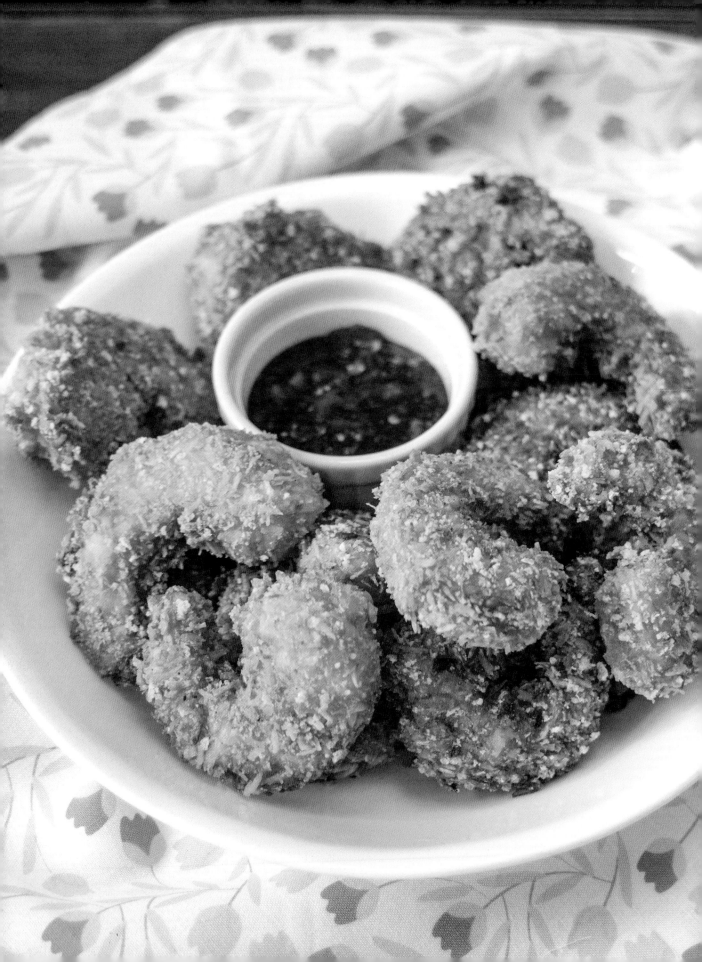

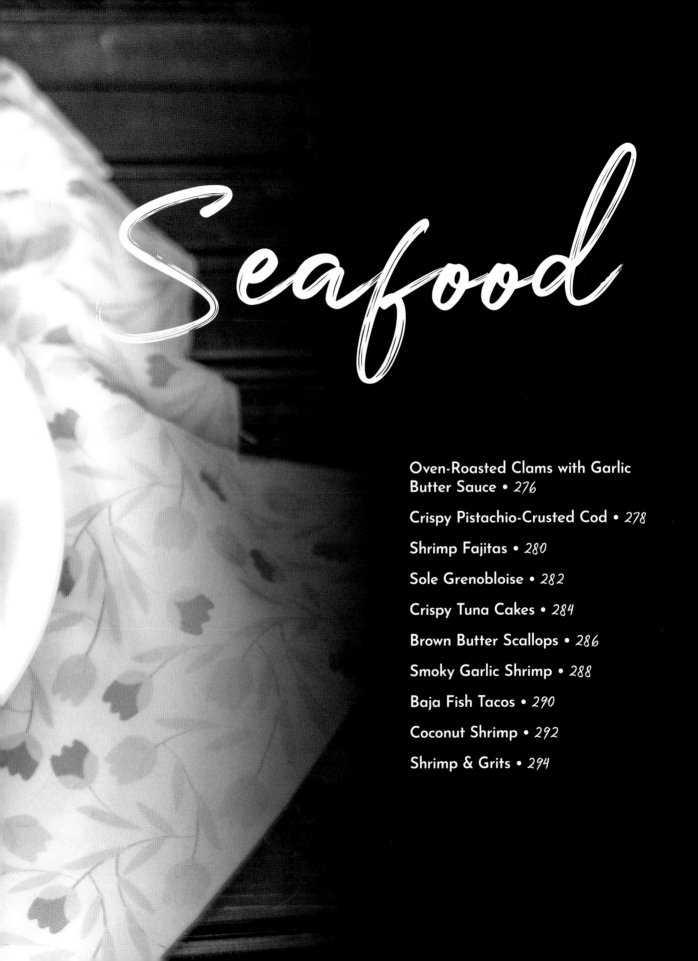

Seafood

OVEN-ROASTED CLAMS
with GARLIC BUTTER SAUCE

SERVES 4

I am a die-hard clam fan! Clam chowder, steamed clams, fried clams—I love them all! I wanted to try something new to give clams even more flavor, so I roasted them in the oven and topped them with a decadent garlic butter–wine sauce. They turned out amazing!

24 cherrystone clams, scrubbed

½ cup (1 stick) unsalted butter

2 cloves garlic, minced

⅓ cup dry white wine

¼ cup chopped fresh parsley

½ teaspoon fine sea salt

¼ teaspoon ground black pepper

Chopped fresh parsley, for garnish (optional)

Note: I only buy clams from a trusted seafood vendor or an upscale grocery store. Be sure all the shells are free of breaks or cracks, and never eat a clam that won't close when touched or knocked or that doesn't open after cooking.

• Preheat the oven to 425°F.

• Place the clams on a large sheet pan and roast until the shells open, about 10 minutes. If any don't open, roast for a few more minutes, and if they still remain shut, then throw them out.

• While the clams are roasting, melt the butter in a small saucepan over medium heat. Add the garlic and sauté until just fragrant, about 2 minutes. Pour in the wine and simmer until it's reduced by half, about 5 minutes. Add the parsley, salt, and pepper and stir to combine. Turn the heat down to low to keep the sauce warm while the clams finish roasting.

• When the clams are ready, use tongs to place them on a serving plate (the shells will be very hot). Spoon the sauce over the clams, garnish with chopped fresh parsley, if desired, and serve immediately.

Variation: OVEN-ROASTED CLAMS WITH LEMON GARLIC BUTTER SAUCE

Swap the juice of 1 lemon for the white wine.

PER SERVING
Calories **274** · Fat **25g** · Total Carbs **1g** · Net Carbs **1g** · Fiber **0g** · Protein **11g**

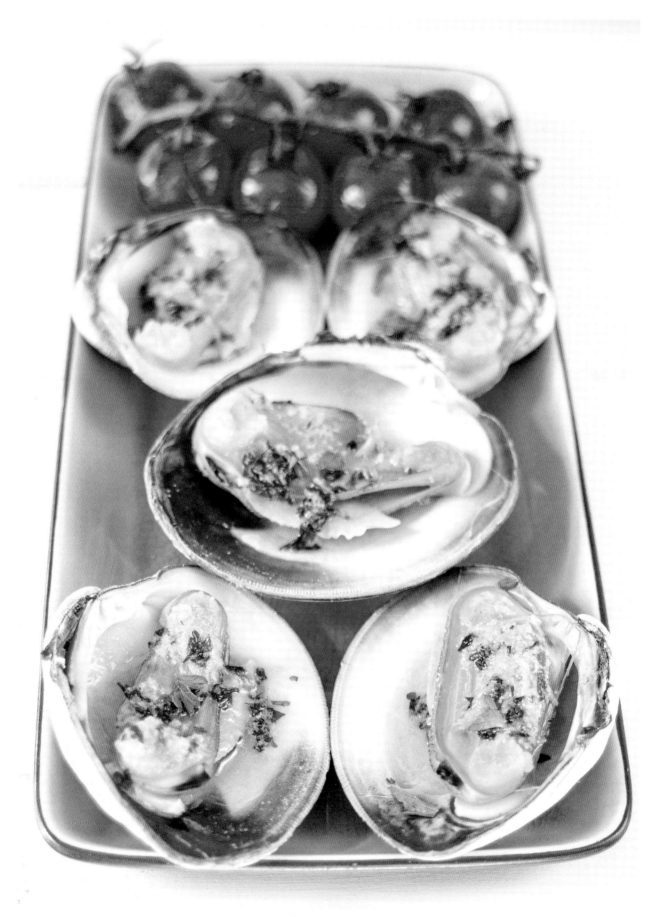

CRISPY PISTACHIO-CRUSTED COD

SERVES 4

Cod is easily my favorite fish. I love that it's meaty yet so flaky and light! When I came up with the idea for this recipe, I knew it would be good, but I wasn't expecting to be blown away. This may just be my favorite recipe in this book. It doesn't need a sauce, but I still always serve this with my Lemon Dill Tartar Sauce (page 72) because I just love it!

4 cod fillets (about 1 pound total)

2 tablespoons unsalted butter

⅔ cup chopped pork rinds (see Note)

¼ cup chopped pistachios

⅛ teaspoon fine sea salt

1 tablespoon chopped fresh parsley

1 teaspoon grated lemon zest

Note : This is the only recipe I have where the pork rinds should just be roughly chopped, not crushed into crumbs.

· Preheat the oven to 425°F.

· Place the cod fillets in an oven-safe 9 by 13-inch baking dish and bake until flaky, about 15 minutes.

· While the fish is baking, melt the butter in a skillet over medium-high heat. Add the pork rinds, pistachios, and salt. Cook, stirring frequently, until the pork rinds and nuts are toasted, about 5 minutes. Remove the pan from the heat and stir in the parsley and lemon zest.

· When the fish is cooked, remove it from the oven and sprinkle it with salt. Put the fillets on 4 plates and divide the topping evenly among the fillets. Serve immediately.

· Store leftovers in an airtight container in the fridge for 2 to 3 days.

Variation : CRISPY MEXICAN COD

Substitute lime zest for the lemon zest and cilantro for the parsley for crispy-crusted cod with a Mexican flair!

PER SERVING
Calories **277** · Fat **18g** · Total Carbs **2g** · Net Carbs **1g** · Fiber **1g** · Protein **26g**

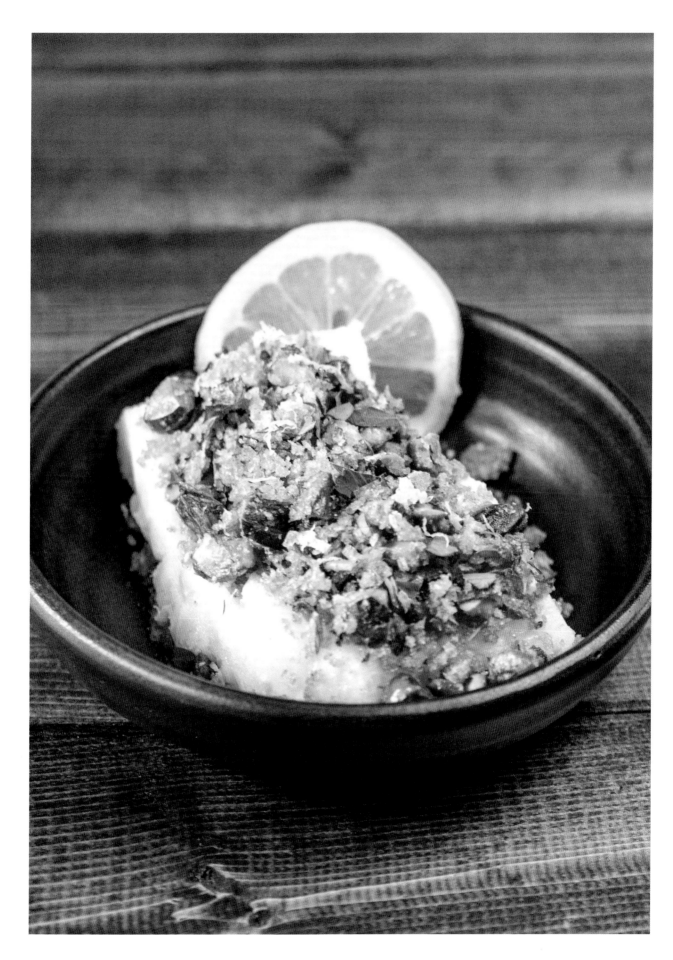

SHRIMP FAJITAS

SERVES 4

I'm a fajita girl! I've always ordered fajitas at Mexican restaurants, and I love that they are just as good eaten with a fork as in a tortilla, making them perfectly keto-friendly. These shrimp fajitas are no exception: wrap them in lettuce or devour them just as they are. Be sure to make my Baja Sauce (page 76) ahead of time to go with them; you'll be so happy you did!

FOR THE FAJITA SEASONING:

½ teaspoon chili powder

½ teaspoon chipotle powder

½ teaspoon fine sea salt

¼ teaspoon blended erythritol-stevia sweetener (see page 46)

¼ teaspoon chicken bouillon powder

⅛ teaspoon cayenne pepper

⅛ teaspoon garlic powder

⅛ teaspoon ground cumin

⅛ teaspoon onion powder

1 pound large shrimp, peeled, deveined, and tails removed

4 tablespoons light olive oil, divided

1 large bell pepper, any color, cut into ½-inch-wide slices

1 batch Baja Sauce (page 76), for serving

• In a large bowl, combine all of the ingredients for the fajita seasoning and mix well. Transfer ½ teaspoon of the seasoning mix to a tiny bowl and set aside. Add the shrimp to the large bowl and toss to coat the shrimp in the seasoning. Cover and set aside to marinate while you cook the peppers.

• Heat 2 tablespoons of the oil in a skillet over medium-high heat and add the bell peppers. Sauté the peppers until they're softened and brown around the edges, about 10 minutes. Sprinkle with the reserved ½ teaspoon of seasoning and stir, then transfer the peppers to a plate.

• Heat the remaining 2 tablespoons of oil in the pan and add the shrimp. Sauté until the shrimp are golden brown and opaque, about 3 minutes per side. Return the peppers to the pan and stir with the shrimp. Serve immediately with the sauce on the side.

• Store leftovers in an airtight container in the fridge for 2 to 3 days.

Variation: STEAK, CHICKEN, OR COMBINATION FAJITAS

Substitute 1 pound thinly sliced flank steak or chicken breast for the shrimp, or use all three proteins for combination fajitas!

PER SERVING
Calories **413** · Fat **33g** · Total Carbs **3g** · Net Carbs **2g** · Fiber **1g** · Protein **25g**

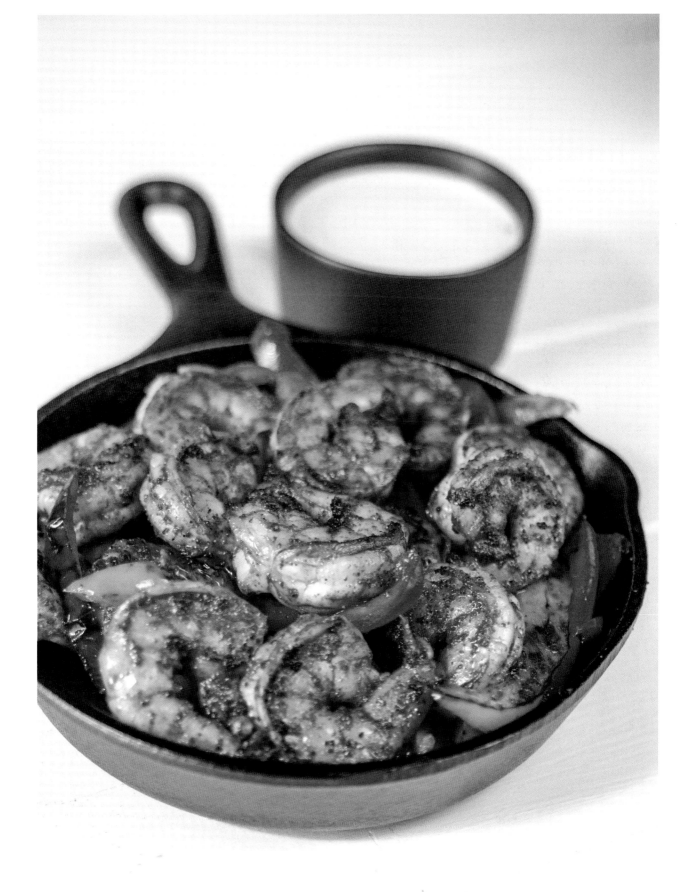

SOLE GRENOBLOISE

MINUTES or LESS

SERVES 4

Fun fact: I had never tried capers until about a year ago! I'm not sure what I was afraid of, but once I tried them, I was hooked. They have the most wonderful briny flavor that pairs just perfectly with fish. This recipe combines capers with lemon and butter, and it is truly marvelous.

4 sole fillets (about 1 pound total)

½ cup (1 stick) unsalted butter

¼ cup capers, drained (reserve the liquid)

2 teaspoons capers liquid

Juice of 1 lemon

2 tablespoons fresh chopped parsley

Fine sea salt and ground black pepper

· Preheat the oven to 425°F.

· Place the sole fillets in an oven-safe 9 by 13-inch baking dish and bake until flaky, about 15 minutes.

· While the fish is baking, melt the butter in a sauté pan over medium-high heat. Add the capers and capers liquid, lemon juice, and parsley and stir to combine.

· Remove the sole from the oven and sprinkle with salt and pepper. Transfer the fillets to a serving dish and pour the butter sauce over the top. Serve immediately.

· Store leftovers in an airtight container in the fridge for 2 to 3 days.

PER SERVING
Calories **313** · Fat **25g** · Total Carbs **2g** · Net Carbs **2g** · Fiber **0g** · Protein **21g**

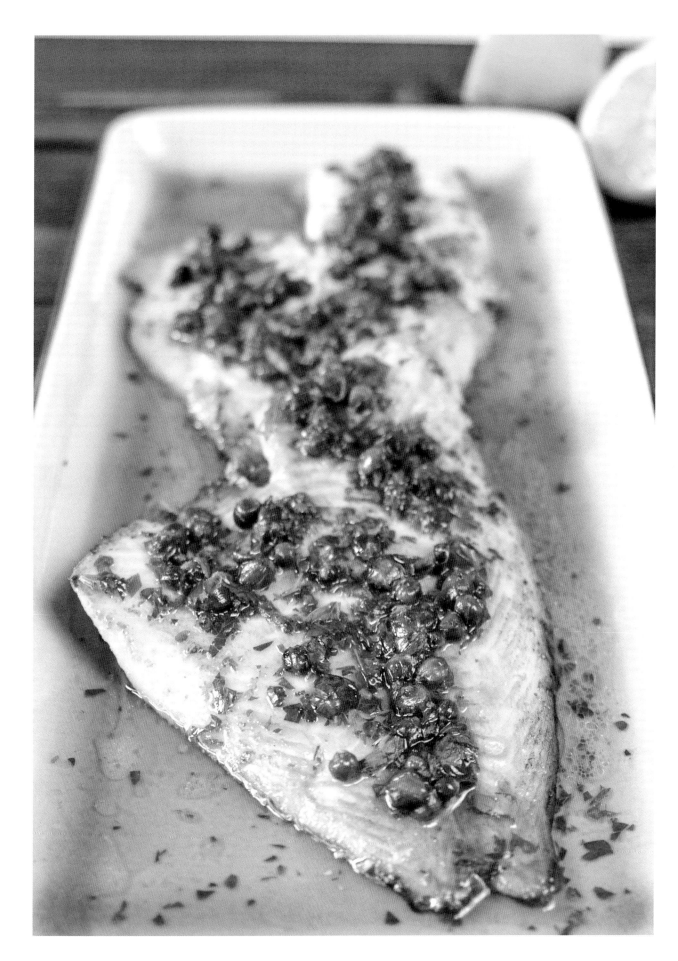

CRISPY TUNA CAKES

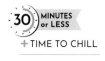

30 MINUTES or LESS

+ TIME TO CHILL

SERVES 4

I've been making these tuna cakes since the start of my keto journey, and I still love them almost three years later. They are quick and easy and so delicious! I always serve these with my Lemon Dill Tartar Sauce (page 72), and it makes them even better!

2 (5-ounce) cans chunk light tuna, drained (see Notes)

⅓ cup crushed pork rinds

¼ cup mayonnaise (see page 43)

2 tablespoons grated Parmesan cheese

2 large eggs

1 teaspoon dried dill weed

⅛ teaspoon fine sea salt

¼ cup ghee (see Notes)

1 batch Lemon Dill Tartar Sauce (page 72), for serving

Sprig of dill, for garnish (optional)

- In a large bowl, mix together all the ingredients except the ghee and sauce until thoroughly combined. Cover the bowl tightly with plastic wrap and refrigerate for 30 minutes.

- After 30 minutes, heat the ghee in a skillet over medium-high heat. Test the heat by adding a tiny bit of the mixture to the ghee. If it starts bubbling immediately, it's ready!

- Make the tuna cakes: Wet a ¼-cup measuring cup or cookie scoop to prevent sticking. (You can also use a 2-tablespoon cookie scoop for mini tuna cakes, my favorite.) Scoop up ¼ cup of the tuna mixture, slightly flatten it with your hand to make a patty, and place it carefully in the hot ghee. Repeat with the remaining mixture to form 4 cakes.

- Once the cakes start to brown, after about 5 minutes, carefully flip them with a rubber spatula and push them down slightly. Fry for another 5 minutes, until the other side starts to brown. (If you want to make the cakes extra crispy, flip them several times—they won't become overcooked or dry.) Serve immediately with the sauce on the side or lightly spooned over the top. Garnish with a sprig of dill if desired.

- Store leftovers in an airtight container in the fridge for 2 to 3 days.

Notes : Even if you prefer albacore tuna, as I do, be sure to use chunk light tuna so the cakes won't be dry.

I like to cook these in ghee because you get a delicious, nutty, brown butter flavor without having to worry about burning the butter while you're getting that nice crispy crust. But if you prefer, you can use 2 tablespoons unsalted butter and 2 tablespoons light olive oil instead of ghee.

For more flavor options, try a variety of dipping sauces, like spicy mayo, chipotle mayo, and even sugar-free ketchup!

PER SERVING
Calories **587** · Fat **53g** · Total Carbs **2g** · Net Carbs **1g** · Fiber **1g** · Protein **24g**

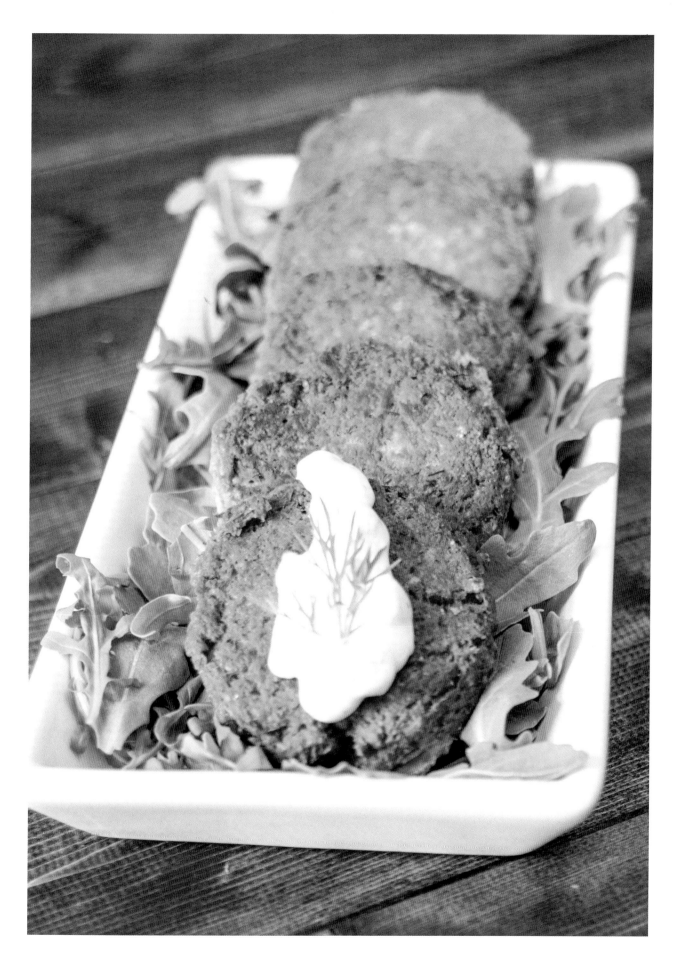

BROWN BUTTER SCALLOPS

SERVES 4

Am I the only one who thinks scallops are almost too good? The texture is so amazing when they are cooked perfectly, and the luscious flavor... Well, I take them one step further here with brown butter. Get your taste buds ready!

1½ pounds sea scallops, side muscle removed (see Notes)

½ teaspoon fine sea salt

¼ teaspoon ground black pepper

2 tablespoons light olive oil

¼ cup (½ stick) unsalted butter

Juice of ½ lemon

Lemon wedges, for serving (optional)

Notes : The side muscle of the scallop is a little rectangle tag that is not edible. Just grab it and pull it off.

It's very important to make sure the scallops are completely dry before you season and fry them—a wet scallop will steam and not brown.

• Dry the scallops well with a paper towel and season them with the salt and pepper.

• Heat the oil in a skillet over medium-high heat. Carefully place the scallops in the hot oil and sear until golden brown, about 3 minutes.

• Carefully flip the scallops and add the butter to the pan. Spoon the butter over the scallops as the other side browns and the butter starts to smell nutty, about 3 minutes more. Squeeze in the lemon juice and swirl it around the pan.

• Plate the scallops and pour the butter sauce over the tops. Serve immediately with lemon wedges, if desired.

PER SERVING
Calories **313** · Fat **20g** · Total Carbs **5g** · Net Carbs **5g** · Fiber **0g** · Protein **26g**

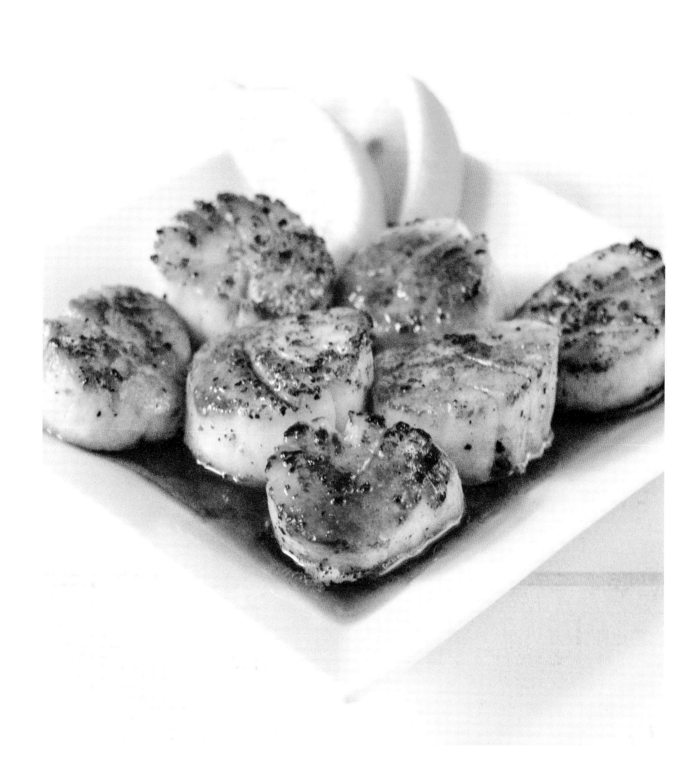

SMOKY GARLIC SHRIMP

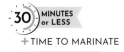

MINUTES or LESS

+ TIME TO MARINATE

SERVES 4

I really love the rich, smoky flavors of the seasonings in this dish, which go so well with the sweet shrimp. These shrimp are even more incredible when served atop my Cauli Risotto (page 184).

FOR THE MARINADE:

1 tablespoon light olive oil

1 teaspoon chipotle powder

1 teaspoon smoked paprika

½ teaspoon fine sea salt

⅛ teaspoon ground white pepper

1 pound large shrimp, peeled, deveined, and tails removed

2 tablespoons light olive oil

2 tablespoons unsalted butter

1 clove garlic, minced

¼ teaspoon chipotle powder

¼ teaspoon smoked paprika

¼ teaspoon fine sea salt

• In a medium-sized bowl, combine all of the marinade ingredients and mix well. Add the shrimp to the bowl and stir to coat. Cover and set aside for 15 minutes to marinate.

• Heat the oil in a large skillet over medium-high heat and add the shrimp. Cook in batches if necessary to avoid crowding the pan. Shallow-fry the shrimp for 2 minutes per side, until opaque, and transfer it to a plate.

• Turn the heat down to medium and melt the butter in the pan. Add the garlic and sauté until fragrant, about 1 minute. Add the chipotle powder, paprika, and salt and stir well.

• Return the shrimp and any juices back to the pan and stir to coat it well in the butter and seasonings. Cook until heated through, about 2 minutes. Plate and serve immediately.

• Store leftovers in an airtight container in the fridge for 2 to 3 days.

Variation: SPICY GARLIC SHRIMP

Add ⅛ teaspoon cayenne pepper to the marinade and the butter sauce to make this a spicy dish.

PER SERVING
Calories **259** · Fat **18g** · Total Carbs **0g** · Net Carbs **0g** · Fiber **0g** · Protein **24g**

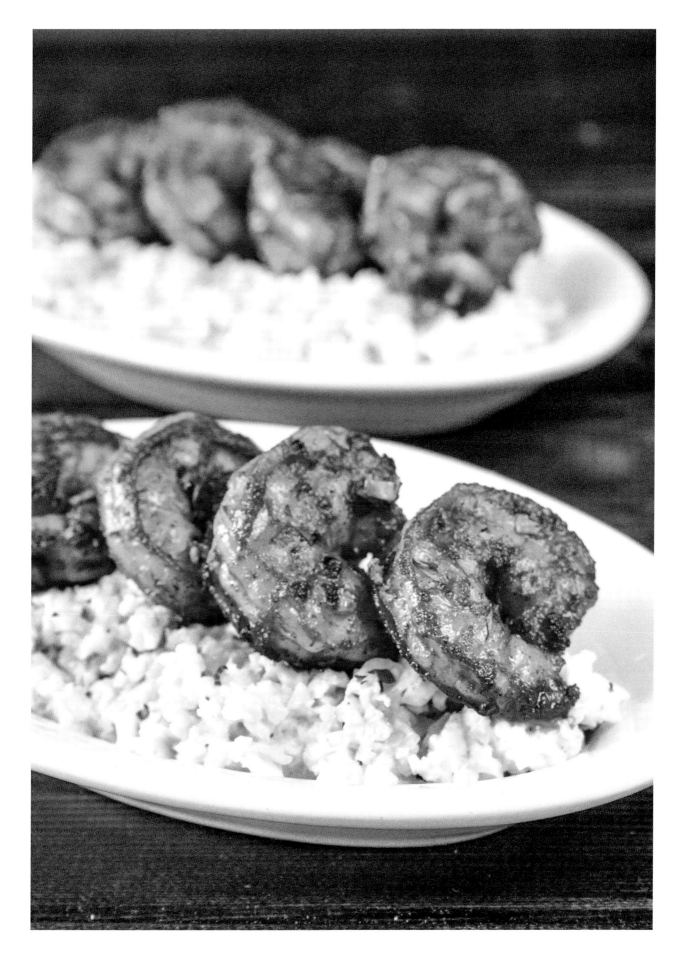

BAJA FISH TACOS

SERVES 4

I just love fish tacos, and this recipe—with tender seasoned cod and mind-blowing Baja Sauce (page 76)—will keep you coming back for more! Be sure to plan in advance so the sauce has time to arrive at its full flavor potential.

1 teaspoon fine sea salt

½ teaspoon chipotle powder

½ teaspoon ground black pepper

½ teaspoon onion powder

½ teaspoon smoked paprika

4 (4-ounce) frozen cod fillets

1 tablespoon light olive oil

FOR SERVING:

1 head Bibb lettuce, leaves separated

2 cups shredded cabbage

1 batch Baja Sauce (page 76)

2 scallions, both white and green parts, sliced

1 Roma tomato, diced

- Preheat the oven to 450°F and line a sheet pan with foil.

- In a small bowl, mix together the salt, chipotle powder, pepper, onion powder and paprika until combined.

- Place the fish fillets on the sheet pan and brush both sides with the oil. Season both sides of fish equally with the seasoning mix. Bake until the fish flakes in the center, about 15 to 20 minutes.

- While the fish is baking, arrange 2 or 3 lettuce leaves on each plate and divide the shredded cabbage equally among them.

- When the fish is done, flake it with 2 forks. Add the fish on top of the cabbage, spoon on the sauce, and sprinkle with the scallions and tomatoes. Serve immediately.

- Store leftovers in an airtight container in the fridge for up to 1 week.

Variation: BLACKENED FISH TACOS

Season the fish with 2 teaspoons of your favorite blackened seasoning instead and add 3 thin slices of avocado to each lettuce wrap.

PER SERVING
Calories **376** · Fat **25g** · Total Carbs **8g** · Net Carbs **5g** · Fiber **3g** · Protein **28g**

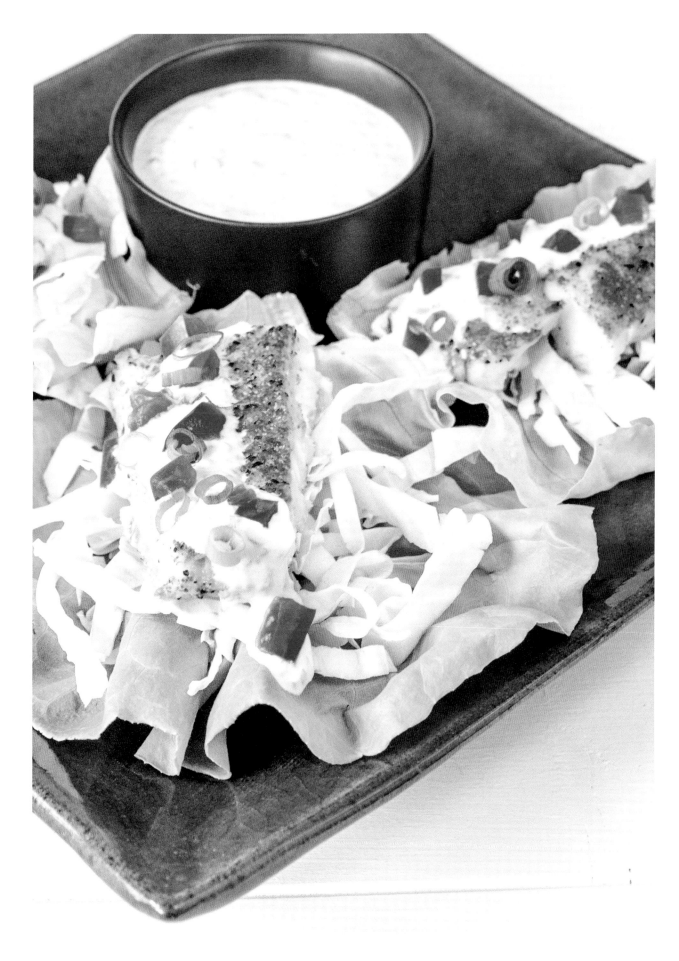

COCONUT SHRIMP

30 MINUTES or LESS

Plump and juicy shrimp coated in crispy coconut breading with a sweet-and-spicy dipping sauce—now that's what I call delicious!

SERVES 4

¼ cup coconut flour, sifted

1 large egg

¾ cup unsweetened shredded coconut

½ cup crushed pork rinds

1 pound large shrimp, peeled, deveined, and tails removed

½ teaspoon fine sea salt

¼ teaspoon ground black pepper

Coconut oil, for frying

FOR THE SAUCE:

¼ cup Sweet Chili Sauce (page 78)

2 tablespoons sugar-free marmalade

Note: To avoid batter buildup on your fingers, use one hand to dip the shrimp in the egg and the other hand to bread them.

• Set up the breading stations: Place the coconut flour in a medium-sized bowl. Whisk the egg in another medium-sized bowl and set it next to the coconut flour. In a large shallow bowl, combine the coconut and pork rinds, then set the bowl next to the egg.

• Season the shrimp with the salt and pepper. Dredge one shrimp in the coconut flour and shake off the excess, then dip it into the egg. Next, lay the shrimp in the breading and, with your hands, scoop the breading on top of the shrimp. Press it down gently, then flip the shrimp and do the same for the other side. Gently knock off any excess breading—but the shrimp should be very well coated. Set the shrimp on a plate and repeat with the remaining shrimp.

• Fill a large sauté pan with ½ inch of oil and heat over medium-high heat. To test the oil temperature, sprinkle in a few pork rind crumbs; if they sizzle, it's ready. Working in batches if necessary to avoid overcrowding the skillet, place the shrimp carefully into the hot oil and fry until golden brown, about 4 minutes, then carefully flip and cook on the other side for another 4 minutes. Transfer the shrimp to a paper towel–lined plate and sprinkle lightly with salt.

• While the shrimp is cooking, make the sauce: In a small saucepan over medium heat, heat the chili sauce and the marmalade, whisking to combine well.

• Serve the shrimp with the sauce on the side for dipping.

• Store leftovers in an airtight container in the fridge for 2 to 3 days.

PER SERVING
Calories **300** · Fat **16g** · Total Carbs **9g** · Net Carbs **5g** · Fiber **4g** · Protein **32g**

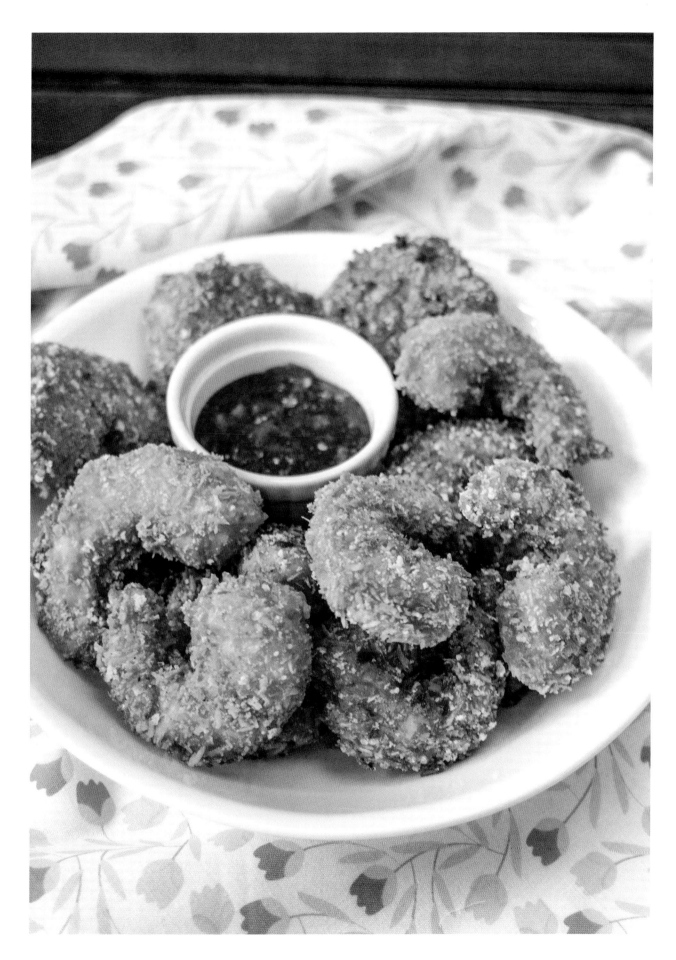

SHRIMP & GRITS

30 MINUTES or LESS

SERVES 4

Just thinking about creamy grits and sweet, luscious shrimp in a smoky rich gravy makes me happy! I had to reinvent this dish to some extent to be truly keto-friendly, but you'll be surprised at just how well the almond flour mimics grits.

4 strips thick-cut bacon, cut into 1-inch pieces

1 pound large shrimp, peeled, deveined, and tails removed

½ teaspoon fine sea salt

¼ teaspoon ground black pepper

FOR THE GRAVY:

1 tablespoon unsalted butter

⅓ cup diced onions

1 clove garlic, minced

2 ounces (¼ cup) cream cheese

¼ cup heavy cream

1 teaspoon Smoky BBQ Rub (page 60)

FOR THE GRITS:

½ cup chicken stock (see page 26)

½ cup heavy cream

⅔ cup almond flour

⅓ cup shredded Colby Jack cheese

2 tablespoons unsalted butter

½ teaspoon fine sea salt

¼ teaspoon ground black pepper

2 scallions, sliced, for garnish

Note: Any kind of cheese can be used in the grits: mild or sharp cheddar, Monterey Jack, pepper Jack, Swiss, and so on.

· Heat a large sauté pan over medium-high heat and drop in the bacon. Fry the bacon until crispy, about 10 minutes. Use a slotted spoon to transfer the bacon to a paper towel–lined plate, leaving the bacon drippings in the pan, and set aside.

· Season the shrimp with the salt and pepper, then add it to the bacon drippings in the pan. Sauté the shrimp until golden brown on both sides, about 3 minutes per side. Use a slotted spoon to move the shrimp to a plate and set aside. Do not wash the pan.

· Make the gravy: Melt the butter in the pan, still over medium-high heat, and add the onions. Sauté the onions until they're translucent and just starting to brown, about 5 minutes. Add the garlic and cook for 3 minutes, until fragrant. Turn the heat down to medium-low and add the cream cheese, heavy cream, and spice rub, then whisk to combine. Keep the gravy over the heat, stirring occasionally, while you make the grits.

· Make the grits: In a medium-sized saucepan over medium heat, heat the chicken stock and cream. Once small bubbles begin to appear, after about 5 minutes, whisk in the almond flour until completely combined. Add the cheese and cook until it has melted and the grits have thickened, about 3 minutes. Add the 2 tablespoons of butter and stir well. Remove from the heat and cover to keep warm.

· Return the shrimp to the pan with the gravy and stir to coat. Cook over medium heat until the shrimp is heated through, about 3 minutes.

· Divide the grits between 4 bowls. Spoon the shrimp and gravy over the grits, then sprinkle it with the reserved bacon and sliced scallions. Serve immediately.

· Store leftovers in an airtight container in the fridge for 2 to 3 days.

Variation: **SAUSAGE, SHRIMP & GRITS**

Substitute 1 pound andouille sausage for the bacon to make an even heartier meal.

PER SERVING

Calories **533** · Fat **42g** · Total Carbs **6g** · Net Carbs **5g** · Fiber **1g** · Protein **33g**

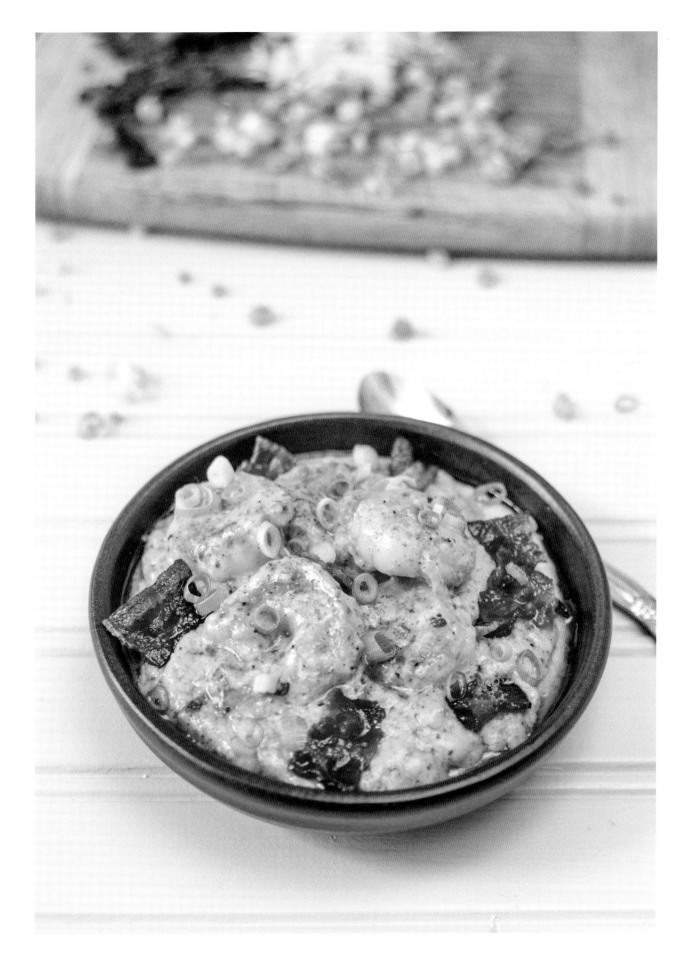

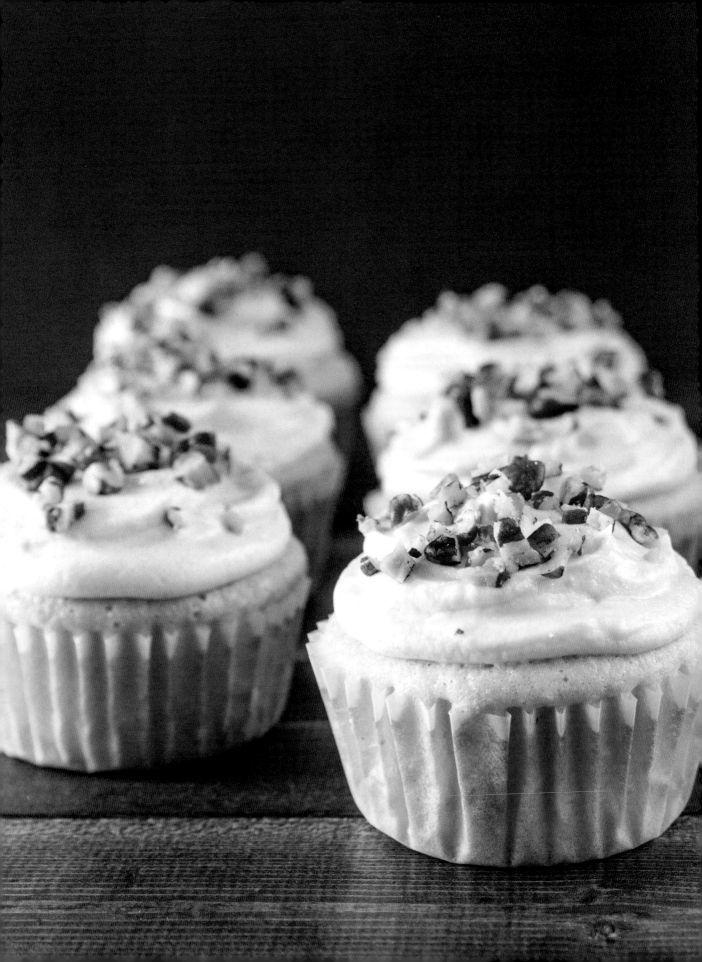

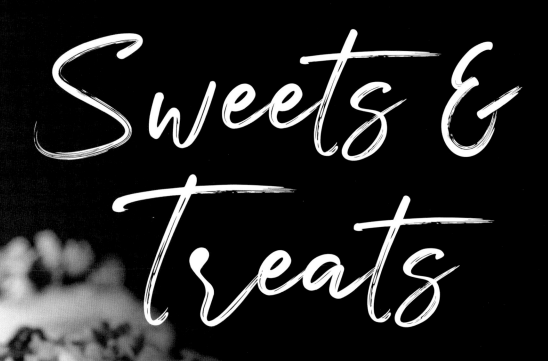

Sweets & Treats

BLUEBERRY COMPOTE

30 MINUTES or LESS

MAKES 1 CUP
(2 tablespoons per serving)

I first made this for my Lemon Cake (page 322), but it's mind-blowingly good on anything you can think of—baked goods, sharp cheese, or even eaten from the jar with a spoon.

2 cups blueberries, fresh or frozen

2 tablespoons water

1 tablespoon blended erythritol-stevia sweetener (see page 46)

1 teaspoon lemon juice

⅛ teaspoon ground cinnamon

Pinch of fine sea salt

¼ teaspoon pure vanilla extract

Note: This compote is a wonderful addition to a cheese plate!

- Combine the blueberries, water, sweetener, lemon juice, cinnamon, and salt in a medium-sized saucepan over medium-high heat and bring to a boil. Turn the heat down to medium-low and simmer until the compote has reduced by half, about 10 minutes.

- Remove the pan from the heat and stir in the vanilla extract. Let cool to room temperature, then pour the compote into a 1-pint glass jar and cover tightly. It can be served warm or chilled.

- Store in the glass jar in the fridge for up to 2 weeks.

Variation: **STRAWBERRY, RASPBERRY, OR MIXED BERRY COMPOTE**

Substitute an equal amount of strawberries or raspberries for the blueberries, or even try a combination of all three!

PER SERVING
Calories **20** · Fat **0g** · Total Carbs **5g** · Net Carbs **4g** · Fiber **1g** · Protein **0g**

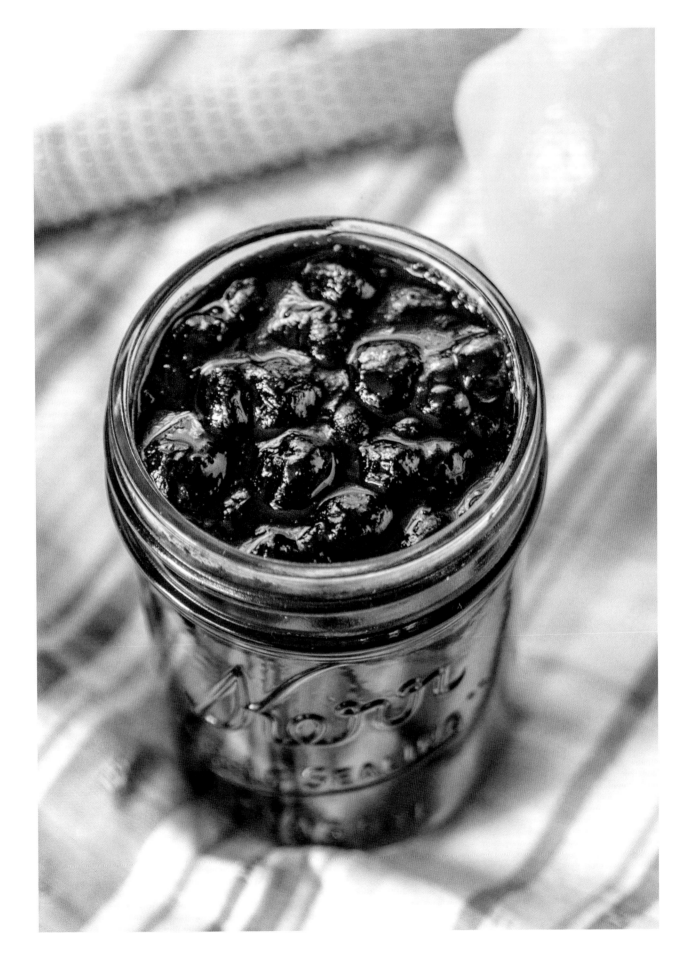

HOT FUDGE

MAKES 3/4 CUP
(3 tablespoons per serving)

This low-carb and delicious hot fudge is perfect drizzled over my Snickerdoodle Frozen Custard (page 316) or your favorite low-carb ice cream. It also makes delicious truffles—see the variation below.

½ cup heavy cream

2 ounces unsweetened chocolate, chopped

¼ cup powdered blended erythritol-stevia sweetener (page 46)

1 teaspoon cocoa powder

¼ teaspoon fine sea salt

1 tablespoon unsalted butter

½ teaspoon pure vanilla extract

• In a medium-sized saucepan over medium-low heat, heat the heavy cream and chocolate until the chocolate melts, stirring frequently. Whisk in the sweetener, cocoa powder, and salt. Bring to a gentle boil, then turn the heat back down to medium-low and simmer until thickened, about 3 minutes.

• Remove the pan from the heat, then stir in the butter and vanilla. Use while still warm.

• Store in an airtight container in the fridge for up to 1 week. Reheat in the microwave on 50 percent power in 20-second increments, stirring after each heating.

Variation : **CHOCOLATE TRUFFLES**

Follow the instructions for making the hot fudge, let cool, then pour it into a shallow 8-inch square glass dish and cover. Refrigerate for 2 hours, until the fudge is semisolid. Using a melon baller or small cookie scoop, scoop out small rounds and place them on a parchment-lined sheet pan. Refrigerate for another 20 minutes, or until the rounds are firm. Roll the rounds in your hands to form them into balls and warm them a bit, then roll them in the coating of your choice, like unsweetened shredded coconut, crushed nuts, or cocoa powder. Store in an airtight container in the refrigerator for up to a week.

PER SERVING
Calories **222** · Fat **21g** · Total Carbs **5g** · Net Carbs **2g** · Fiber **3g** · Protein **5g**

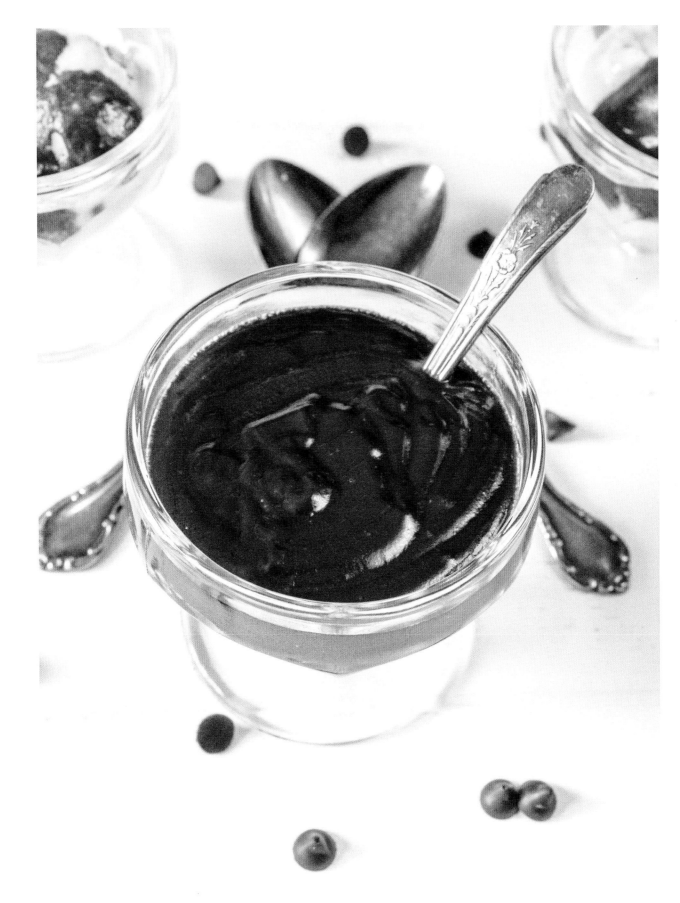

CHOCOLATE CHIPS

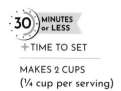

30 MINUTES or LESS

+ TIME TO SET

MAKES 2 CUPS
(¼ cup per serving)

I like making my own sugar-free chocolate and chocolate chips because I can control which sweetener is used (see page 46 for more on sweeteners). Bonus: they are a lot cheaper! I used to pour this mixture onto a parchment-lined sheet pan to cool and then chop it into chunks, but now you can find cute little chocolate chip molds to make perfectly sized bites of chocolate. Either way works, though!

2 ounces cocoa butter

1½ ounces unsweetened chocolate, chopped

¼ cup powdered blended erythritol-stevia sweetener (see page 46)

2 tablespoons cocoa powder, sifted

¼ teaspoon fine sea salt

½ teaspoon pure vanilla extract

· Melt the cocoa butter and chocolate in a double boiler. Alternatively, fill a saucepan with a few inches of water and bring it to a boil. Turn the heat down to low and set a glass bowl over the saucepan. (Be sure that the water does not touch the bottom of the bowl or the chocolate will get too hot and turn into a lumpy mess.) Melt the cocoa butter and chocolate in the bowl.

· Whisk in the sweetener, cocoa powder, and salt until completely dissolved and the mixture is smooth, about 3 minutes. Remove the pan from the heat and whisk in the vanilla extract.

· Let the chocolate mixture cool slightly, then pour it into chocolate chip molds or onto a parchment-lined sheet pan. Refrigerate until completely solid, about 30 minutes, before unmolding or chopping up the chocolate.

· Store in an airtight container in the refrigerator for up to 1 week.

Variation: FLAVORED CHOCOLATE

Try replacing the ½ teaspoon of vanilla extract with a flavor extract to make flavored chocolate, like orange, raspberry, or mint!

PER SERVING
Calories **81** · Fat **8g** · Total Carbs **2g** · Net Carbs **1g** · Fiber **1g** · Protein **1g**

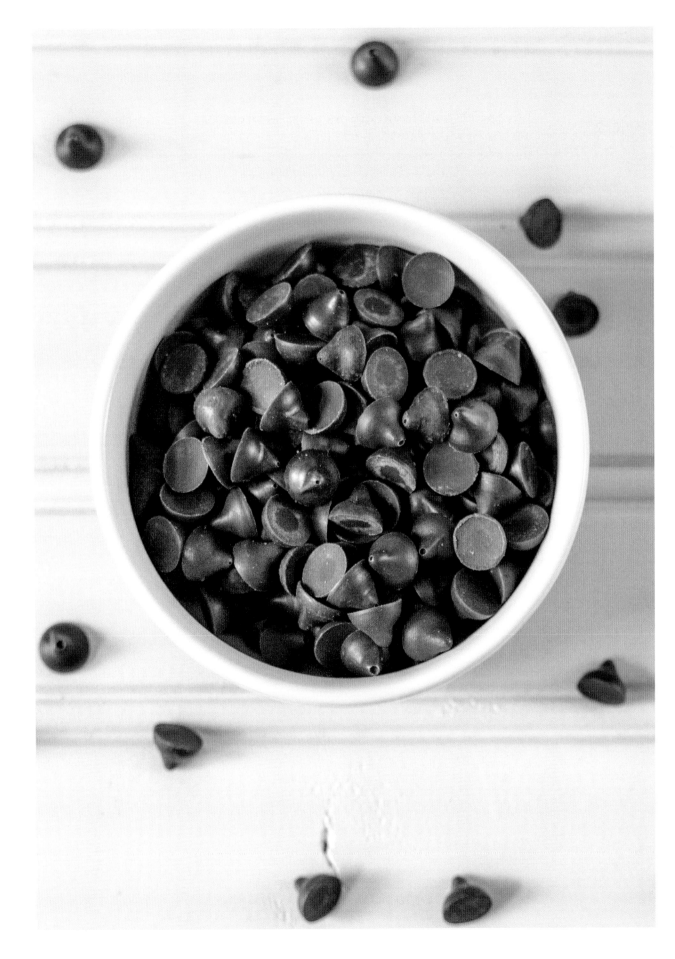

CHOCOLATE COOKIE CRUMBS

MAKES 2 CUPS
(¼ cup per serving)

A recipe just for cookie crumbs? Yes! Chocolate cookie crumbs have so many uses: they're the base for my Frozen Peanut Butter Pie (page 306), a very important component in my Cookies & Cream Parfait (page 308), and even a delicious topping on my Snickerdoodle Frozen Custard (page 316).

1 large egg yolk

2 tablespoons blended erythritol-stevia sweetener (see page 46)

2 tablespoons unsalted butter, softened

½ teaspoon pure vanilla extract

1 cup blanched almond flour

2 tablespoons cocoa powder

¼ teaspoon baking soda

¼ teaspoon fine sea salt

• Preheat the oven to 325°F and line a large sheet pan with parchment paper.

• In a medium-sized bowl, whisk together the egg yolk, sweetener, butter, and vanilla until creamy and smooth. Set aside.

• In a small bowl, combine the almond flour, cocoa powder, baking soda, and salt and stir until well blended. Add the dry ingredients to the wet ingredients and stir until well mixed.

• Using a rubber spatula or your hand, spread the dough onto the parchment-lined sheet pan in an even layer that's about ⅛ inch thick. Bake for 8 minutes, or until it starts to become crispy at the edges, then remove from the oven and pull the parchment paper onto potholders on the countertop to cool.

• Once the cookie has cooled and become crispy, break it up into crumbs. Store in an airtight container in the fridge for up to 2 weeks or in a sealed bag in the freezer for up to 2 months.

Variation: CRISPY CHOCOLATE COOKIES

If you'd rather make crispy cookies than use the recipe for crumbs, form the dough into a cylinder and wrap it in plastic wrap. Refrigerate for 30 minutes, then cut into slices and place the slices 2 inches apart on the parchment paper–lined sheet pan. Bake in a preheated 325°F oven for 8 minutes, or until crispy around the edges.

Variation: VANILLA COOKIE CRUMBS

To make vanilla cookie crumbs, just omit the cocoa powder. (And for vanilla cookies, follow the variation for Crispy Chocolate Cookies, above, without cocoa powder.)

PER SERVING
Calories **119** · Fat **11g** · Total Carbs **2g** · Net Carbs **0g** · Fiber **2g** · Protein **4g**

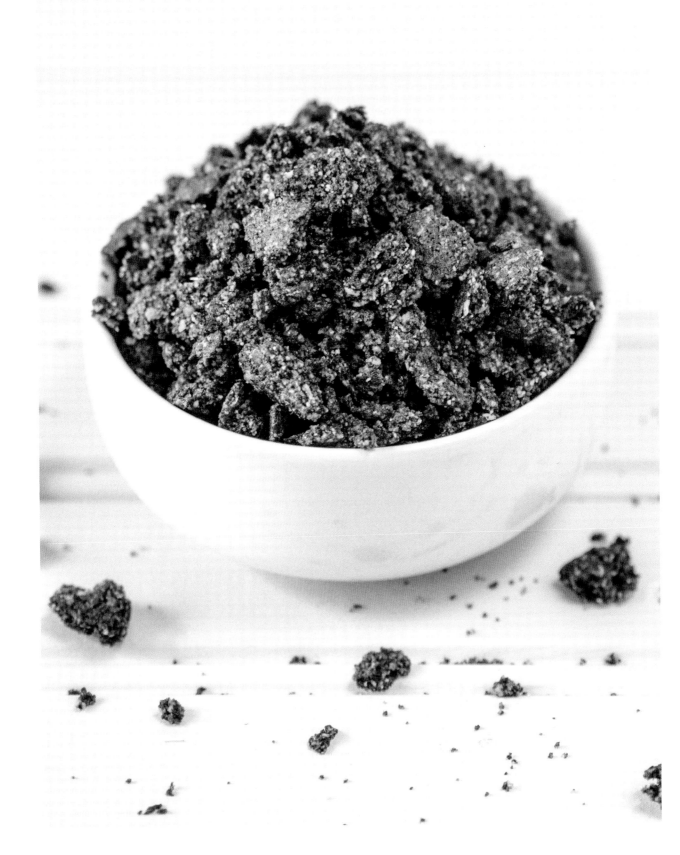

FROZEN PEANUT BUTTER PIE

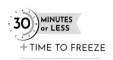

MINUTES or LESS

+TIME TO FREEZE

MAKES ONE
9-INCH PIE
(8 servings)

This is a sinfully rich frozen peanut butter pie with a chocolate cookie crust. It's even more wonderful topped with my Hot Fudge (page 300).

FOR THE CRUST:

1 cup Chocolate Cookie Crumbs (page 304)

⅓ cup finely chopped toasted pecans (see Notes)

2 tablespoons unsalted butter, melted

Pinch of fine sea salt

FOR THE FILLING:

4 ounces cream cheese (½ cup), room temperature

½ cup heavy cream

½ cup natural crunchy peanut butter, room temperature (see Notes)

¼ cup powdered blended erythritol-stevia sweetener (see page 46)

½ teaspoon pure vanilla extract

Pinch of fine sea salt

Hot Fudge (page 300), for drizzling (optional)

- In a medium-sized bowl, mix together all of the crust ingredients until well blended. Press the crust into the bottom and up the sides of a 9-inch pie pan. Place in the freezer to set while you make the filling.

- In a large bowl, combine all the filling ingredients. Using a hand mixer on medium speed, mix until thick and creamy. Spread the filling on the pie crust and drizzle with hot fudge, if desired. Cover with plastic wrap and freeze for at least 5 hours or overnight.

- Before slicing and serving, let the frozen pie sit at room temperature for 10 minutes.

- Store, covered, in the freezer for up to 1 week.

Switch It Up :

Try it with different nut butters, like almond, pecan, or cashew!

Notes : Toast the chopped pecans in a small dry skillet over medium heat, shaking frequently, until nutty and golden, about 5 minutes.

If you prefer, you can substitute natural creamy peanut butter for the crunchy.

This recipe will also make 2 smaller 4-inch pies instead of 1 full 9-inch pie.

PER SERVING
Calories **323** · Fat **31g** · Total Carbs **5g** · Net Carbs **2g** · Fiber **3g** · Protein **8g**

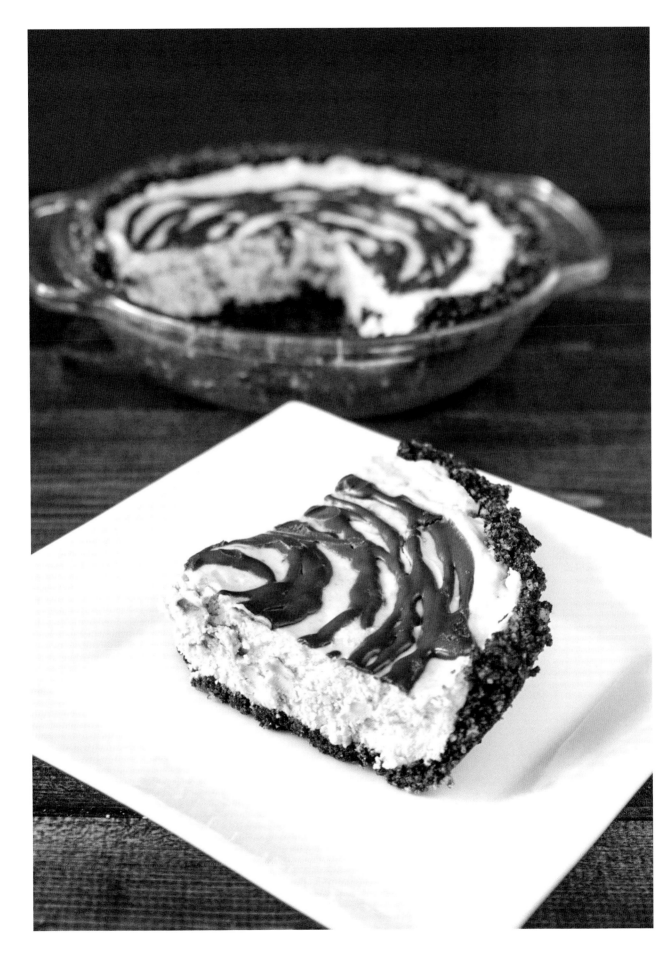

COOKIES & CREAM PARFAIT

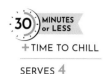

30 MINUTES or LESS
+ TIME TO CHILL
SERVES 4

This creamy and delicious pudding-like dessert will knock your socks off! Layer after layer of smooth cream and chocolate cookie crumbs will satisfy even the pickiest sweet tooth. This is a great recipe to make ahead—it's best after sitting overnight in the fridge.

1½ cups heavy cream, divided

½ cup powdered blended erythritol-stevia blend sweetener (see page 46), divided

⅛ teaspoon fine sea salt

2 large egg yolks

1 tablespoon unsalted butter

1 teaspoon pure vanilla extract

4 ounces cream cheese (½ cup), room temperature

1 cup Chocolate Cookie Crumbs (page 304)

• Whisk together 1 cup of the cream, ¼ cup of the sweetener, and the salt in a medium-sized heavy-bottomed saucepan over medium heat and heat until the mixture comes to a light boil, stirring frequently.

• Temper the eggs: Whisk the egg yolks in a medium-sized bowl until pale yellow, then slowly drizzle in a ladle of the hot cream mixture while whisking.

• Whisk the tempered eggs into the cream mixture and cook, stirring frequently, until thickened, about 5 minutes.

• Remove the pan from the heat and add the butter and vanilla extract, stirring to combine. Transfer the pudding to a large bowl, cover, and refrigerate for 2 hours to cool and set.

• Once the pudding is set, use a hand mixer on high speed to beat the remaining ½ cup of cream in a medium-sized bowl until soft peaks form. Set aside and clean the beaters.

• Place the cream cheese and remaining ¼ cup of sweetener in a separate medium-sized bowl and use the hand mixer on medium speed to beat them together until well combined. Add the pudding and mix with the hand mixer on the lowest speed just until combined. Carefully fold the whipped cream into the pudding-and-cream-cheese mixture.

• Assemble the parfaits: Use 8-ounce mason jars for individual servings, or assemble in just one medium-sized straight-edged clear trifle bowl. Place a layer of cookie crumbs in the bottom of the containers, followed by a layer of the pudding mixture. Repeat until all the pudding mixture and crumbs have been used.

• Cover the containers with plastic wrap and chill in the fridge for at least 3 hours or overnight. Serve cold.

• Store, covered, in the fridge for up to 1 week.

PER SERVING
Calories **583** · Fat **56g** · Total Carbs **5g** · Net Carbs **3g** · Fiber **2g** · Protein **9g**

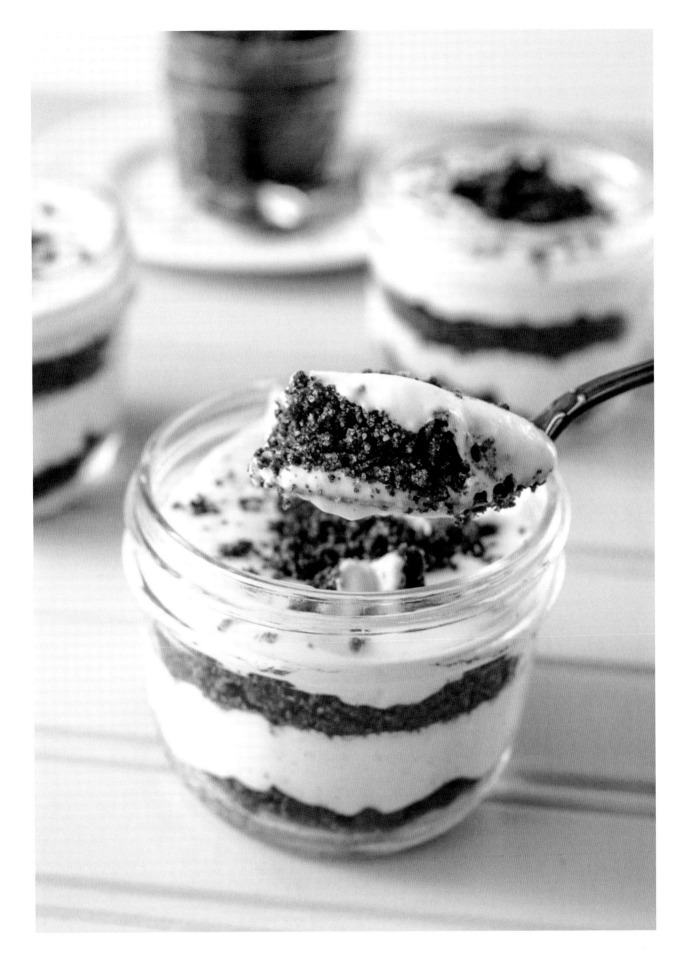

LEMON-LIME POSSET

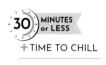

30 MINUTES or LESS

+ TIME TO CHILL

SERVES 4

This classic English dessert is truly a magic three-ingredient recipe. Citrus fruit, cream, and sweetener together create a plush texture and bright tart flavor. It does need time to chill and set in the fridge, so plan ahead for this one.

2 cups heavy cream

½ cup granulated erythritol (see page 46)

Pared zest of 1 lemon

Pared zest of 1 lime

Pinch of fine sea salt

3 teaspoons lemon juice

3 teaspoons lime juice

Grated lime and lemon zest, for garnish

Fresh whipped cream, for serving

- Heat the cream, erythritol, zest, and salt in a saucepan over medium heat, stirring frequently, until it comes to a light boil. Turn the heat down to medium-low and simmer gently, stirring frequently, until thickened, about 5 minutes.

- Remove from the heat and stir in the citrus juice. Strain the liquid through a fine-mesh sieve into 4 ramekins. Discard the solids.

- Refrigerate the ramekins, uncovered, for 30 minutes, then cover and continue chilling for at least 2 hours, until set. Garnish with grated zest and serve cold with fresh whipped cream.

- Store covered in the refrigerator for 2 to 3 days.

Switch It Up:

Try using all lemon or all lime and top with fresh berries.

PER SERVING INCLUDING WHIPPED CREAM
Calories **465** · Fat **55g** · Total Carbs **4g** · Net Carbs **4g** · Fiber **0g** · Protein **3g**

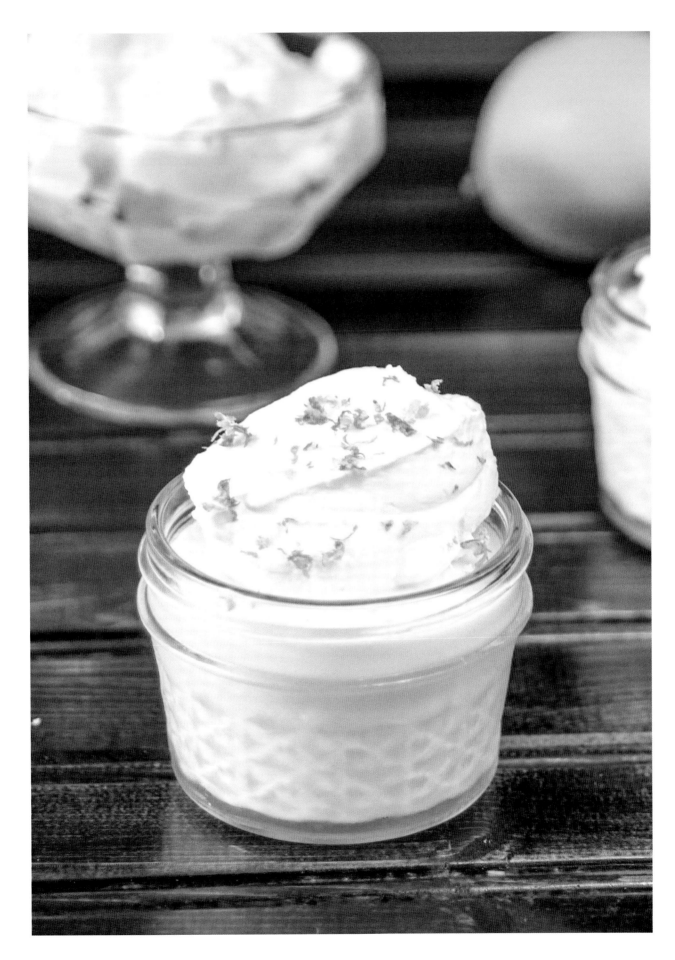

DARK CHOCOLATE POTS DE CRÈME

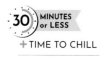

30 MINUTES or LESS

+ TIME TO CHILL

SERVES 4

With its rich dark-chocolate flavor and luxuriously creamy texture, this French dessert will quickly become a favorite. It tastes like pure elegance, but it couldn't be easier to make. It does require chilling before serving, so be sure to plan ahead for this recipe.

1 cup heavy cream

½ cup plain, unsweetened almond milk

⅓ cup granulated erythritol (see page 46)

3 tablespoons cocoa powder, sifted

2 teaspoons strong brewed coffee

¾ teaspoon fine sea salt

3 large egg yolks

1 tablespoon unsalted butter

1 teaspoon pure vanilla extract

Fresh whipped cream, for serving

Sugar-free chocolate sprinkles or chocolate shavings, for garnish (optional; see Note)

- Whisk together the cream, almond milk, erythritol, cocoa powder, coffee, and salt in a medium-sized heavy-bottomed saucepan over medium heat and heat until the mixture comes to a light boil, stirring frequently.

- Temper the eggs: Whisk the egg yolks in a medium-sized bowl until pale yellow, then slowly drizzle in a ladle of the hot cream mixture while whisking.

- Whisk the tempered eggs into the cream mixture and continue to cook, stirring frequently, until thickened, about 5 minutes.

- Remove the pan from the heat and add the butter and vanilla extract, stirring to combine. Divide the mixture evenly between 4 ramekins.

- Refrigerate the ramekins, uncovered, for 30 minutes, then cover and continue chilling for at least 2 hours, until set. Serve cold with fresh whipped cream. Garnish with sugar-free chocolate sprinkles, if desired.

- Store, covered, in the refrigerator for 2 to 3 days.

Switch It Up:

Try substituting other flavored extracts for the vanilla—dark chocolate, orange, raspberry, mint...

Note: You can buy my own brand of sugar-free chocolate sprinkles at The Sprinkle Company, etsy.com/shop/thesprinklecompany.

PER SERVING INCLUDING THE WHIPPED CREAM
Calories **334** · Fat **34g** · Total Carbs **4g** · Net Carbs **3g** · Fiber **1g** · Protein **4g**

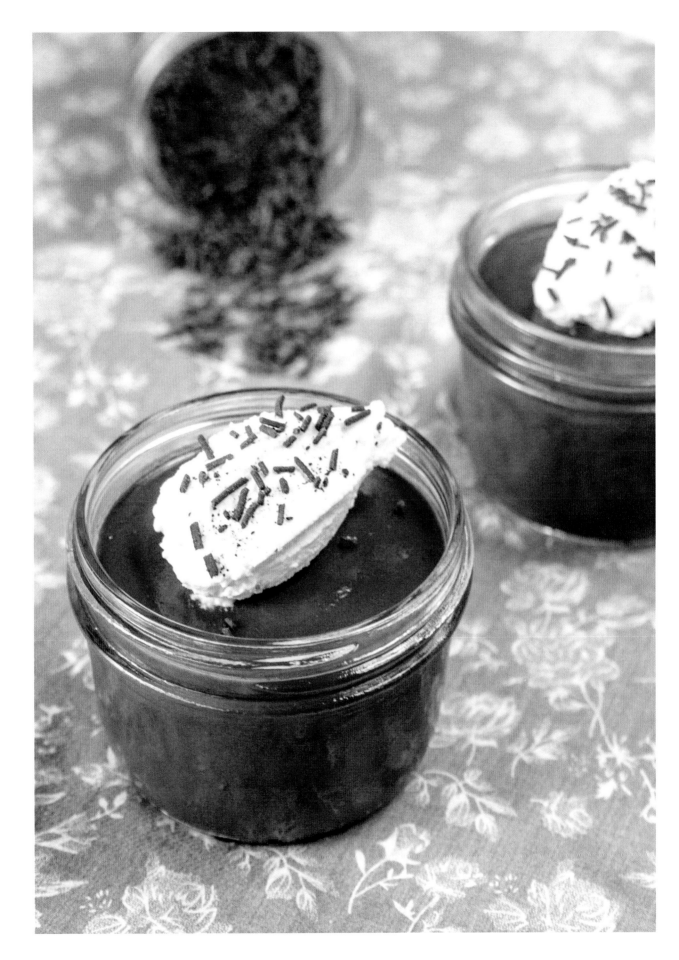

THUMBPRINT COOKIES

MAKES 1 DOZEN COOKIES
(1 per serving)

Thumbprint cookies have always been a favorite in my family. The beauty of these cookies is they can be filled with just about anything—I've used strawberry and raspberry preserves and my Hot Fudge (page 300) here, but my Blueberry Compote (page 298) would also work beautifully, as would other sugar-free preserves, like apricot or blackberry.

FOR THE COOKIES:

1 tablespoon powdered blended erythritol-stevia sweetener (see page 46)

1 tablespoon unsalted butter, softened

1 large egg

1 teaspoon pure vanilla extract

¼ cup natural smooth almond butter, room temperature

2 ounces cream cheese (¼ cup), room temperature

½ cup pecan meal (see Note)

⅛ teaspoon fine sea salt

FOR THE FILLING:

1 tablespoon sugar-free strawberry or raspberry preserves

1 tablespoon Hot Fudge (page 300)

Note : If you're unable to find pecan meal, just pulse ¾ cup raw pecan halves in a food processor or blender until finely ground.

- Preheat the oven to 350°F and line a large sheet pan with parchment paper.

- In a medium-sized bowl, using a whisk, cream together the sweetener and butter until smooth. Whisk in the egg and vanilla, followed by the almond butter and cream cheese. Stir in the pecan meal and salt until completely combined.

- Using a 2-tablespoon cookie scoop, drop rounds of dough 2 inches apart onto the parchment-lined sheet pan. Bake for 8 minutes, until the cookies are just set but not browned.

- Remove the cookies from the oven and gently press the bottom of a teaspoon into the top of each cookie to create a well. Return the cookies to the oven and bake until golden brown, about 5 minutes.

- Remove the cookies from the oven and set on a baking rack to cool. Once cooled, fill each cookie well with ½ teaspoon of either preserves or chocolate.

- Store in an airtight container in the fridge for up to 1 week.

Switch It Up :

Thumbprint fillings are pretty limitless. Try different kinds of sugar-free preserves, lemon curd, caramel, or even maple syrup with pieces of bacon!

PER SERVING
Calories **82** · Fat **8g** · Total Carbs **2g** · Net Carbs **1g** · Fiber **1g** · Protein **2g**

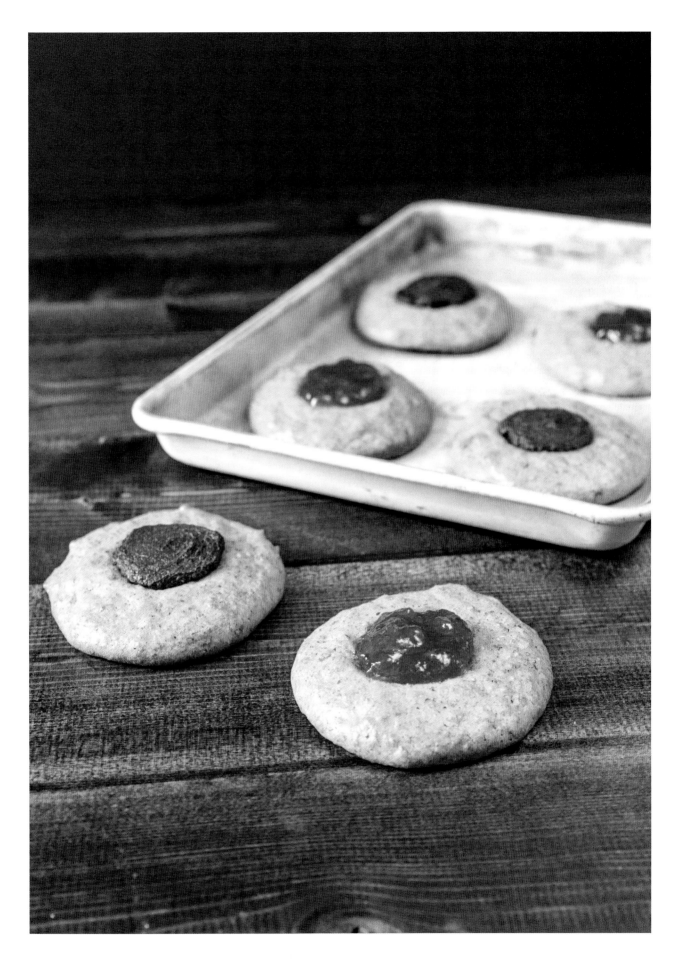

SNICKERDOODLE FROZEN CUSTARD

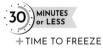

MINUTES or LESS

+TIME TO FREEZE

SERVES 4

Frozen custard is so rich and creamy, and this snickerdoodle version is no exception. It has cinnamon sweetness with a touch of salt, just like the cookie!

1½ cups heavy cream

1½ cups plain, unsweetened almond milk

¾ cup powdered blended erythritol-stevia sweetener (see page 46)

1 teaspoon ground cinnamon, plus more for garnish if desired

1 teaspoon fine sea salt

4 large egg yolks

1 teaspoon pure vanilla extract

Switch It Up :

To add mix-ins, freeze the custard to the soft-serve stage, about 2 hours. Then stir in your mix-in of choice, like my Chocolate Chips (page 302) or Chocolate Cookie Crumbs (page 304).

• Whisk together the cream, almond milk, sweetener, cinnamon, and salt in a medium-sized heavy-bottomed saucepan over medium heat and heat until the mixture comes to a light boil, stirring frequently.

• Temper the eggs: Whisk the egg yolks in a medium-sized bowl until pale yellow, then slowly drizzle in a ladle of the hot cream mixture while whisking.

• Whisk the tempered eggs into the cream and continue to cook, stirring frequently, until thickened, about 5 minutes.

• Remove the pan from the heat and stir in the vanilla extract. Transfer the custard mixture to a large bowl, cover, and refrigerate for 2 hours.

• Follow the manufacturer directions for your ice cream machine. Alternatively, transfer the mixture to a 9 by 5-inch loaf pan and cover with plastic wrap, then freeze until the custard is solid but scoopable, about 5 hours. (If you use a loaf pan, set it out for 15 to 20 minutes before serving so it's more scoopable.) Garnish with ground cinnamon before serving, if desired.

• Store in the freezer for up to 1 week.

PER SERVING
Calories **378** · Fat **38g** · Total Carbs **4g** · Net Carbs **3g** · Fiber **1g** · Protein **5g**

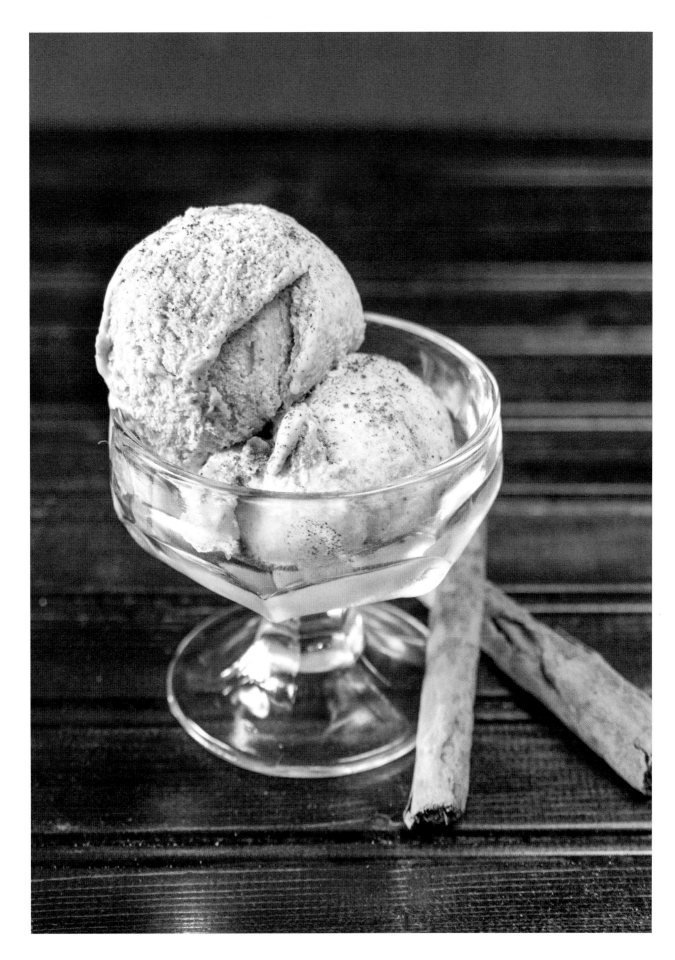

COCONUT CUPCAKES

 1 HOUR or LESS

MAKES 8 CUPCAKES
(1 per serving)

This is one of the first keto cakes I ever made, and it's still a family favorite years later. The coconut cake is dense and buttery, and the frosting is creamy, light, and bursting with coconut flavor.

FOR THE CUPCAKES:

½ cup unsalted butter, softened

¼ cup blended erythritol-stevia sweetener (see page 46)

3 large eggs

½ teaspoon pure vanilla extract

½ cup unsweetened coconut flakes

½ cup coconut flour, sifted

½ teaspoon baking soda

½ teaspoon fine sea salt

FOR THE FROSTING:

¼ cup powdered blended erythritol-stevia sweetener (see page 46)

1½ ounces cream cheese (3 tablespoons), room temperature

3 tablespoons unsalted butter, softened

1 tablespoon heavy cream

½ teaspoon pure vanilla extract

Pinch of fine sea salt

¼ cup unsweetened coconut flakes, for topping

Switch It Up:
Add ½ cup of Chocolate Chips (page 302).

- Preheat the oven to 350°F and line 8 wells of a standard-size 12-well muffin tin with paper liners.

- In a large bowl, whisk together the butter and sweetener until smooth and creamy. Add the eggs and vanilla, whisking well to combine.

- In a medium-sized bowl, combine the coconut flakes, coconut flour, baking soda, and salt and stir to combine. Add the dry ingredients to the wet ingredients and stir until well mixed.

- Divide the batter evenly between the lined muffin wells and lightly press down on the tops with the back of a spoon or your fingers to smooth. Bake for 20 minutes, or until a toothpick inserted in the middle of a cupcake comes out clean.

- While the cupcakes are baking, make the frosting: In a large bowl, beat together all the frosting ingredients with a hand mixer on medium speed until light and fluffy.

- Remove the cupcakes from the oven and let cool completely before frosting. Top with coconut flakes.

- Store in an airtight container in the fridge for up to 1 week.

Variation : COCONUT LOAF CAKE

This can also be made as a loaf cake: Mix the batter as directed above and put it in a greased 9 by 5-inch loaf pan. Bake in a preheated 350°F oven for 20 minutes, or until a toothpick inserted in the middle comes out clean. Allow to cool before frosting.

PER SERVING
Calories **241** · Fat **23g** · Total Carbs **5g** · Net Carbs **2g** · Fiber **3g** · Protein **4g**

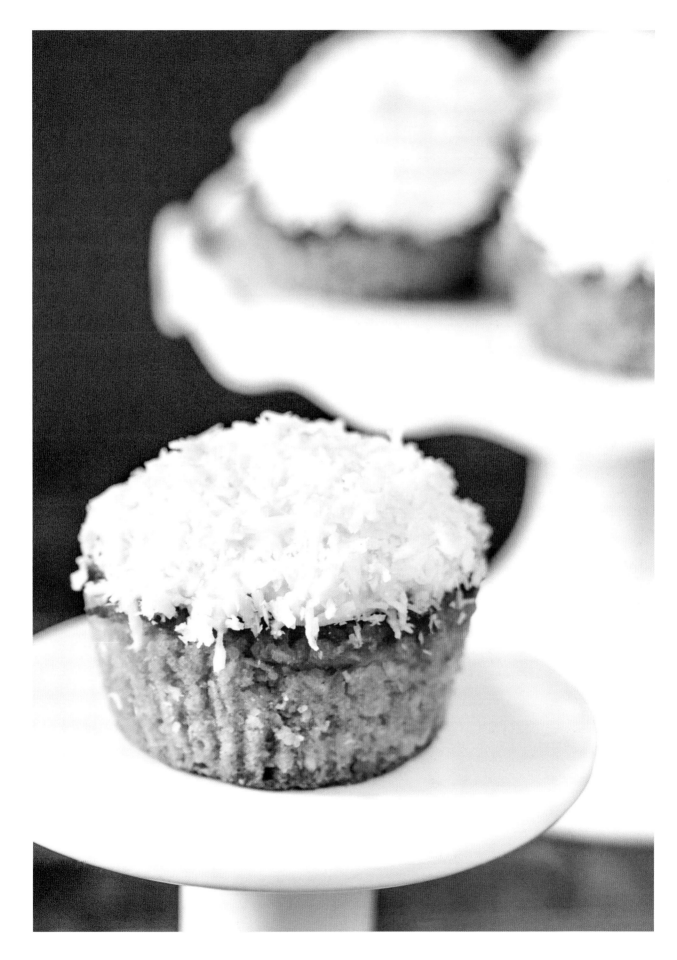

BANANA CUPCAKES
with SWEET BROWN BUTTER FROSTING

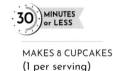

30 MINUTES or LESS

MAKES 8 CUPCAKES
(1 per serving)

My great-grandmother always made me banana bread when I was growing up, and I'm still nostalgic for the taste of banana bread. I was so happy when I came up with these keto-friendly cupcakes. They have that same banana flavor and are light and fluffy, with a decadent brown butter–cream cheese frosting and topped with toasted pecans. You'll love them even if you're not nostalgic for banana bread.

⅓ cup unsalted butter, softened

⅓ cup blended erythritol-stevia sweetener (see page 46)

3 large eggs

¼ cup full-fat sour cream

1 teaspoon banana extract

1¼ cups blanched almond flour

1 teaspoon baking powder

¼ teaspoon fine sea salt

FOR THE FROSTING:

2 tablespoons unsalted butter

2½ ounces cream cheese (¼ cup plus 1 tablespoon), room temperature

2 tablespoons powdered blended erythritol-stevia sweetener (see page 46)

½ teaspoon pure vanilla extract

Pinch of fine sea salt

¼ cup chopped toasted pecans, for garnish (see Note)

Note : *Toast the chopped pecans in a small dry skillet over medium heat, shaking frequently, until nutty and golden, about 5 minutes.*

• Preheat the oven to 325°F and line 8 wells of a standard-size 12-well muffin tin with paper liners.

• Make the brown butter for the frosting: Heat the 2 tablespoons of butter in a heavy-bottomed saucepan over medium heat, swirling occasionally, until the butter smells nutty and the milk solids are just starting to turn golden brown, about 5 minutes. Transfer to a bowl and set aside on the countertop to cool and solidify while you make the cupcakes.

• Make the cupcakes: In a large bowl, whisk together the butter and sweetener until smooth and creamy. Add the eggs, sour cream, and banana extract and whisk until well combined.

• In a medium-sized bowl, combine the almond flour, baking powder, and salt and stir to combine. Add the dry ingredients to the wet ingredients and stir until well mixed.

• Using a ⅓-cup measuring cup, fill each lined well of the muffin tin with ⅓ cup of batter. Bake for 15 minutes, or until a toothpick inserted in the middle of a cupcake comes out clean.

• While the cupcakes are baking, make the frosting: In a large bowl, combine the brown butter, cream cheese, sweetener, vanilla, and salt. Using a hand mixer on medium speed, whip the ingredients together until light and fluffy.

• Remove the cupcakes from the oven and let cool completely before frosting. Garnish with the toasted pecans.

• Store in an airtight container in the fridge for up to 1 week.

PER SERVING
Calories **302** · Fat **29g** · Total Carbs **3g** · Net Carbs **1g** · Fiber **2g** · Protein **7g**

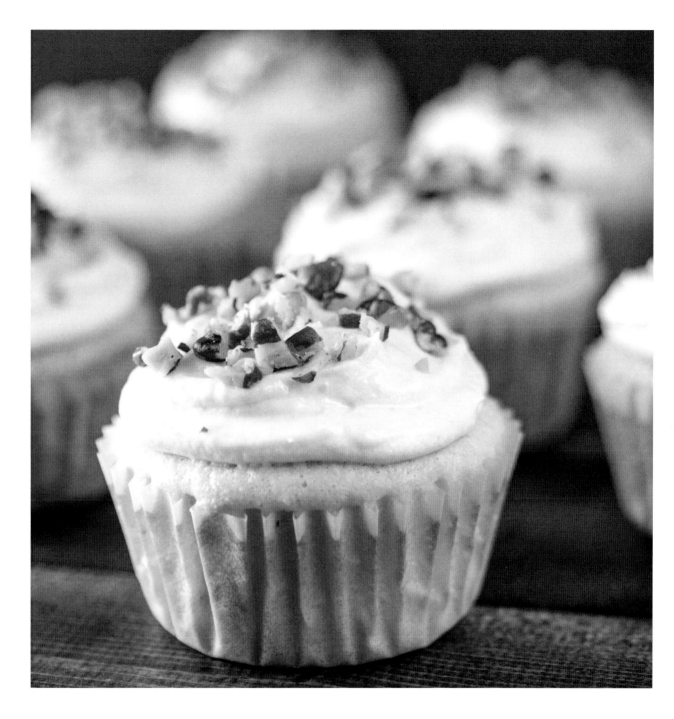

Variation : BANANA CAKE WITH SWEET BROWN BUTTER FROSTING

Double the ingredients and make a two-layer cake instead!

Mix the batter as directed and divide it evenly between 2 greased 8-inch cake pans. (I recommend putting a piece of parchment at the bottom of both pans.)

Bake in a preheated 325°F oven for 25 minutes, or until a toothpick inserted in the middle comes out clean. Set aside to cool.

Once the cakes are completely cooled, place one cake on a serving plate or cake stand and spread half of the frosting on top. Place the other cake on top of the frosted cake and spread the rest of the frosting over the top. Slice and serve.

LEMON CAKE

1 HOUR or LESS

MAKES ONE
DOUBLE-LAYER
9-INCH CAKE
(12 servings)

When I decided to go keto, I knew I had to find a way to make a low-carb version of my favorite lemon cake. It turned out better than I could have imagined. It has a dense, tangy lemon cake bottom and a sweet lemon cheesecake-like top. This cake is wonderful topped with Blueberry Compote (page 298).

FOR THE CAKE LAYER:

½ cup (1 stick) unsalted butter, softened

¼ cup powdered blended erythritol-stevia sweetener (see page 46)

3 large eggs

1 tablespoon grated lemon zest

1 tablespoon lemon juice

½ teaspoon pure vanilla extract

½ cup coconut flour, sifted

½ teaspoon baking soda

½ teaspoon fine sea salt

FOR THE CHEESECAKE LAYER:

1 (8-ounce) package cream cheese, room temperature

⅓ cup powdered blended erythritol-stevia sweetener (see page 46)

2 large eggs

1 tablespoon grated lemon zest

1 tablespoon lemon juice

· Preheat the oven to 325°F. Coat the sides and bottom of a 9-inch square baking dish with nonstick cooking spray.

· Make the cake layer: Using a hand mixer on medium speed, beat together the butter and sweetener in a large bowl until thick and creamy. Add the eggs, lemon zest, lemon juice, and vanilla extract, then beat again until thoroughly combined.

· In a small bowl, whisk the coconut flour, baking soda, and salt until well mixed. Add the dry ingredients to the wet ingredients and stir until well combined and a thick dough forms.

· Spread the dough into the greased baking dish and push down on the top using the back of a spatula until it's evenly distributed and the bottom of the dish is completely covered.

· Make the cheesecake layer: Using a hand mixer on medium-high speed, in a large bowl, beat the cheesecake layer ingredients together until creamy, then pour the mixture on top of the dough.

· Bake for 30 to 40 minutes, until the top is no longer jiggly and is starting to become golden.

· Remove from the oven and let cool before slicing.

· Wrap leftovers tightly in plastic wrap and store in the refrigerator for up to 1 week. To freeze, wrap in plastic wrap, then in foil. It will keep in the freezer for up to 1 month. Thaw in the fridge overnight.

PER SERVING
Calories **186** · Fat **17g** · Total Carbs **4g** · Net Carbs **2g** · Fiber **2g** · Protein **5g**

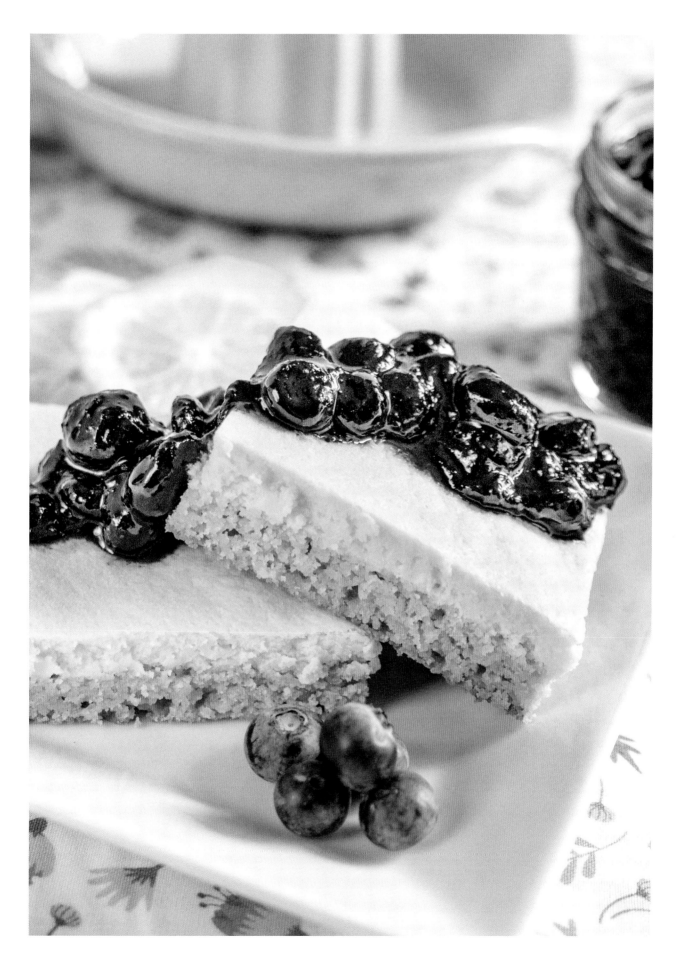

GERMAN CHOCOLATE CAKE

1 HOUR or LESS

MAKES ONE
DOUBLE-LAYER
8-INCH CAKE
(8 servings)

German chocolate cake just screams decadence to me! This dense and delicious chocolate cake is topped with the most divine coconut-and-pecan frosting.

½ cup blended erythritol-stevia sweetener (see page 46)

½ cup unsalted butter, softened

4 large eggs

¼ cup full-fat sour cream

1 teaspoon pure vanilla extract

1½ cups blanched almond flour

⅓ cup cocoa powder, sifted

1 teaspoon baking powder

¼ teaspoon fine sea salt

FOR THE FROSTING:

½ cup heavy cream

½ cup powdered blended erythritol-stevia sweetener (see page 46)

¼ teaspoon fine sea salt

2 large egg yolks

½ cup unsweetened shredded coconut

⅓ cup chopped toasted pecans (see Notes)

3 tablespoons unsalted butter, softened

1 teaspoon pure vanilla extract

• Preheat the oven to 325°F and grease two 8-inch cake pans. (I recommend adding a piece of parchment to the bottoms as well.)

• In a large bowl, whisk together the sweetener and butter until smooth and creamy. Add the eggs, sour cream, and vanilla extract and whisk until well combined.

• In a medium-sized bowl, combine the flour, cocoa powder, baking powder, and salt and stir until well combined. Add the dry ingredients to the wet ingredients and stir until well mixed.

• Divide the batter evenly between the 2 prepared pans. Bake for 25 minutes, or until a toothpick inserted into the center of each cake comes out clean. Remove from the oven and set aside to cool.

• While the cakes are baking, make the frosting: Place the cream in a large saucepan over medium heat and whisk in the sweetener and salt until completely dissolved.

• In a medium-sized bowl, whisk the egg yolks until creamy and pale yellow. Whisking continuously, ladle in about ⅓ cup of the hot cream mixture to temper the eggs. Whisk the tempered eggs into the cream mixture.

• Continue cooking, stirring occasionally, until the mixture has thickened, about 5 minutes. Remove the pan from the heat and add the coconut, pecans, butter, and vanilla. Stir until well combined.

• Once the cakes are completely cooled, place one cake on a serving plate or cake stand and spread half of the frosting on top. Place the remaining cake on top of the frosted cake and spread the rest of the frosting over the top. Slice and serve.

• Store leftovers in an airtight container in the fridge for up to 1 week.

PER SERVING
Calories **454** · Fat **44g** · Total Carbs **8g** · Net Carbs **3g** · Fiber **5g** · Protein **11g**

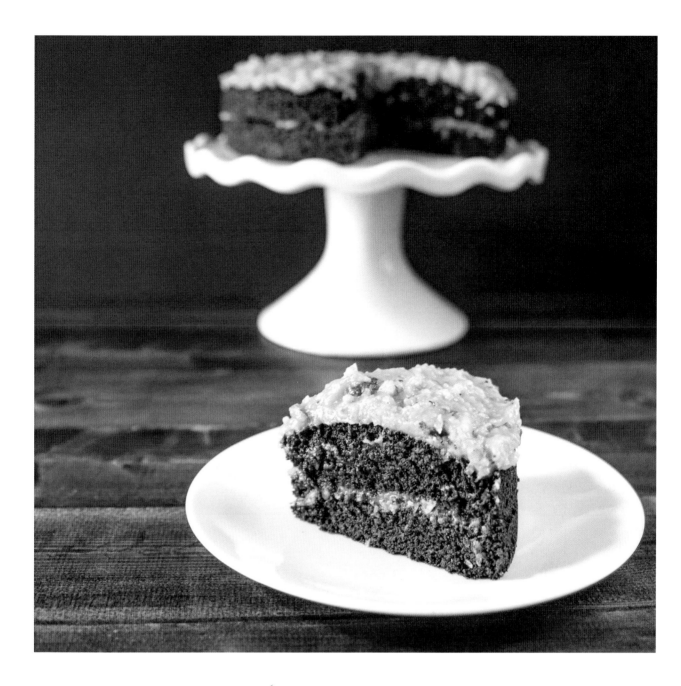

Notes : Toast the chopped pecans in a small dry skillet over medium heat, shaking frequently, until nutty and golden, about 5 minutes.

If you'd like to frost the sides of the cake, double the frosting.

For added decadence, chill a batch of my Hot Fudge (page 300) and whip it with a hand mixer on medium speed until light and fluffy, then use it to frost the sides of the cake.

Variation : GERMAN CHOCOLATE CUPCAKES

Line 8 wells of a standard-size 12-well muffin tin with paper liners. Instead of pouring the batter into 2 pans, divide it evenly among the wells, filling each about two-thirds full. Bake in a preheated 325°F oven for 25 minutes, or until a toothpick inserted into the middle of a cupcake comes out clean. Allow to cool completely. Using a piping bag with a large hole or a plastic bag with one corner snipped off, fill each cupcake with 1 tablespoon of cooled Hot Fudge (page 300). Top with the coconut pecan frosting.

So there I am, 156 steps up this beautiful lighthouse in Daytona Beach, Florida—exactly halfway to the top. I can't breathe, my legs are cramped, and sweat is rolling down my face and back. I'm too far up to go back down and too far down to make it to the top. I'm in full-blown panic mode. The disappointed look from my son and the worried looks from the people passing us in the stairwell made this my rock bottom. I knew I needed to change my life. I joined a CrossFit gym and adopted the Paleo diet. It was an amazing jumping-off point. I lost 40 pounds rather quickly, but as with most diets, I hit a wall. I turned to Nicole in the desperate hope of finding something that would help me get back on track. She talked about the keto diet and all the amazing effects it has on your body. It was like magic—within the first month I dropped another 20 pounds, and I've been off to the races ever since.

To date, I've lost 110 pounds. I never could've imagined being this successful with any diet, but keto is the lifestyle for me. I've tried almost every recipe from Nicole's website and her Instagram page. They're easy to make and amazingly delicious. It's easy to get bored with the same four or five things on the menu every week, but her recipes have made it possible for me to stay on my path. For next summer, I'm booking a trip back to that same lighthouse, where I will not only make it to the top, but I'll run up the stairs, blaring the Rocky theme song through my earbuds!

—Noah Shaffer O'Neill, @itsaketothing

I was overweight and tired all the time, and I took medication for high blood pressure. I also had what I thought was Hashimoto's and hyperthyroidism. I was thirty-six, way too young to be sick and tired all the time. I knew it was time to finally do something about the extra pounds I was carrying around. I started my low-carb weight-loss journey in April 2015. Along with eating low-carb, I was working out almost every day at home with DVDs and my treadmill. I was determined to lose weight and stick to my new eating habits. As the scale started moving down and results were starting to show from my hard work, my motivation and dedication continued to grow.

All was well until I was diagnosed with thyroid cancer in November 2015. What the doctors once thought was Hashimoto's turned out to be something that terrified me. The day I was told my diagnosis, I was not prepared to hear the word cancer. My world stopped and thoughts of my kids growing up without me filled my head. It was a scary time in my life. Not long after, Nicole told me about keto and her weight-loss experience, along with keto's many health benefits. Her progress was inspiring, and I was very interested in trying the same foods she was making and creating.

Keto has been one of the easiest diets I have been on. Nicole's recipes make it even easier, and they do not disappoint! My kids love the food we make, and I have some pretty picky eaters. In total I have lost 45 pounds, and I feel amazing. I've also stopped taking medications that I had been on for years. I continue to work on my health and fitness daily, working out at my gym five or six days a week. I consider myself a constant work in progress.

—Emily Headley, @lowcarbandlovingfit

Pre-keto, I had PCOS symptoms, prediabetic bloodwork, and high blood pressure. I was constantly hungry. My energy level ranged from tired to lethargic. My sugar cravings were raging. It wasn't until I changed my eating habits by upping my fats and limiting my carbs to 20 grams a day that I realized how much carbs had been affecting my body!

I started keto to lose weight after everything else I tried had failed. Two years later, I'm living a keto lifestyle because of how I feel! I've lost 45 pounds and maintained that loss. All my health markers are within the normal range. I don't ever wake up starving, I don't have dips in my energy, and I don't even have the desire for sugary treats! This is crazy to me because when I first read about keto, I thought, "No way will a foodie like myself be able to only eat 20 net carbs a day!" Now I'll consume no more than 10 net carbs a day.

I've been following Nicole's blog for quite a few years already. I know that part of my keto success was finding recipes that were so tasty and satisfying, I didn't miss carbs or feel like I was missing out on anything. She has so many awesome recipes that are just as yummy as dishes that were loaded with carbs. I never felt like I was on a diet. When I think of keto recipe bloggers, I think of Nicole as one of the first pioneers. Her recipes are consistently outstanding. The instructions are always clear and easy to follow and perfect for all cooking levels. I have some of the harshest food critics in my house, but when I make them one of her recipes, they always love it and are blown away when I tell them, "Oh, by the way...that was keto."

–Chastity Nieves, @chastity.loves.keto

It can be so confusing starting a ketogenic lifestyle and eliminating carbohydrates. I was lost after I was diagnosed with PCOS and my doctor recommended keto as a treatment. I found Nicole on Instagram, and it was my ketogenic starting point. She has so many amazing recipes, and she herself has had great success with weight loss on keto. I started to screenshot all her meals and recipes and used her as my meal planner. Nicole's recipes have been a huge part of my keto journey. Having Nicole take the guesswork out of figuring what to cook was and is still a lifesaver for me. Her recipes are so delicious, satisfying, easy to follow, and simple to make, with normal ingredients.

The ketogenic lifestyle has changed me. It is the lost key I was looking for that unlocked me from the hopelessness of obesity. I have lost over 100 pounds and I'm so close to a healthy BMI, something I never thought possible. If you are feeling defeated, depressed, anxious, overwhelmed, and trapped by obesity, I understand completely. Take back your power and control of your life by introducing yourself to the ketogenic lifestyle. Nicole has already prepared the recipes—just cook them up and enjoy the satisfying and delicious meals. In six months, you'll be celebrating your weight loss. You got this, and I am so happy you are changing your life!

–Shauna Dell, @peekabooitsme_

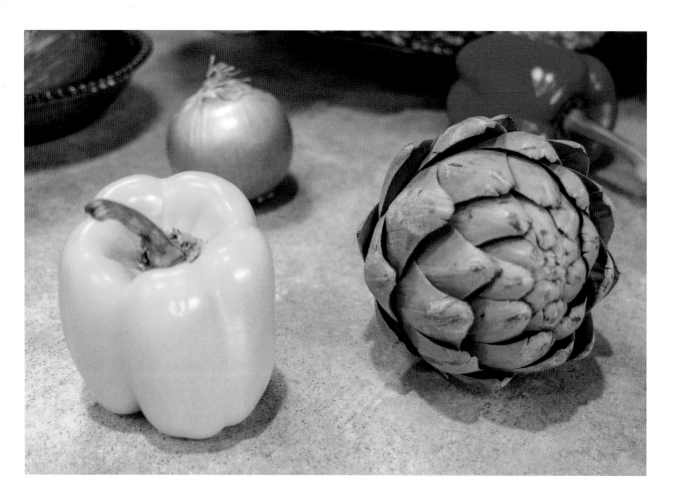

ACKNOWLEDGMENTS

First and foremost, I want to send a huge THANK YOU to the entire keto community for being so supportive and inspiring over the past three years. I wouldn't be where I am today without all of you cheering me on each day. It is truly a blessing to be involved with such a tight-knit and caring group of people, and I'm eternally grateful to be a part of this community.

To the entire Victory Belt crew: I cannot thank you enough for all of the amazing things you've done to make this book as incredible as it is. Erich—Thank you for taking a chance on me and making me believe in myself. Lance—Your Photography 101 is top-notch, and I'm so thankful for all you've taught me and all the great advice you've given me. Susan—I can barely put into words how much your friendship means to me and how endlessly helpful and encouraging you've been. Thank you for always being there when I needed you. Erin—Your attention to detail during the editing process was awesome, and you made it such an enjoyable process. Thank you! The design team—You have truly outdone yourselves with the gorgeous design of my book, and I'm so very thankful for all of you.

My kiddos, Makenzie and Cameron—I appreciate your tasting every single one of these recipes and giving them two thumbs up! Thank you for always believing in me and pushing me to be my best every day. I love you both to the moon and back, and I couldn't be prouder of you if I tried.

Emily—I know you're "not even trying to think about a pork rind," but I couldn't have picked a better best friend to have for over twenty-five years. Thank you for always being my support system and for letting me use your home for various photo shoots. I know it's taken a long time, but I finally forgive you for the fish earring debacle!

Korey—Thank you for always believing in me and for all your endless research on the healthiest ways to eat—keto being the last and best.

Maryam—Your friendship means the absolute world to me. You have the most caring heart of anyone I've ever met, and I'm so blessed to know you. I am beyond thankful to have you in my life and in my corner.

Noah—Thank you for being my biggest cheerleader through the years and always making me laugh until I can't breathe. Plus, you're pretty good about seeing that light at the end of the tunnel, and I will always appreciate that.

Chastity—I honestly don't know what I would do without you most days. You make me laugh and keep me focused, and I cannot thank you enough. I look forward to all of our upcoming adventures together!

Mom & Dad—Thank you so much for supporting my keto lifestyle and trying my keto recipes! I appreciate everything you've both done for me throughout the years.

Michael & Katie—Thank you for always having keto-friendly foods available at get-togethers and for giving me the sweetest and most adorable niece and nephew.

And last but not least…

Indie Lou & Bella Marie—You both stayed by my side through this entire process. Even though you were both endlessly hoping for a piece of dropped food, I couldn't imagine life without you.

RECIPE INDEX

Dressings, Sauces & Seasonings

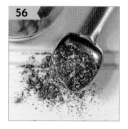
56

Taco Seasoning

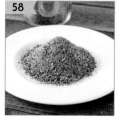
58

Cajun Seasoning

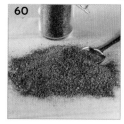
60

Smoky BBQ Rub

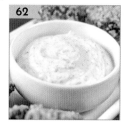
62

Ranch Dressing

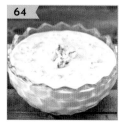
64

Blue Cheese
Dressing

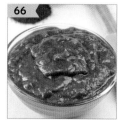
66

Chipotle
BBQ Sauce

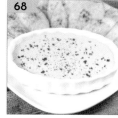
68

Bloom Sauce

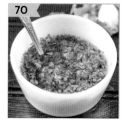
70

Cilantro Chimichurri

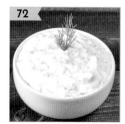
72

Lemon Dill
Tartar Sauce

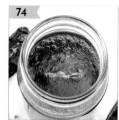
74

Authentic
Enchilada Sauce

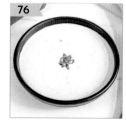
76

Baja Sauce

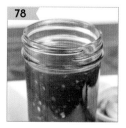
78

Sweet Chili Sauce

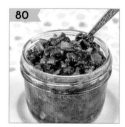
80

Bacon Onion Jam

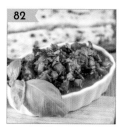
82

Italian Salsa

Appetizers & Snacks

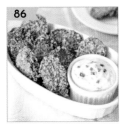
86
Zucchini Fritte

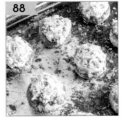
88
Stuffed Mushrooms

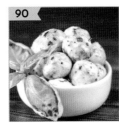
90
Marinated
Mozzarella Bites

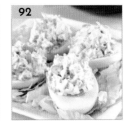
92
Ham & Chives
Stuffed Eggs

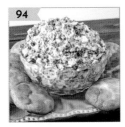
94
Spinach Dip

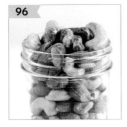
96
Roasted Nuts

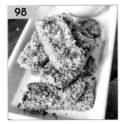
98
Fried Jalapeño
Mozzarella Bites

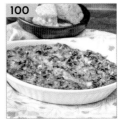
100
Olive Dip

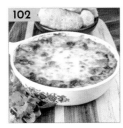
102
Queso Fundido

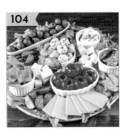
104
Antipasto Platter

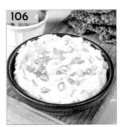
106
Garlic Chive
Cheese Spread

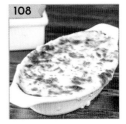
108
Shrimp &
Lobster Dip

Breads, Crackers & Pizza

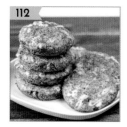
112

Best-Ever Flax Buns

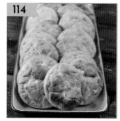
114

Buttery Slider Buns

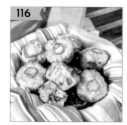
116

Three-Cheese
Jalapeño Muffins

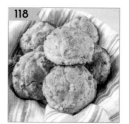
118

White Cheddar
Chive Biscuits

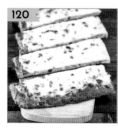
120

Cheesy Garlic
Butter Breadsticks

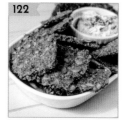
122

Bacon Seed
Crackers

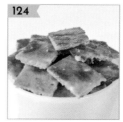
124

Chewy Cheese Bites

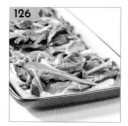
126

Steak Pizza with
Zesty Aioli

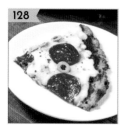
128

Crispy Personal
Pizzas

Salads

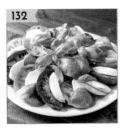

132

Heirloom Caprese Salad

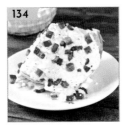

134

Blue Cheese Wedge Salad

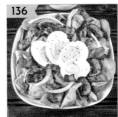

136

Spinach Salad with Warm Bacon Dressing

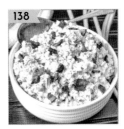

138

Bacon Broc-Cauli Salad

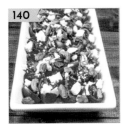

140

Grape Tomato Salad with Feta & Pistachios

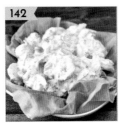

142

Classic Shrimp Salad

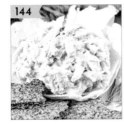

144

Lemon Tarragon Chicken Salad

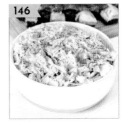

146

Sweet Dijon Coleslaw

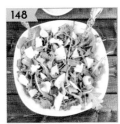

148

Parmesan Arugula Salad

Soups & Stews

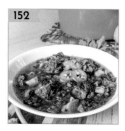

152

Albondigas Soup

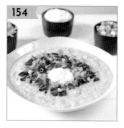

154

Loaded Cauli Leek Soup

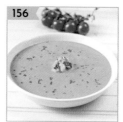

156

Lobster Bisque

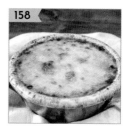

158

French Onion Soup

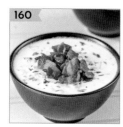

160

Bacon Clam Chowder

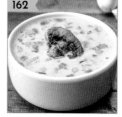

162

Golden Mushroom Soup

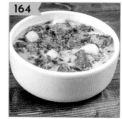

164

Creamy Steak Soup

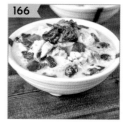

166

Chicken Bacon Poblano Soup

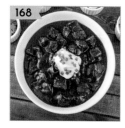

168

Chili con Carne

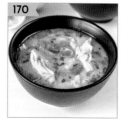

170

Avgolemono

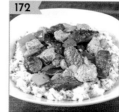

172

Gumbo

Veggies & Sides

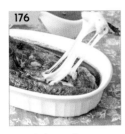
176

Chile Rellenos

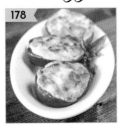
178

Parmesan Broiled Tomatoes

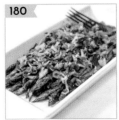
180

Crispy Shallot & Bacon Asparagus

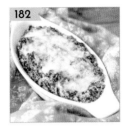
182

Gruyère Spinach Gratin

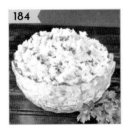
184

Cauli Risotto

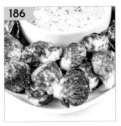
186

Roasted Brussels Sprouts with Balsamic Mayo

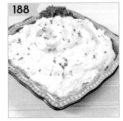
188

Best-Ever Cauli Mash

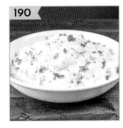
190

Spaghetti Squash Alfredo

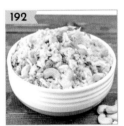
192

Cashew Fried Cauli Rice

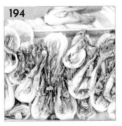
194

Lemon Garlic Baby Bok Choy

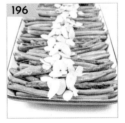
196

Toasted Almond Haricots Verts

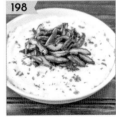
198

Cauli Puree with Crispy Shiitake Mushrooms

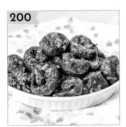
200

Garlic Butter Roasted Mushrooms

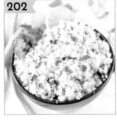
202

Cilantro Lime Cauli Rice

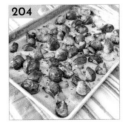
204

Garlic Roasted Radishes

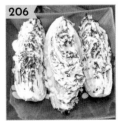
206

Grilled Napa Cabbage with Creamy Dressing

Beef

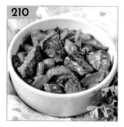

210

Beef Bourguignon

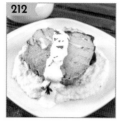

212

Garlic Roast Beef
with Horseradish
Cream

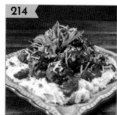

214

Cheesy Meatball
Marinara

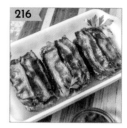

216

BBQ Bacon
Mini Meatloaves

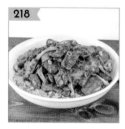

218

Mongolian Beef

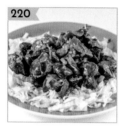

220

Beef Stroganoff

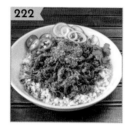

222

Barbacoa

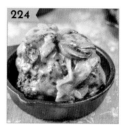

224

Salisbury Steak

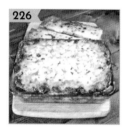

226

Bolognese Zucchini
Lasagna

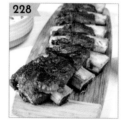

228

Oven-Roasted
Beef Ribs

Poultry

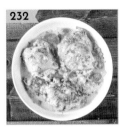

232

French Country Stew

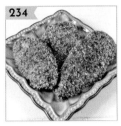

234

Pecan Chicken

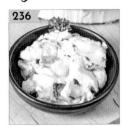

236

Chicken Pot Pie

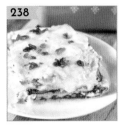

238

Chicken Bacon Swiss Lasagna

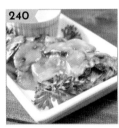

240

Fully Loaded Chicken

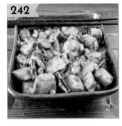

242

Kung Pao Chicken

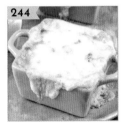

244

Green Chile Chicken Casserole

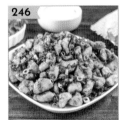

246

Indian Chicken

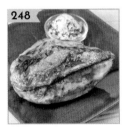

248

Chipotle Lime Chicken with Charred Scallion Butter

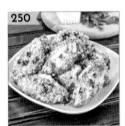

250

Parmesan Garlic Wings

Pork

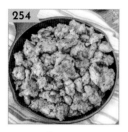
254
Hot Italian Sausage

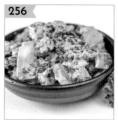
256
Cajun Alfredo
Sausage Skillet

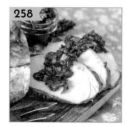
258
Roast Pork Loin
with Bacon Onion
Jam

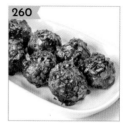
260
Szechuan Meatballs

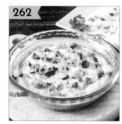
262
Quiche Lorraine

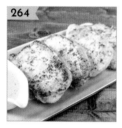
264
Creamy Dijon
Pork Chops

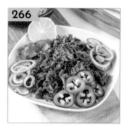
266
Carnitas

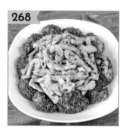
268
Spicy Garlic Pork
with Stir-Fried
Broccoli

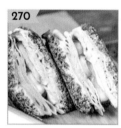
270
Cuban Sandwiches

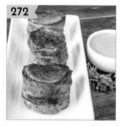
272
Bacon-Wrapped
Pork Medallions
with Maple
Chipotle Cream

Seafood

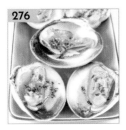

276

Oven-Roasted Clams with Garlic Butter Sauce

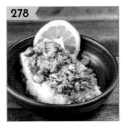

278

Crispy Pistachio-Crusted Cod

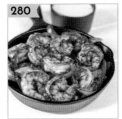

280

Shrimp Fajitas

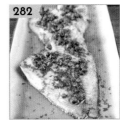

282

Sole Grenobloise

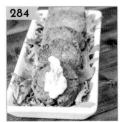

284

Crispy Tuna Cakes

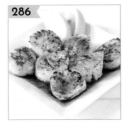

286

Brown Butter Scallops

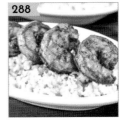

288

Smoky Garlic Shrimp

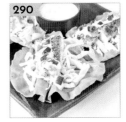

290

Baja Fish Tacos

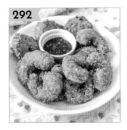

292

Coconut Shrimp

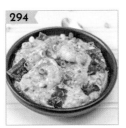

294

Shrimp & Grits

Sweets & Treats

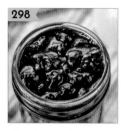
298
Blueberry Compote

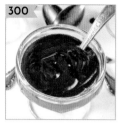
300
Hot Fudge

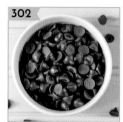
302
Chocolate Chips

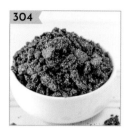
304
Chocolate Cookie Crumbs

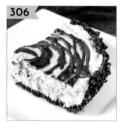
306
Frozen Peanut Butter Pie

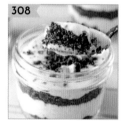
308
Cookies & Cream Parfait

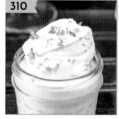
310
Lemon-Lime Posset

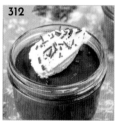
312
Dark Chocolate Pots de Crème

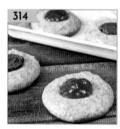
314
Thumbprint Cookies

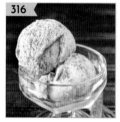
316
Snickerdoodle Frozen Custard

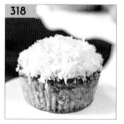
318
Coconut Cupcakes

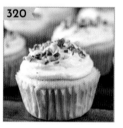
320
Banana Cupcakes with Sweet Brown Butter Frosting

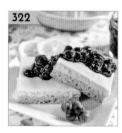
322
Lemon Cake

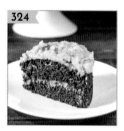
324
German Chocolate Cake

GENERAL INDEX